Current Issues i

Current Issues in Cardiology

Management Strategies

Edited by

JEAN R McEWAN

Senior Lecturer and Consultant Cardiologist,
University College London Medical School, London, UK

BMJ Publishing Group

© BMJ Publishing Group 1998

First published in 1997
by the BMJ Publishing Group, BMA House, Tavistock Square,
London WC1H 9JR

British Library Cataloguing in Publication Data

A catalogue record for this book is available
from the British Library

ISBN 0-7279-1010-8

Typeset by Apek Typesetters Ltd, Nailsea, Bristol
Printed and bound in Great Britain by Latimer Trend, Plymouth

Contents

Contributors

CJ Bulpitt
Professor of Geriatric Medicine, Division of Geriatric Medicine, Imperial College School of Medicine, London

AJ Camm
Department of Cardiological Sciences, St George's Hospital Medical School, London

MR Cowie
Wellcome Research Fellow, Department of Cardiac Medicine (Clinical Epidemiology Group), Imperial College School of Medicine at the National Heart and Lung Institute, London

NC Davidson
Specialist Registrar in Cardiology, Regional Cardiothoracic Unit, Freeman Hospital, Newcastle on Tyne

AE Fletcher
Reader in Epidemiology, Department of Epidemiology and Population Sciences, London School of Hygiene and Tropical Medicine, London

MM Gallagher
Research Fellow in Clinical Cardiology, Department of Cardiological Sciences, St George's Hospital Medical School, London

SMC Hardman
Senior Lecturer, University College London Medical School and Honorary Consultant Cardiologist, University College London Hospitals and the Whittington Hospital, London

WS Hillis
Reader in Medicine and Therapeutics and Consultant Cardiologist, Department of Medicine and Therapeutics, Gardiner Institute, Western Infirmary, Glasgow

DR Holdright
Consultant Cardiologist, Department of Cardiology, University College London Hospitals, London

JR McEwan
Senior Lecturer and Consultant Cardiologist, Hatter Institute and Centre for Cardiology, University College London Medical School, London

AG Ravi Kishore
Consultant Cardiologist, Mediciti Hospital, Hyderabad, India, Department of Cardiological Sciences, St George's Hospital Medical School, London
JM Ritter
Professor of Clinical Pharmacology, United Medical and Dental Schools of Guy's and St Thomas' Hospitals, London
AD Struthers
Professor of Clinical Pharmacology, Department of Cardiology, Ninewells Hospital and Medical School, Dundee
GR Thompson
Professor of Clinical Lipidology, MRC Lipoprotein Team, Clinical Sciences Centre, Hammersmith Hospital, London
P Yiu
MRC/RCS Training Fellow, Hatter Institute and Centre for Cardiology, University College London Medical School, London

Preface

Cardiovascular diseases remain the commonest cause of death in the western world and in the past 10 years large clinical trials have defined new effective treatments. The sheer numbers of patients that succumb to such diseases means that they will most often be cared for by their general practitioner or a general physician, who nevertheless will be required to have the expert opinion and evidence to determine the appropriate management. In this book we have addressed common cardiovascular problems where there have been substantial breakthroughs in determining effective management.

The subjects considered range from the now relatively complex management of the acute myocardial infarction through to sensible interpretation of symptoms and investigations of cardiovascular disease in low risk women. In each chapter there is critical appraisal of trial-based evidence, then an attempt to define the management strategy for that condition, based on the current state of knowledge. Rapid advances in interventional cardiology (angioplasty and stenting) and early transfer of patients back to referring sources after cardiac surgery make knowledge of the procedures and the subsequent outcome, essential for general practitioners and physicians. Particular attention is given to modification of the risk factors of hypertension and hyperlipidaemia with guidance on interpretation of measurements outside the "normal" range.

Finally, since management strategies have to be distilled into treatment protocols I have provided a skeleton to be padded according to further advances in knowledge, in the form of the Acute Cardiology Handbook that I use to guide my own junior staff.

I am grateful to all the contributors, particularly to those who had to revise their chapters (more than once!) because of new information becoming available during the collation of the book. The treatments for these common disorders continues to be defined, and remaining current in our knowledge is a major responsibility of all physicians.

1: Assessment and treatment of cardiovascular risk and disease in women

A FLETCHER, DR HOLDRIGHT AND JR McEWAN

Cardiovascular risks in women

Epidemiology

Cardiovascular diseases (CVD) are an important cause of mortality and morbidity in women in the United Kingdom. In this review we will consider risk modification with respect to cardiovascular disease as a whole, but investigation and treatment of coronary disease in particular.

The CVD rates are lower at all ages for women compared to men but the actual number of CVD deaths each year is greater in women (136,000 in England and Wales) compared with men (126,000) since women numerically outnumber men in the population, especially in old age when most deaths occur.[1] The difference between the male and female rate is greatest at younger ages. For example, at ages 45–64 the female rate is 20% of the male rate; the difference attenuates with increasing age to 44% (ages 65–74), 58% (ages 75–84) and 80% (aged 85 +). There are also differences between men and women in the relative contribution of different causes of CVD death. Strokes contribute to one third of CVD deaths in women compared to one fifth in men while ischaemic heart disease contributes to two thirds of deaths in men and one fifth in women.

The higher risk of CVD for men compared to women is mainly due to the increased risk of coronary artery disease, while male and female stroke rates are much closer at all ages.

Cardiovascular risk factors in women

Until relatively recently most research and health promotion activities have focused on middle aged men. Evidence on risk and protective factors for CVD in women is variable. For some factors, such as blood pressure, there is a large body of data from both observational studies and

1

Table 1.1 Coronary risk factors present in male or female patients presenting as either angina or myocardial infarction (adapted from Murabito et al.[2] with the publishers' permission)

Risk factor	Angina	MI
Men (age years)	61	62
Cholesterol mmol/L	6·19	6·07
Diabetes %	10	8
Hypertension %	35	34
Smokers	57	58
Women (age years)	64	69
Cholesterol mmol/L	6·71	7·01
Diabetes %	12	22
Hypertension %	49	51
Smokers	22	45

randomised controlled trials, while for factors such as cholesterol and hormone replacement therapy, evidence exists primarily from observational data. The prevalence of the various risk factors differs between men and women, diabetes and hypertension being more common in women, particularly when the presentation of the CVD is as a myocardial infarct[2] (Table 1.1).

Blood pressure

In most populations, blood pressure rises with age in both men and women. Systolic pressure rises throughout life while diastolic pressure tends to plateau around the sixth decade. At younger ages, blood pressure in women is lower than in men, but after the menopause the rate of rise of systolic pressure with age is greater in women than in men, leading to a higher prevalence of isolated systolic hypertension in older women. Several observational studies in women have demonstrated the importance of both systolic and diastolic pressure and isolated systolic hypertension in predicting strokes and coronary heart disease.[3-6] At all ages, the risk is lower for women compared with men, although the relative risk associated with a particular level of blood pressure is the same in women as in men, i.e. a sustained blood pressure which doubles a man's risk of stroke or MI will also double a woman's risk of developing these diseases.

The majority of placebo controlled trials of antihypertensive agents have included women[7-14] and in some trials in elderly people,[7-9] the majority of participants were women.

The results from trials of antihypertensive treatment show consistent evidence for the benefits of active therapy on stroke events in both men and women, with the magnitude of reduction of around 40% agreeing with the epidemiological predictions. The results for coronary heart disease are less certain and there are no data in women alone suggesting a benefit on CHD, while both the MRC studies[11,12] showed results consistent with no effect.

Because women have lower absolute risks of CHD than men, it is probable that the trials lacked the power to detect the benefits predicted from the observational studies of around 26%.

Recommendations for the management and treatment of hypertension in women, as in men, need to take account of the absolute risk for the patient, either by level of blood pressure alone or by the presence of concomitant risk factors.

Standard antihypertensive therapies are the same for both men and women (see Chapter 3) but with some limitation due to specific side effects. For example, hirsutism induced by minoxidil limits its acceptability to women, even in severe hypertension, and stress incontinence may be troublesome with either α-blockers such as prazocin or doxazocin (lax pelvic muscles in the elderly means greater dependence on adrenergic-influenced bladder neck sphincter for continence) or when an angiotensin converting enzyme inhibitor induces a cough. On the other hand potency problems with β-blockers or thiazide diuretic use in men are not usually a consideration when these drugs are used by women.

Weight loss, reduction in sodium intake, increased physical activity, and reduction of excessive alcohol intake are the principal non-pharmacological approaches which should be implemented in male and female patients with mild hypertension (<105 mmHg diastolic or systolic 140–160 mmHg).

Cholesterol

As with blood pressure, total cholesterol rises with age in both men and women. Women have lower cholesterol values at younger ages, but a sharp rise occurs in the fifth decade so that from age 50 onwards the average cholesterol level in women is higher than in men.[15] A pooled overview of data from 25 populations showed a strong consistent association between total cholesterol and CHD for women less than 65 years.[16a] There was no evidence that the relative risks were different in men compared with women; the pooled relative risk of CHD for a cholesterol level of 6·2 mmol/L or above compared with levels of 5·2 and below was 1·7 in men and 2·4 in women. In older women the evidence was less strong and not consistent between studies; the pooled relative risk was 1·12. The data for older men were more consistent but again the relative risks were weaker than at younger ages, the pooled relative risk for older men being 1·3. Although the magnitude of the relative risk tends to be lower at older ages, population-attributable risks are higher in elderly people since absolute risk is greater and high cholesterol levels are more prevalent.

There are fewer data on the relationship of other lipid fractions to CHD. In the pooled overview, HDL cholesterol inversely predicted CHD in both middle aged men and women and in older women but less convincingly for older men. LDL cholesterol predicted CHD mortality in middle aged men and women but the prediction was less consistent across the studies. Triglyceride levels showed a strong and consistent relationship with CHD in middle aged and older women but the evidence was weaker in men. HDL cholesterol and triglycerides show a strong inverse correlation and it remains controversial whether triglycerides independently predict CHD.

The evidence supporting pharmacological lipid lowering therapy and current directives are reviewed in Chapter 5. Few women have been included in many of the trials discussed; some specifically excluded women. Certainly their lower susceptibility to the measured end points of cardiac event or death means that more female subjects would have been required than has been necessary to show benefit in males. It is uncertain whether results of cholesterol lowering as part of primary prevention trials carried out in middle aged men can be extrapolated to women and in particular to elderly women.

The 4S study[16b] was a trial of secondary prevention, examining cholesterol lowering with simvistatin after a first myocardial infarction; 18·5% of participants were women. The relative risk of death was 0·7 (95% confidence interval [CI] 0·58–0·85) and the risk of major coronary events was 0·66 (95% CI 0·59–0·75). Subgroup analysis showed no effect on total mortality between treatment and placego group women, risk 1·12 (95% CI 0·65–1·93), but the risk of a major coronary event was reduced to 0·65 (95% CI 0·47–0·91). The CARE study also examined postinfarct lowering of lipids, this time using pravastatin, in patients with average cholesterols (<6·3 mmol/L);[16c] 576 women were included in the study. Pravastatin reduced the risk of further cardiac events by 24% (95% CI 9–36) in the whole population and in females the reduction was 46% (95% CI 22–62). No effects were seen in total mortality. Women with coronary artery disease have certainly identified themselves as being at high risk of further events and have a higher mortality following the initial myocardial infarct (see below). Secondary prevention in women should include lipid lowering and is probably relevant at all levels of total cholesterol.[16d] Further trials are now encouraging adequate female participation, including the Antihypertensive and Lipid Lowering Treatment to Prevent Heart Attack (ALLHAT) in the US, which will recruit patients of all ages, and a factorial trial in the UK which will determine the effects of lipid lowering treatments and vitamin E supplementation in men and women up to the age of 79 years. In the meantime, general recommendations for managing high blood cholesterol can be followed.

There are some limited data to indicate that total, HDL and LDL cholesterol can be modified by dietary interventions, but that the magnitude of effect in women is less than in men.[17] Obesity is associated with high levels of total cholesterol and low levels of HDL cholesterol. Beneficial effects on HDL cholesterol occur when obese people lose weight.[18] There is consistent evidence that smoking lowers HDL cholesterol and this effect may be more pronounced in women than men.

In summary, while the relative risk increase due to elevated cholesterol is the same in middle aged men and women, the evidence of a harmful effect of a high cholesterol is not strong in older women. Primary cholesterol lowering therapy needs to be tailored not to the absolute cholesterol level but to the individual and the risk factor profile. Lipid lowering as part of secondary preventive measures is equally applicable to women as well as men.

Smoking

While the prevalence of smoking is falling, the rate of decline is less in women, particularly in the younger age groups. Knowledge of the adverse effects of smoking on cardiovascular diseases continues to grow. In women smoking has been shown to be a risk factor for CHD, subarachnoid and ischaemic stroke[19-21] and the adverse risk persists into old age.[22, 23] Cessation of smoking reduces the risk of CHD and stroke but few studies in women have compared the time since giving up with reduction in risk. In the Nurses Health Study, in predominantly middle aged women, stroke risk declined soon after cessation and had largely disappeared 2–4 years later[20] (Figure 1.1). Many studies have examined CHD risk in ex-smokers by time since cessation but most of these have been exclusively in men.[24a] A review of these studies concluded that CHD risk is reduced in former smokers compared with those who continue to smoke and that the risk declines rapidly within a year after stopping smoking with up to 50% reduction in the excess risk of smoking. The remaining decline is more gradual and the risk reaches that of non-smokers 10–15 years after cessation. The review concluded that the findings were similar for both men and women and extended to older people, including those with CHD. However, a case controlled study of women after a first myocardial infarct suggested that the relative risk of 3·5 (95% CI 3·0–4·4) in smokers dissipates more rapidly in women after cessation of smoking, with risk indistinguishable from lifelong non-smokers after three years of abstinence.[24b] As absolute risks are higher in older people the benefits of stopping smoking even late in life can be considerable.

Diabetes

The impact of diabetes on CHD in women is considerable with relative risks up to fivefold compared with non-diabetic women described.[25-28] The increased risk is proportionately greater than observed for men with diabetes compared with non-diabetic men, so that diabetic women have a mortality from CHD very similar to that of men. Diabetic women have also been shown to be at increased risk of stroke.[29-31] Diabetics have higher

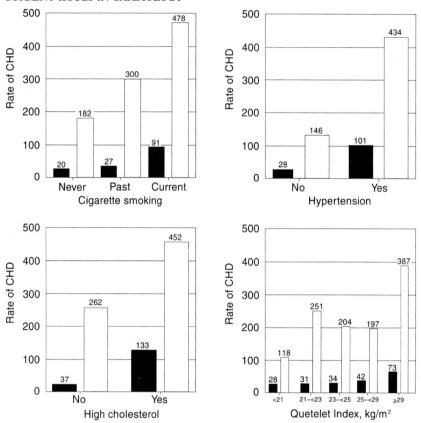

Fig 1.1   Age adjusted rates of non-fatal myocardial infarction and fatal coronary heart disease (CHD) (combined) per 100,000 person-years in relation to diabetes status, as modified by the presence or absence of other coronary risk factors. Solid bars indicate non-diabetic subjects; shaded bars, diabetic subjects. Manson JE, Colditz GA, Stampfer MJ *et al.* A prospective study of maturity-onset diabetes mellitus and risk of coronary heart disease in women. *Arch Intern Med* 1991; **151:** 1141–7.

blood pressure levels, are more obese and have higher cholesterol levels and triglyceride levels and lower HDL cholesterol than non-diabetics, which may be explained by an underlying metabolic or genetic disturbance such as hyperinsulinaemia. The presence of these cardiovascular risk factors alone does not appear to explain the increased risk associated with diabetes although these concomitant risk factors greatly amplify the risks (Figure 1.1). In practice, this means that the significance of hyperlipidaemia in a female diabetic is similar to that in a man. This justifies more aggressive attempts to lower cholesterol in these particular female patients.

Management of concomitant risk factors, and in particular weight control, is the principal non-pharmacologic strategy to reduce CVD risk in diabetic women.

Obesity

Obesity is related to CVD mortality since it increases blood pressure, predisposes to diabetes and adversely affects lipids. Whether obesity has additional and independent effects on CVD is uncertain and in a sense irrelevant since the biological consequences of obesity are considerable enough. The Nurses Health Study found that in women with a BMI of 29 or more, 70% of coronary events could be attributed to obesity.[32] However, even mild to moderate levels of obesity exerted an adverse effect with 40% of all coronary events in the study population being attributed for hypertension, diabetes and cholesterol levels, which may represent additional adverse effects on other variables, such as fibrinolytic activity.

In the age group 65–74, lean elderly women with no history of weight loss were at the lowest mortality risk.[33] Body fat distribution may be more important than actual weight. Waist–hip ratio has been shown to be an independent predictor of mortality in both middle aged[34] and older women.[35, 36] The benefits of weight loss on subsequent mortality in both middle aged and elderly people are more difficult to identify because most observational studies have not been able to distinguish voluntary from disease induced weight loss.[37] Weight loss and increased exercise remain sensible advice for both men and women.

Socioeconomic factors

The British Longitudinal Study, using descriptors of socioeconomic status such as housing tenure and car ownership in addition to occupation or husband's occupation, has described a strong inverse gradient between measures of socioeconomic status and mortality, including cardiovascular disease in women.[38] Differences in mortality by socioeconomic indicators are only in part explained by differences in the distribution of risk factors. The Scottish Heart Study found that body mass index, triglycerides and HDL cholesterol were most important in accounting for the effect of socioeconomic differences in CHD in women but the effect of housing tenure persisted after all other traditional risk factors had been taken into account, with women living in rented accommodation experiencing a 50% excess of CHD risk compared to women in owner occupier accommodation.[39]

Other nutritional factors, such as intake of fresh food and vegetables, are known to vary by socioeconomic status, with the poorest groups having the lowest intakes of possible protective factors.[40] Opportunities and incentives for healthy lifestyles such as increased physical activity and weight loss are also lower in the more socially disadvantaged groups. Access to health care has been shown to be markedly influenced by the social class of the patient for a variety of conditions.

Our understanding of the socioeconomic variations in cardiovascular disease mortality is incomplete. Ensuring that women from lower socio-economic groups receive similar investigations and attention to lifestyle changes is one way to ensure equity of health care provision.

Protective factors against cardiovascular disease in women

Evidence for protective factors against cardiovascular disease, both pharmacological and lifestyle, is accumulating.

Exercise

There is consistent evidence from observational studies, a few of which have included women, that physical activity reduces CHD risk.[41] Reasons for the inverse association between physical activity and coronary heart disease include its effect in raising HDL cholesterol and reducing body weight as well as its blood pressure lowering effect and impact on glucose tolerance. Recent studies on exercising women demonstrate that the benefits on HDL are proportional to the amount of exercise undertaken. The greater the regular exercise level, the greater risk factor improvement seen at levels of exercise higher than current recommendations.[42]

Alcohol

Moderate alcohol intake, 1–2 drinks daily, protects against CHD and ischaemic stroke but increases the risk of subarachnoid haemorrhage.[43] Even moderate alcohol consumption may increase breast cancer risk. In the Nurses Health Study, consumption of 3–9 drinks weekly was associated with a 30% excess breast cancer risk and for more than nine drinks a week a 60% increase in risk (Table 1.2).[43] Excess alcohol consumption, more

Table 1.2 Relative risk of major illnesses among women according to level of alcohol intake (g/day), Nurses Health Study (adapted from Colditz,[43] with permission)

	Alcohol intake (g/day)				
	Never drink (reference category)	0.0–1.4	1.5–4.9	5.0–14.9	≥15
Coronary heart disease	1·0	0·7	0·5	0·6	0·6
Stroke	1·0	0·9	0·6	0·6	0·9
Ischaemic	1·0	0·7	0·4	0·3	0·5
Subarachnoid	1·0	2·4	2·9	3·7	2·6
Breast cancer	1·0	1·0	0·9	1·3	1·6
Gallstones	1·0	1·0	0·9	0·8	0·7
Diabetes	1·0	0·9	0·8	0·8	0·6
Hypertension[a]	1·0	0·9	1·1	1·5	1·7

[a]For hypertension only, the categories for alcohol intake are, from left to right, never drink, 0·1–9·9 g/day; 10–19·9 g/day; 20–29·9 g/day, and 30 g/day.

than six drinks daily, does more harm than good since the beneficial effects on CHD are outweighed by adverse effects on other causes of death. At present the evidence continues to support general recommendation of 1–2 drinks daily as the optimum intake but, for any individual, the risks and benefits of alcohol intake depend on the absolute risks of different causes of mortality and hence their individual risk profile for CHD and breast cancer.

Vitamin E

A possible protective effect of antioxidant vitamins on atherosclerosis has been suggested by laboratory work, ecological comparisons, case control and cross-sectional studies and, more recently, by prospective studies.[44]

In the WHO MONICA Project highly significant and large inverse correlations were described between vitamin E concentrations and IHD mortality rates in 16 European populations[45] and weaker correlations for carotene and vitamin C.[46] In cross-sectional studies in Finnish populations no relationships were found between plasma vitamins C, E or retinol and CHD[47] while the Scottish Heart Health Study of men and women aged 40–59 years showed significantly lower risks in the highest quintile of dietary β-carotene, vitamins C, E and A for men with undiagnosed CHD but only weak evidence for a protective effect for women.[48a] Opposite trends were observed for men with diagnosed CHD.[49]

The effects of dietary supplementation with antioxidant vitamins have been examined in several studies, notably the Alpha Tocopherol Beta Carotene Prevention Study, but only men (29,133 male smokers)[48b] participated. A weak effect of vitamin E (risk 0·91, 95% CI 0·83–0·99) and no significant effect of vitamin A on the development of angina were reported.

A protective effect of vitamin E on CHD risk was observed in the Nurses Health Study but most of the benefit was due to vitamin E supplementation (for at least two years) rather than dietary intake.[49] Weak trends were also seen for vitamin E supplementation and reduced ischaemic stroke and CVD mortality. It must be noted that this was an observational study rather than a randomised trial. Multivitamin and vitamin C use were not associated with any reductions in risk, suggesting the operation of a specific protective effect of vitamin E rather than selection of health conscious individuals. Vitamin and mineral supplement use was not associated with decreases in mortality or any major cause-specific mortality in over 10,000 men and women aged 25–74 years in NHANES I; however, the study was not able to investigate supplements of specific vitamins or minerals.[50] The recently pubished Cambridge Heart Antioxidant Study showed a beneficial effect of vitamin E supplements post-MI in men and women, supporting its secondary prevention role in this group with confirmed coronary disease.[51] Only a small number of women were recruited, however, precluding direct comparisons in women.

The hypothesis for a protective effect of vitamin E on CHD risk is currently being tested in three randomised controlled trials, two of which include women.

Aspirin

Evidence for the benefit of low dose aspirin in the primary prevention of CHD in men has been examined in two randomised trials in British and American doctors[52] (see Chapter 3). No such randomised trials have been conducted in women. Observational data from the Nurses Health Study found a lower risk of CHD in women who took 1–6 aspirins weekly compared to women who did not take aspirins regularly. No benefit was seen with increased aspirin consumption or for any effect on ischaemic or haemorrhagic stroke.[53a] Another observation study reported on the effects of aspirin use in participants in the Bezafibrate Infarction Prevention Study. The 45% of women who reported regular aspirin ingestion had a reduced cardiovascular risk of 0·61 (95% CI 0·38–0·97) and all-cause mortality risk of 0·66 (95% CI 0·47–0·93) compared with those not using aspirin. Women who were older, diabetic or had evidence of existing coronary disease benefited most.[53b]

Oestrogens

For postmenopausal women there is substantial evidence that oestrogen replacement therapy is associated with a lower risk of coronary heart disease,[54a] with an overall estimate of 44% reduction in CHD. In nearly all these studies unopposed conjugated oestrogen without progestin was given, though a recent report from the Nurses Health Study demonstrated that taking oestrogens combined with progestin reduced the risk of coronary events to 0·39 (95% CI 0·19–0·78), in comparison to women who used no hormones.[54b] This compared favourably to use of oestrogen alone, which gave a risk of 0·6 (95% CI 0·43–0·83).

Oestrogens have beneficial effects on a range of cardiovascular risk factors. Most noticeably, they increase HDL cholesterol and lower LDL cholesterol and plasma levels of plasminogen activator inhibitor type 1 (PAI-1), which inhibits fibrinolysis, are reduced by 50% with enhancement of systemic fibrinolysis.[54c]

Adverse effects of unopposed oestrogens on endometrial cancer risk make it unlikely that unopposed oestrogen will be prescribed other than for women without uteri.

The risks and benefits of modern combination therapies such as oestrogen and progestin need to be fully evaluated in a randomised trial evaluating their long term effects on cardiovascular disease, osteoporotic fractures and breast cancer. Current trials examining these issues are underway in other countries and in preparation in the UK. The results of

Table 1.3   Prevalence of angiographically documented coronary artery disease as a function of symptoms (adapted from Chatman et al.[54])

Symptom	% Prevalence of coronary artery disease	
	Men	Women
Definite angina	93	72
Probable angina	66	36
Non-specific chest pain	14	6

these trials will not be available for a further 10–15 years. In the meantime hormone replacement therapy may be given as indicated for the symptomatic relief of menopausal symptoms after careful consideration of the medical history of the patient for possible contraindications. Hypertension, hyperlipidaemia, diabetes or established coronary or cerebrovascular disease are not contraindications to hormone replacement therapy.

The presentation, diagnosis and treatment of coronary disease in women

Presentation

Typical angina pectoris is strongly predictive of significant ($>70\%$ narrowing) coronary disease in women as well as men[55] (Table 1.3). Angina is the most common presentation of women subsequently confirmed as having coronary artery disease[2] (Table 1.4). In men the high prevalence of coronary disease in the population means there is still a 14% chance of significant coronary disease even if the presenting chest pain is quite atypical, but in women presenting similarly, coronary obstructions will be found in only about 6%.[55]

In trying to assess the risks and benefits of investigations, the individual risk factor profile is important in women. The prevalence of coronary diseases is lower in women than in men at all ages, but particularly before the menopause. Therefore the premenopausal woman with atypical pain and a good risk factor profile (no family history of premature coronary disease, normal cholesterol, non-smoker and not diabetic) can be confidently reassured.

After the menopause, the rate of rise of coronary disease is steeper in

Table 1.4   Initial clinical presentation of coronary heart disease (adapted from Murabito et al.[2] with the publishers' permission)

CHD presentation	Men %	Women %
Angina	32	47
Unstable angina	6	7
Recognised MI	30	18
Silent MI	16	14
CHD death	16	14

11

women than in men but the mean age at first presentation is around 10 years older in women than men. Older women with chest pain must be evaluated carefully.

One group that must be considered at high risk are diabetic women, insulin dependent or independent. As stated earlier, diabetes is a strong risk factor for cardiovascular disease in women of all ages. Chest pain may not feature prominently or may be atypical. Myocardial dysfunction and associated cardiac failure may be the presentation of the combination of large and small vessel disease. All diabetics, incuding women of all ages, require careful assessment whenever coronary disease is suspected.

Myocardial infarction is less commonly the first presentation of coronary disease in women than in men. However, perhaps reflecting their older age at presentation, the prognosis post-MI is considerably worse.[56] In a recent Framingham report, two-year mortality was 35% in women compared to 24% in men, with age adjustments to take account of the older age of females at presentation; by 10 years, age adjusted mortality was 53% for men and 69% for women. The instigation of secondary preventive measures and a search for evidence of prognostically significant coronary disease cannot be neglected in female patients.

Non-invasive investigation of chest pain in women

Exercise testing of patients with typical chest pain is a useful confirmatory test of the presence of significant coronary disease and may give information of prognostically significant disease. In men with typical pain, an abnormal exercise test (> 1 mm ST depression) is highly predictive of coronary disease but the prevalence of coronary disease in males with typical pain is such that even a negative exercise test will be associated with significant coronary disease in more than half of them[57] (Table 1.5). In women, on the other hand, 25% of those with typical pain and a positive exercise test will not have coronary disease that can be considered to

Table 1.5   Correlation between exercise test, history and angiographic data in patients without previous MI (adapted from Detry et al.[56])

History of typical chest pain	Exercise test	Presence of CAD %
Men		
Yes	Abnormal	98
	Normal	56
No	Abnormal	33
	Normal	11
Women		
Yes	Abnormal	75
	Normal	17
No	Abnormal	17
	Normal	8

account for their symptoms. In the absence of typical symptoms and without a positive exercise test, the chance of significant coronary disease is low (<8%) and if the patient is premenopausal and without other major risks the chance of there being important coronary disease is even lower.

SPET thallium scintigraphy during exercise or pharmacological stress testing is more sensitive than a standard treadmill exercise test for reversible ischaemia and haemodynamically significant coronary disease in women and the patient may avoid coronary arteriography.[58]

Coronary arteriography

Persistent typical symptoms in both genders certainly justify coronary arteriography, particularly if exercise tolerance is low. The lower potential for positive findings in women means that the risks of the procedure have to be carefully weighed against potential benefits of an anatomical diagnosis. Some patients are relieved by confirmation of normal coronary anatomy but a surprisingly high percentage of women will still cling to antianginal therapy, despite a demonstration of no or minimal coronary disease.[59]

It has been suspected for several years that women are underinvestigated and undertreated for their coronary disease. Tobin et al.[60] reported that men with abnormal thallium perfusion scans were 10 times more likely to be investigated further than women with similar abnormalities. A recent study from the UK examined referral of men and women for coronary arteriography and bypass grafting following a hospital admission related to ischaemic heart disease. Despite study limitations imposed by the source of the data (hospital discharge diagnosis), it seemed that women were less likely than men to be either investigated or treated surgically, even when the influence of age at presentation is taken into account.[61]

It may be that, at least for chronic stable angina pectoris diagnosis and treatment, the referral rate for investigation is appropriately different for men and women. A recent report of a review of management strategy of 410 (280 male, 130 female) patients attending an American academic department suggested that there were gender-related differences in the referral rate for angiography. The referral rate reflected the history, examination and exercise test result and the decision making process was influenced by the recognised difference in disease prevalence between the sexes but this was deemed appropriate.[62]

Further studies from the USA suggest that after a myocardial infarction women are just as likely as men to be offered arteriography,[63, 64] supporting the concept that once a woman is firmly identified as having coronary disease she should be treated no differently from a man.

Surgical and endovascular interventions

Results of both coronary artery bypass grafting and percutaneous transluminal coronary angioplasty (PTCA) are poorer in women than

13

men.[65, 66] Surgical mortality is higher (almost double) and relief of symptoms less common in women. Procedural mortality and complication rates for PTCA are higher for women than men.[66] While physical size of the coronary arteries is felt to account for some of the discrepancy, much of the difference may be due to the older age and wider spectrum of risk factors experienced (particularly diabetes and hypertension) and more complicated disease (unstable symptoms). The different referral patterns for intervention for women may be appropriate to the different short and long term results. Women with high risk coronary disease (main stem disease, proximal LAD disease or three vessel disease with left ventricle impairment) should be and probably are referred appropriately for surgery.[64] Symptomatic benefit and good long term results of surgery for other indications should not be underestimated but it is correct to consider carefully the risks and benefits to the individual patient, male or female.

Heart failure

The major trials of ACE inhibitor therapy have included women who have made up around 20% of the study populations.[66-70] The studies were not designed to have sufficient power to allow gender comparisons so subgroup analysis must be viewed in this light. For example, in the SAVE Study the overall risk of all causes of mortality was reduced by 19% (95% CI 3–32) and cardiovascular death and morbidity by 24% (95% CI 13–34), but in females the reduction was only 2% (95% CI −53–37) all-cause mortality and 4% (95% CI 32–30) for cardiovascular death and morbidity.[69] In the SOLVD Study, no gender specific analysis was reported but there was a 16% (95% CI 5–36) reduction in all-cause mortality and 22% (95% CI 6–35) in death due to progressive heart failure in the total population, which included 20% females. The wide confidence limits illustrate the lack of power of the study to accurately reflect female response to this therapy. In general, ACE inhibitors should be used in the treatment of both females and males with the expectation of worthwhile benefit (see Chapter 7).

Digoxin treatment (as additional treatment to ACE inhibitor therapy) continues to excite interest. In a recent study, 22% of the participants were female.[71] The follow-up was for a mean duration of 37 months. Patients were assigned to digoxin or placebo as an adjunct to other antifailure treatment. No gender specific analysis was reported, but the results for the whole population (6800 patients) indicated that despite no effect (neither favourable nor detrimental) on mortality, there was a reduction in the rate of hospitalisation overall and for worsening heart failure in those on active therapy for heart failure, risk ratio 0·72 (95% CI 0·66–0·79) and overall 0·92 (95% CI 0·87–0·98). The current evidence supports the use of digoxin in chronic heart failure with persisting symptoms despite ACE inhibitors and diuretics.

Amlodipine has now been examined as adjuvant therapy to ACE inhibitors in severe heart failure.[72] A reduction in fatal and non-fatal events of 31% (95% CI 2–51) and in death of 46% (95% CI 21–63) was seen in patients with non-ischaemic cardiomyopathy, but no effects for those with ischaemic heart disease. Subgroup analysis of the 20% of female participants did reveal a reduction in mortality, risk ratio 0·62 (95% CI 0·40–0·96).

Summary

Cardiovascular disease is the major cause of death in women as well as men of the Western world. Standard risk factor modification applies to women as well as men, though evidence from clinical trials of the benefits of pharmacological lipid lowering does not exist. At this time it would seem appropriate to treat hyperlipidaemic women with a poor risk factor profile or documented coronary disease with lipid lowering drugs as well as diet if the cholesterol is high.

Diabetes is a major risk factor for coronary disease in women. Diabetic patients who present with chest pain even before the menopause require careful evaluation. Coronary artery disease presents only infrequently before the menopause in women without a high risk profile (such as diabetes, family history of premature coronary disease or hyperlipidaemia). Such women with atypical chest pain should be reassured of their good cardiovascular outlook.

Observational data suggest that oestrogen replacement therapy helps to postpone the rise in prevalence of coronary disease seen in women after the menopause. While prospective data and proper randomised trial results are pending it would seem appropriate to advise oestrogen (or cyclical oestrogen/progestogen) therapy for menopausal symptoms and bone disease, in the absence of contraindications, with a fair degree of confidence in added cardiovascular protection. Cardiovascular disease such as hypertension or ischaemic heart disease does not contraindicate postmenopausal hormone replacement.

Women with angina-like symptoms after the menopause and younger women with an adverse risk profile should be referred for a cardiology opinion and investigation. After a myocardial infarction women as well as men should be assessed non-invasively or invasively if appropriate to define their risk of future events. Coronary artery bypass grafting and PTCA should be offered to women when the benefits are perceived to outweigh any risks to the individual patient.

All currently proven therapies for the treatment of heart failure (ACE inhibitors, digoxin and amlodipine) would appear to be equally applicable for female as well as male patients and there is some suggestion that amlodipine has greater advantages for women.

15

1 Office of Population Censuses and Surveys *Mortality statistics 1991*. Series DH2 no 18. London: HMSO.

2 Murabito JM, Evans JC, Larson MG, Levy D. Prognosis after the onset of coronary heart disease. An investigation of the difference in outcome between the sexes according to initial coronary disease presentations. *Circulation* 1993; **88**: 2548–55.

3 Stamler J, Rhomberg P, Schoenberger JA *et al*. Multivariate analysis of the relationship of seven variables to blood pressure. Findings of the Chicago Heart Association Detection Project in Industry, 1967–1972. *J Chron Dis* 1975; **28**: 527–48.

4 Higgins M, Keller JB, Ostrander LD. Risk factors for coronary heart disease in women: Tecumseh Community Health Study, 1959 to 1980. In: Eaker E, Packard B, Wenger N *et al*. eds. *Coronary heart disease in women*. New York: Haymarket Doyma, 1987.

5 Dawber T. *The Framingham Study. The epidemiology of atherosclerotic disease*. Cambridge: Harvard University Press, 1980.

6 Bush TL, Criqui MH, Cowan LD *et al*. Cardiovascular disease mortality in women: results from the Lipid Research Clinics Follow-up Study. In: Eaker E, Packard B, Wenger N *et al*. eds. *Coronary heart disease in women*. New York: Haymarket Doyma, 1987.

7 Amery A, Birkenhager W, Brixko R *et al*. Efficacy of antihypertensive drug treatment according to age, sex, blood pressure and previous cardiovascular disease in patients over the age of 60. *Lancet* 1986; **ii**: 589–92.

8 Coope J, Warrender TS. Randomised trial of treatment of hypertension in elderly patients in primary care. *Br Med J* 1986; **293**: 1145.

9 Dahlof B, Lindholm LH, Hanson L, Schersten B, Ekbom T, Wester P-O. Morbidity and mortality in the Swedish trial in old patients with hypertension (STOP-hypertension). *Lancet* 1991; **338**: 1281–5.

10 Systolic Hypertension in the Elderly Program Cooperative Research Group. Implications of the Systolic Hypertension in the Elderly Programme. *Hypertension* 1993; **21**: 335–43.

11 Medical Research Council Working Party. MRC trial of treatment of mild hypertension: principal results. *Br Med J* 1985; **291**: 97.

12 Medical Research Council Working Party. MRC trial of treatment of hypertension in older adults: principal results. *Br Med J* 1992; **304**: 405–12.

13 Hypertension Detection and Follow-up Programme Co-operative Group. Five year finding of the Hypertension Detection and Follow-up Programme I. Reduction in mortality in persons with high blood pressure, including mild hypertension. *JAMA* 1979; **242**: 2562–71.

14 Report by the Management Committee. The Australian therapeutic trial in mild hypertension. *Lancet* 1982; **i**: 1261–7.

15 Kronman RA, Cain KC, Ye Z, Omenn GS. Total serum cholesterol levels and mortality risk as a function of age. *Arch Intern Med* 1993; **153**: 1065–73.

16a Manclio TA, Pearson TA, Wenger NK *et al*. Cholesterol and heart disease in older persons and women. Review of an NHLBI Workshop. *Ann Epidemiol* 1992; **2**: 161–76.

16b Scandinavian Simvistatin Survival Study. Randomized trial of cholesterol lowering in 4444 patients with coronary heart disease: the Scandinavian Simvistatin Survival Study. *Lancet* 1994; **344**: 1383–9.

16c Sacks FM, Pfeffer MA, Moye LA *et al*. The effect of pravastatin on coronary events after myocardial infarct in patients with average cholesterol levels. *N Engl J Med* 1996; **335**: 1001–9.

16d Scandinavian Simvistatin Survival Study Group. Baseline serum cholesterol and treatment effect in the Scandinavian Simvistatin Survival Study (4S). *Lancet* 1995; **345**: 1274–5.

17 Krisk Etherton PM, Krummel D. Role of nutrition in the prevention and treatment of coronary heart disease in women. *J Am Diet Assoc* 1993; **93**: 987–93.

18 Follick MJ, Abrams DB, Smith TW, Henderson LO, Herbert R. Contrasting short and long term effects of weight loss on lipoprotein levels. *Arch Intern Med* 1984; **144**: 1571–4.

19 Hammond EC, Garfinkel L. Coronary heart disease, stroke and aortic aneurysms, factors in the etiology. *Arch Environ Health* 1969; **19**: 167–82.

20 Kawachi I, Colditz GA, Stampfer MJ *et al*. Smoking cessation and decreased risk of stroke in women. *JAMA* 1993; **269**: 232–6.

21 Shapiro S, Weinblatt E, Frank CW, Sager RV. Incidence of coronary heart disease in a

population insured for medical care (HIP). *Am J Public Health* 1969; **59**: 1–107.

22 La Croix AX, Lang J, Scherr P *et al.* Smoking and mortality among older men and women in three communities. *N Engl J Med* 1991; **324**: 1619–25.

23 Aronow WS, Herzig AH, Fritzner E, D'Alba P, Ronquillo J. 40 month follow-up of risk factor correlated with new coronary events in 708 elderly patients. *JAGS* 1989; **37**: 501–6.

24a US Department of Health and Human Services. *The health benefits of smoking cessation.* Publication No CDC 90–8416. Washington DC: Department of Health and Human Services.

24b Rosenberg L, Palmer JR, Shapiro S. Decline in the risk of myocardial infarction among women who stop smoking. *N Engl J Med* 1990; **322**: 213–17.

25 Butler WJ, Ostrander LD, Carman WJ, Lamphiear DE. Mortality from coronary heart disease in the Tecumseh Study. *Am J Epidemiol* 1985; **121**: 541–7.

26 Barrett-Connor E, Wingard DL. Sex differentials in ischaemic heart disease mortality in diabetics. *Am J Epidemiol* 1983; **118**: 489–96.

27 Pan WH, Cedres LB, Liu K *et al.* Relationship of clinical diabetes and asymptomatic hyperglycaemia to risk of coronary disease mortality in men and women. *Am J Epidemiol* 1986; **123**: 504–16.

28 Heyden S, Heiss G, Bartel Hames CG. Sex differences in coronary mortality among diabetics in Evans County, Georgia. *J Chron Dis* 1980; **33**: 265–73.

29 Barrett-Connor E, Khaw K. Diabetes mellitus: an independent risk factor for stroke? *Am J Epidemiol* 1988; **128**: 116–23.

30 Kannel WB, McGee DL. Diabetes and cardiovascular disease: the Framingham Study. *JAMA* 1979; **241**: 2035–38.

31 Manson J, Colditz GA, Stampfer MJ *et al.* A prospective study of maturity-onset diabetes mellitus and risk of coronary heart disease and stroke in women. *Arch Intern Med* 1991; **151**: 1141–7.

32 Manson JE, Colditz GA, Stampfer MJ *et al.* A prospective study of obesity and risk of coronary heart disease in women. *N Engl J Med* 1990; **322**: 882–9.

33 Rumpel C, Harris TB, Madans J. Modification of the relationship between the Quetelet Index and mortality by weight-loss history among older women. *Ann Epidemiol* 1993; **3**: 343–50.

34 Lapidus L, Bengtsson C, Larsson B, Penmert K, Sjostrom L. Distribution of adipose tissue and risk of cardiovascular diseases and death. A 12 year follow up of participants in the population study of women in Gothenburg, Sweden. *Br Med J* 1984; **289**: 1257–61.

35 Prineas RJ, Folsom AR, Kaye SA. Central adiposity and increased risk of coronary artery disease mortality in older women. *Ann Epidemiol* 1993; **3**: 35–41.

36 Folsom AR, Kaye SA, Sellers TA *et al.* Body fat distribution and 5 year risk of death in older women. *JAMA* 1993; **269**: 438–47.

37 Kushner RF. Body weight and mortality. *Nutr Rev* 1993; **51**: 127–36.

38 Office of Population Censuses and Surveys. *Longitudinal study sociodemographic mortality differentials 1971–1975.* (Fox AJ, Goldblatt PO, eds). London: HMSO, 1982.

39 Woodward W, Shewry MC, Smith WCS, Tunstall-Pedoe H. Social status and CHD. *Prev Med* 1992; **21**: 136–48.

40 Black D, Morris JN, Smith C, Townsend P. *Inequalities in Health.* The Black Report. Ed. Townsend P, Davidson N. London: Penguin, 1990.

41 Powell KE, Thompson PD, Caspersen CJ, Kendrick JS. Physical activity and the incidence of coronary heart disease. *Annu Rev Public Health* 1987; **8**: 253–87.

42 Williams PT. High density lipoprotein cholesterol and other risk factors for coronary heart disease in female runners. *N Engl J Med* 1996; **334**: 1298–303.

43 Colditz GA. A prospective assessment of moderate alcohol intake and major chronic diseases. *Ann Epidemiol* 1990; **1**: 167–77.

44 Gey KF. Prospects for the prevention of free radical disease, regarding cancer and cardiovascular disease. *Br Med Bull* 1993; **49**: 679–99.

45 Gey KF, Puska P, Jordan P, Moser UK. Inverse correlation between plasma vitamin E and mortality from ischaemic heart disease in cross cultural epidemiology. *Am J Clin Nutr* 1991; **53**: 326S–334S.

46 Gey KF, Moser UK, Jordan P, Stahelin EB, Eicholzer M, Ludin E. Increased risk of

cardiovascular disease at suboptimal plasma levels of essential antioxidants. *Am J Clin Nutr* 1993; **57**: 778S–789S.

47 Salonen JT, Salonen R, Seppanen K *et al.* Relationship of serum selenium and antioxidants to plasma lipoproteins, platelet aggregability and prevalent ischaemic heart disease in Eastern Finnish men. *Atherosclerosis* 1988; **170**: 155–60.

48a Bolton Smith C, Woodward M, Tunstall Pedoe H. The Scottish Heart Health Study. Dietary intake by food frequency questionnaire and odds ratio for coronary heart disease risk. II. The antioxidant vitamins and fibre. *Eur J Clin Nutr* 1992; **46**: 85–93.

48b Rapola JM, Virtamo J, Haukka JK *et al.* Effect of vitamin E and beta carotene on the incidence of angina pectoris. A randomized, double-blind, controlled trial. *JAMA* 1996; **275**: 693–8.

49 Stampfer MJ, Hennekens CH, Manson JE, Colditz GA, Rosner B, Willett WC. Vitamin E consumption and the risk of coronary disease in women. *N Engl J Med* 1993; **328**: 1444–9.

50 Kim I, Williamson DF, Byers T, Koplan JP. Vitamin and mineral supplement use and mortality in a US cohort. *Am J Public Health* 1983; **83**: 546–50.

51 Stephens NG, Parsons A, Schofield PM *et al.* Randomised controlled trial of vitamin E in patients with coronary disease: Cambridge Heart Antioxidant Study (CHAOS). *Lancet* 1996; **347**: 781–6.

52 Hennekens CH, Buring JE, Sandercock P, Collins R, Peto R. Aspirin and other antiplatelet agents in the secondary and primary prevention of cardiovascular disease. *Circulation* 1989; **80**: 749–56.

53a Manson JE, Stampfer MJ, Colditz GA *et al.* A prospective study of aspirin use and primary prevention of cardiovascular disease in women. *JAMA* 1991; **266**: 521–7.

53b Harpaz D, Benderly M, Goldbourt U, Kishon Y, Behar S for the Israeli BIP Study Group. Effect of aspirin on mortality in women with symptomatic or silent myocardial ischaemia. *Am J Cardiol* 1996; **78**: 1215–19.

54a Stampfer MJ, Colditz GA. Oestrogen replacement therapy and coronary heart disease: a quantitative assessment of the epidemiologic evidence *Prev Med* 1991; **20**; 47–63.

54b Grodstein F, Stampfer MJ, Manson JE. Postmenopausal estrogen and progestin use and the risk of cardiovascular disease. *N Engl J Med* 1996; **335**: 453–61.

54c Koh KK, Mincemoyer R, Bui MN. Effects of hormone replacement therapy on fibrinolysis in postmenopausal women. *N Engl J Med* 1997; **386**: 683–90.

55 Chaitman BR, Bourassa MG, Davis K *et al.* Angiographic prevalence of high risk coronary artery disease in patient subsets (CASS). *Circulation* 1981; **64**: 360–7.

56 Greenland P, Reicher Reiss H, Goldbourt U, Behar S and the Israeli SPRINT Investigators. In hospital and 1-year mortality in 1524 women after myocardial infarction: comparison with 4315 men. *Circulation* 1991; **83**: 484–91.

57 Detry JMR, Kapita BM, Cosyns J, Sottiauk B, Brassuer LA, Rousseau MF. Diagnostic value of history and maximal exercise electrocardiography in men and women suspected of coronary heart disease. *Circulation* 1977; **56**: 756–761.

58 Chae SC, Heo J, Iskandrian AS, Wasserleben V, Cave V. Identification of extensive coronary artery disease in women by exercise single-photon emission computed tomographic (SPET) thallium imaging. *J Am Coll Cardiol* 1993; **21**: 1305–11.

59 Sullivan AK, Holdright DR, Wright CA, Sparrow JL, Cunningham D, Fox KM. Chest pain in women: clinical, investigative and prognostic features. *Br Med J* 1994; **308**: 883–6.

60 Tobin JN, Wassertheil-Smollers, Wexler JP *et al.* Sex bias in considering coronary bypass surgery. *Ann Intern Med* 1987; **107**: 19–25.

61 Petticrew M, McKee M, Hones J. Coronary artery surgery: are women discriminated against? *Br Med J* 1993; **306**: 1164–6.

62 Mark DB, Shaw LK, DeLong ER, Califf RM, Pryor DB. Absence of sex bias in the referral of patients for cardiac catheterisation. *N Engl J Med* 1994; **330**: 1101–6.

63 Krumholz HM, Douglas PS, Lauer MS, Pasternack R. Selection of patients for coronary arteriography and coronary revascularisation early after myocardial infarction: is there evidence for gender bias? *Ann Intern Med* 1992; **116**: 785–90.

64 Bickell NA, Pieperks, Lee *et al.* Referral patterns for coronary artery disease treatment: gender bias or good clinical judgement? *Ann Intern Med* 1992; **116**: 791–7.

65 Loop FD, Golding LR, Macmillan JP, Cosgrove DM, Lytle BW, Sheldon WC. Coronary

artery surgery in women compared with men: analysis of risks and long term results. *J Am Coll Cardiol* 1983; **1**: 383–90.

66 Fisher LD, Kennedy JW, Daris KB *et al.* Association of sex, physical size and operative mortality after coronary artery bypass in the Coronary Artery Surgery Study (CASS). *J Thorac Cardiovasc Surg* 1982; **84**: 334–41.

67 Cowley MJ, Mullin SM, Kelsey SF *et al.* Sex differences in early and long term results of coronary angioplasty in the NHLBI PTCA Registry. *Circulation* 1985; **71**: 90–7.

68 The Consensus Trial Study Group. Effect of enalapril on mortality in severe congestive heart failure. *N Engl J Med* 1987; **316**: 1429–35.

69 Pfeffer MA, Braunwald E, Moyé LA *et al.* Effect of captopril on mortality and morbidity in patients with left ventricular dysfunction after myocardial infarction. Results of survival and ventricular enlargement trial. *N Engl J Med* 1992; **327**: 669–77.

70 The SOLVD Investigators. Effect of enalapril on survival in patients with reduced left ventricular ejections, fractions and congestive heart failure. *N Engl J Med* 1991; **325**: 292–302.

71 The Digitalis Investigation Group. The effect of digoxin on mortality and morbidity in patients with heart failure. *N Engl J Med* 1997; **336**: 525–33.

72 Packer M, O'Connor CM, Ghali JK *et al.* Effect of amlodipine on morbidity and mortality in severe chronic heart failure. *N Engl J Med* 1996; **335**: 1107–14.

2: Acute treatment of myocardial infarction

WS HILLIS

Introduction

Coronary artery disease, with its clinical presentations of angina pectoris, myocardial infarction and sudden death, remains the main cause of premature morbidity and mortality in developed countries. Observational studies show a reduction in deaths from coronary artery disease in some populations, suggesting that preventive programmes targeted at risk factor modification for atheroma may be influential[1] but the treatment of acute myocardial infarction remains a major medical challenge with over 250,000 patients annually in the United Kingdom. The major clinical trials have demonstrated that the new treatment protocols have a significant effect on the morbidity and mortality associated with myocardial infarction. New protocols of acute and long term pharmacological management are in current use. This chapter will review the clinical trials and end with a summary of the author's interpretation of the currently available evidence translated into a treatment protocol.

Early management strategies

The early management of patients with acute myocardial infarction recognises that most deaths occur within the first hour of onset and are usually due to ventricular fibrillation.[2] Patient education is required to reduce the time to presentation and should be undertaken in subjects with high risk, including those with multiple risk factors or previous ischaemic heart disease events. Inherent delays are recognised between the onset of symptoms and treatment administration, including patient delay in recognising the severity of illness, prehospital delay including physician attendance delay, treatment administration and ambulance transfer. A dual response of physician and ambulance attendance is beneficial. In-hospital delays secondary to the performance of diagnostic tests and mechanisms for treatment administration are being addressed. Integrated services should be developed with the provision of ambulances containing appropriate equipment for resuscitation including defibrillators, oxygen and suction apparatus, endotracheal tubes and appropriate cardiac drugs. In-hospital triage times should be minimised with appropriate fast tracking systems.

Analgesia

Adequate analgesia is often not given out of hospital, although it is recognised by all that pain relief is mandatory in the treatment of acute

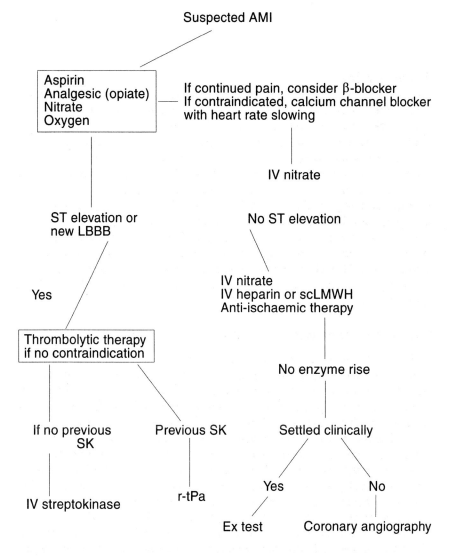

Fig 2.1   Early management of acute myocardial infarction.

myocardial infarction. Pain relief reduces central sympathoadrenal discharge and therefore reduces myocardial oxygen requirement by acting as a mild venous and arteriolar dilator.[3]

Morphine and diamorphine remain the drugs of choice as those with mixed agonist activity may lead to increased peripheral vascular resistance.[4] Diamorphine has widespread clinical acceptance in the United Kingdom and is rapidly hydrolysed to monoacetyl morphine; comparative studies suggest that it is superior to morphine as it provides analgesia, has fewer side effects and haemodynamic effects and early complete relief of pain.[5] When given to supine patients in the absence of cardiac dysfunction, diamorphine has little effect on heart rate, rhythm or arterial pressure. The combined venous and arteriolar dilating action may be helpful in reducing left ventricular filling pressure and afterload but hypotension may occur in 2–8%, particularly when there is hypovolaemia. It may be secondary to a direct depressant action on the vasomotor centre or due to histamine release[6] and may require reversal with head tilting, fluid replacement or the use of pressor agents. Other clinical problems include respiratory depression in about 1% with opiates[7] and vomiting, secondary to stimulation of the chemoreceptor trigger zones for emesis, occurs in 20–30%. This latter side effect may be blocked by metoclopramide. Cyclizine should be avoided as it may counteract the beneficial haemodynamic effects of the opiates. Additional gastrointestinal problems include reduced gastric motility which may reduce absorption of cardioactive drugs given by the oral route and enhanced biliary tract contraction may occur. Direct stimulation of the vagal nucleus may cause bradycardia and may require reversal by atropine, particularly in patients where parasympathetic imbalance may occur, seen with inferior infarcts and mediated by the Bezold–Jarrisch reflex.[8]

Adjunctive analgesic therapeutic options

Sublingual nitrates may be effective in the alleviation of chest pain by coronary vasodilation and systemic venous dilating action. GTN should be avoided in the presence of marked hypotension or in patients with inferior infarcts with right ventricular involvement where preload reduction should be avoided.[9] Further IV administration of nitrates should be continued with routine blood pressure monitoring.

β-adrenoreceptor blocking compounds given in the early phase may reduce the need for analgesia.[10] Clinical indications include those with tachycardia and hypertension. β-blockers should be avoided in the presence of cardiac failure or hypotension.

Oxygen therapy has traditionally been given. However, the new application of pulse oximetry may confirm those with a specific need. In the presence of arterial hypoxaemia, 2–4 L/min of 100% oxygen should be delivered by mask or nasal prongs. Although ST elevation is reduced with oxygen suggestive of infarct size reduction, little evidence is available to show an impact on long term survival.[11]

Antiarrhythmic drugs

Following the introduction of monitoring of patients during the early phase of acute myocardial infarction, a high incidence of complex ventricular extrasystoles and R-on T beats were identified. The presence of such arrhythmias provide an unacceptably low sensitivity and specificity in identifying patients at risk of ventricular fibrillation. The prophylactic suppression of ventricular arrhythmias by class I antiarrhythmic therapy is therefore no longer utilised and indeed may have been associated with an increased risk of bradycardiac and asystolic events.[12, 13]

Thrombolytic therapy in acute myocardial infarction

Following the introduction of coronary care units, the in-hospital mortality for acute myocardial infarction was reduced from 30% to 10–15%. The continued resistant mortality was secondary to myocardial damage. With the recognition of coronary thrombus as the causal problem in coronary artery occlusion, thrombolytic agents were used to obtain coronary artery reperfusion. The agents with widespread use in clinical practice include streptokinase (SK), anistreplase and tissue plasminogen activator (TPA). The role of aspirin is addressed in Chapter 3.

Streptokinase

SK is a single chain protein produced from group 'C' β-haemolytic streptococci. It complexes plasminogen or plasmin and converts additional plasminogen molecules to active lys plasmin and combines directly to fibrin, activating fibrin bound plasminogen in an environment relatively free from the inhibitors α_2 antiplasmin and α_2 macroglobulin. SK has a short half life of 16 minutes which may represent complexing to circulating antibody, and a longer elimination half life for SK, SK activator complexes and SK fragments (83 min). The clearance half life of functionally active SK plasminogen and SK plasminogen complex is shorter (23 min).

Streptococcal infection or SK therapy stimulates antistreptokinase antibodies. Antibody production occurs within five days of exposure and increasing titre peaks at 2–3 weeks, with a variable return to pretreatment level. Recent observations have confirmed significant SK resistance present for up to four years.[14–16] The continued presence of IgG and IgE SK antibodies may lead to an increased risk of adverse reactions such as hypotension or anaphylaxis. These observations of SK resistance antibody formation suggest that therapy should not be repeated for up to one year following treatment and it may be in some that SK may be given once

23

only.[17] Alternatively it may be that a loading dose of Sk may be given to neutralise the antibodies, followed by a standard therapeutic dose.

SK infusion leads to a variable hyperplasminaemia. Its duration is variable, depending on the rate of plasminogen activation, concentration of α_2 antiplasmin and α_2 macroglobulin and the rate of clearance of plasmin. Hyperplasminaemia degrades circulating fibrinogen and coagulation factors V and V2I, leading to a lytic state and an induced coagulation defect. Fibrinogen degradation products are also produced and exert an antithrombotic action and inhibit fibrin polymerisation. Hypofibrinogenaemia reduces blood viscosity and may favour increased flow in the microvasculature and may also reduce peripheral vascular resistance.[18] The associated anticoagulant effect means that SK may be given without adjunctive heparin.

Anistreplase

Anistreplase or eminase is an acylated plasminogen streptokinase complex in which the active serine site is temporarily inactivated by a reaction with the anisoyl group of a special reversible acylating agent p-amidinophenyl p-anisate hydrochloride (APAN). This acylation renders the molecule catalytically inert in serum and it evades the normal plasma inhibitors.[19] Its main advantage was its use by bolus injection. SK is complexed to lys plasminogen to bind to fibrin through its fibrin binding kringles. The lysine fibrin binding sites are structurally and functionally separate from the catalytic centre. Following bolus injection there is a very marked gradient for its diffusion into thrombus. Deacylation then occurs by hydrolysis with generation of plasminogen activator in a linear fashion. Deacylation begins immediately after injection. Initial studies demonstrated a prolonged half life of 105–120 minutes in human blood, and further plasma clearance *in vivo* confirmed a half life of some 90 minutes.[20] Anistreplase has shown strong binding affinity to preformed human plasma clots *in vitro*. When used clinically, systemic fibrinogenolytic activity is seen with similar changes in coagulation factors V and V2I and hypofibrinogenaemia and reduced plasma viscosity similar to that obtained with SK. Anistreplase has found its main use in community administration, where a simplified regimen is required.[21]

Tissue plasminogen activator

TPA is a 529 amino acid single chain serine protease. It is available in a mainly single chain form (alteplase). TPA is characterised by a low efficiency of plasminogen activation in the absence of fibrin and has a marked acceleration of this activation in the presence of fibrin, where the one chain molecule is quickly converted to the two chain variety.[22] TPA in blood originates from vascular endothelial cells. Several active protease inhibitors are contained in several forms (PAI-1, PAI-2) and have been found in endothelial cell cultures, placental tissue, and in plasma. TPA is removed by hepatic clearance with a half life of only a few minutes.[23] Once bound to fibrin, a longer functional dynamic half life is evident but its short half life has led to anxieties concerning coronary artery reocclusion.[24] The administration of TPA has varied with the use of the single chain or two chain structures. Most clinical studies have been performed using actylise given by a decremental infusion. Following clinical studies of efficacy using coronary artery patency and observations of complications including intracranial haemorrhage, a dose of 100 mg has been established. When given by front loading with a 15 mg bolus, 50 mg over 30 minutes and 35 mg given over a further 60 minutes, a very high degree of coronary artery patency can be achieved, with resulting major benefits in left ventricular function and mortality.[25]

Urokinase

Urokinase is a trypsin like serine protease and is a direct plasminogen activator with specific affinity for fibrin. As a human glycoprotein, it is not antigenic, has minor haemodynamic effects and a bolus dose regimen may allow its use as an alternative to tissue plasminogen activator. Currently urokinase is not in routine clinical use in the UK, but has been extensively applied in the US by infusion locally into the coronary arteries, particularly after acute procedure related occlusion.[26]

Clinical studies with thrombolysis in acute myocardial infarction

Fletcher et al.[27] described the initial use of SK in acute myocardial infarction. Subsequently thrombolytic regimes have aimed to produce persistent coronary artery reperfusion to improve left ventricular function and hence to reduce mortality. Widespread application of intracoronary thrombolysis is impractical and high dose, brief, intravenous infusions were introduced and an empirical infusion regimen of 1·5 MU of SK given over 60 minutes has been the standard widely accepted therapy.[28] Using this technique, patency rates of 55–84% have been reported. Following these observations with SK, similar studies have been performed using the different routes of administration for both anistreplase and TPA.

Comparative trials of SK and TPA have shown a difference in efficiency for early coronary artery recanalisation, early patency measured by coronary angiography at 90 minutes after start of therapy being 22% with placebo, 53% with SK, 75% with TPA, and up to 85% with accelerated regimen.[25, 28, 29] The other thrombolytic agents are probably intermediate in their efficacy. A catch-up phenomenon occurs with SK within three hours so that the patency of infarct related coronary arteries with both agents is 75–80% at three hours.[25]

Functional changes following thrombolysis

Serial assessments of left ventricular function performed both invasively and non-invasively show beneficial changes with successful thrombolysis. ST elevation is the usual admission criterion for most thrombolytic studies. Rapid sequential changes occur following reperfusion with accelerated pattern of R wave loss and Q wave development. Early ST reversal is often associated with reperfusion or occurs in patients with a good prognosis in terms of left ventricular function and subsequent clinical events. The distribution and degree of R wave loss and Q wave development is less in reperfused than non-reperfused patients and QRS scoring systems have confirmed evidence of myocardial salvage.[30, 31]

Following successful thrombolysis, an early peak of cardiac enzyme release occurs in reperfused subjects and established modelling techniques have shown reduction in infarct size in the ISAM Study[32] and in the Netherlands Interuniversity Study.[33]

Improvement in left ventricular function is quantitatively small. Serial improvements in radionuclide global ejection fraction at day 10 compared with day 1 in reperfused cases show an increase of 5% compared with deterioration of 3% in controls.[29]

Mortality studies for thrombolytic therapy in acute myocardial infarction

In 1985, Yusuf et al.[34] performed a meta-analysis of previously conducted appropriately designed randomised clinical studies of thrombolytic agents in the treatment of acute myocardial infarction. Although the individual studies were small, the overview produced a highly significant ($22 \pm 5\%$, $p < 0.001$) reduction in the odds of reinfarction. Reduction in mortality in individual studies was small and it was clear that large, prospective randomised trials were required.

Placebo controlled studies

The GISSI Study[35, 36] randomised 11,811 patients in 176 Italian coronary care units to unblinded SK or standard therapy within 12 hours of symptoms. Patients were stratified into three-hour time blocks from 0 to 12 hours. Thirty-five percent of patients were >65 years, with 10% >75 years of age. The in-hospital mortality at 21 days was reduced (10·7% versus 13%). In patients treated within one hour, the mortality was reduced by 47%. The mortality was reduced in those treated up to six hours from onset and was particularly marked in those with anterior infarcts. The one-year survival data confirmed the in-hospital benefit.

The ISIS 2 Study[37] randomised 17,187 patients in 417 hospitals and evaluated the separate and combined effects of intravenous SK and oral aspirin 160 mg on mortality in patients with symptoms of up to 24 hours duration. Using SK alone, mortality was reduced from 12% to 9·2%, a 25% reduction. Reduction was greatest for those randomised within four hours, but was still significant in those randomised between five and 24 hours. Aspirin therapy alone showed a reduction of mortality of 23% in five weeks and combined therapy showed a mortality reduction of 42%. Combined treatment was associated with an excess tendency for major bleeds of 0·3% and excess of disabling strokes of 0·1%. The combination was associated with fewer infarctions, cardiac rupture or in-hospital cardiac arrest.

The AIMS Study group[38, 39] reported on the 12-month mortality data on 1258 patients randomised in a double blind placebo controlled trial of anistreplase. At 30 days, 40 (6%) of 625 patients treated with anistreplase had died, compared with 77 (12%) of 634 patients on placebo. Mortality reduction was 50·5%. The survival benefit was still observed at 12 months: 69 (11%) patients treated with anistreplase died, compared with 112 (18%) patients given placebo, odds reduction 43%, p = 0·0007, 95% confidence intervals, 21–59%. The effects on mortality were not related to the time between the onset of symptoms and treatment or to any patient characteristic. In addition, the major complications of acute myocardial infarction were less frequent in patients treated with anistreplase than in controls. Haemorrhage was more common, but usually minor. In this study, concomitant aspirin therapy was not administered.

The 1988 ECSG Trial[40] examined the effects of TPA on left ventricular function and mortality. Both showed a significant improvement in those patients treated within three hours.

The ASSET Study[41] randomised 5011 patients within five hours of symptoms to TPA or placebo and all received heparin for 24 hours. There was a reduction in mortality at 30 days of 26% (9·8% versus 7·2%) in favour of the TPA group. Although ECG entry criteria were not required, in those retrospectively confirmed to have myocardial infarction, the mortality difference was greater (13% versus 9%). Similar reductions in mortality were seen in patients treated within three hours and between three and five hours.

This series of studies confirmed without doubt the benefits of intravenous thrombolysis in acute MI.

Comparative studies of mortality following thrombolysis

GISSI-2[42] was a direct comparative study of the effects of SK or alteplase (TPA) on mortality and left ventricular function. Of 389,086 patients screened, 12,490 entered this multicentre randomised open trial. Patients received either SK 1·5 MU over 30–60 minutes or 100 mg of TPA infused over three hours. Half of the patients were randomised to receive 12,500 units subcutaneous heparin twice daily starting 12 hours after the commencement of thrombolytic therapy, until hospital discharge. All patients had oral aspirin 325 mg a day and atenolol 5–10 mg given by IV injection. The combined endpoint was the number of patients who died, plus late extensive left ventricular damage or clinical heart failure. Left ventricular damage was assessed from electrocardiographic techniques and from echocardiography.

The overall mortality was 8·8%. There was no difference in the four treatment groups with regard to the combined endpoint or its components. There were more strokes with TPA (70 versus 54), but more major bleeds with SK (34 versus 61), while TPA had fewer allergic reactions and hypotension. The overall stroke rate was 1·1% in the TPA group compared to 0·9% in the SK group – no significant difference in either haemorrhagic or ischaemic strokes.

The International Study Group

It was decided following GISSI-2 that mortality alone should be anlaysed in a larger study population and the International Study Group was formed, with the primary endpoint of comparing the effects on the in-hospital and six-month mortality rates. The second objective was the evaluation of postthrombolytic treatment of heparin on mortality and the safety of the different drug regimens.[43]

Eight thousand four hundred and one patients were randomised, 4108 to TPA and 4203 to SK; 4198 patients were allocated to subcutaneous heparin, 4209 had no heparin. There was good matching of the groups and therapy was given in a high percentage of patients. In the acute phase, atenolol was administered intravenously in 23% of patients and these were matched for SK, TPA, heparin, and no heparin. Diagnosis at discharge or death was acute myocardial infarction in 94·9%, angina pectoris in 3·4%, and other 1·7%. Angioplasty or coronary artery bypass surgery was performed in 2·1% and 2·1% of patients respectively. The incidence of death and other major clinical events are similar to those of the GISSI-2 Trial, the only exception being a higher overall incidence of reinfarction and stroke. The stroke total was 68 (1·6%) in TPA and 44 (1%) in SK. Haemorrhagic strokes were 25 (0·6%) versus 15 (0·4%). The in-hospital reinfarction rate was similar. Similar mortality rates were shown in males and females, patients below or above 70 years of age, patients treated within or after three hours from onset of symptoms or in patients with/without previous myocardial infarction. For both agents there was an excess of strokes in patients over 70 years. More allergic reactions and hypotension were seen with SK. The overall incidence of stroke was low, although more strokes were reported with TPA, but the frequency of confirmed haemor-rhagic stroke was similar for TPA and SK. Streptokinase and heparin treatment were both independently associated with a higher incidence of major bleeds, the highest frequency being observed in patients treated with both SK and heparin. These major bleeds, however, were not responsible for an excess of deaths. Minor bleeding complications were more frequently seen with TPA.

ISIS-3 Study

This study was performed as a multicentre (936 hospitals) international collaboration in 46,092 patients and was a comparative study of streptokinase 1·5 MU IV, r-TPA using duteplase (two chain) and anistreplase 30 U.[44] All patients received aspirin with further randomisation to heparin, 12,500 U bd. The mortality rates for those patients receiving SK, TPA and APSAC were similar at 35 days (10·5%, 10·3%, 10·6%). The incidence of probable cerebral haemorrhage, however, was higher for both TPA and APSAC (0·75, 0·65) compared with SK (0·35).[44]

Several issues have been raised regarding interpretation of the study as two chain TPA (duteplase) was used and the regimen used had little previous exposure.

GUSTO Study

In the GUSTO Study,[25] four treatment regimens were assessed in 41,021 patients treated within six hours of the onset of symptoms. One group was studied with accelerated doses of TPA with IV heparin, two patient groups were treated with SK with either subcutaneous or intravenous heparin and a further group with combination therapy with TPA, SK, and IV heparin. On comparing the study groups, the mortality was reduced in the patients treated with TPA compared to the three groups using SK. The addition of IV heparin did not improve efficacy of SK, but increased the number of strokes. The maximum benefits of r-TPA were seen in patients with anterior infarction and the maximum stroke incidence, which was increased in the TPA group, occurred in the over 75s. There has been widespread discussion concerning the results of this trial. In a subset of patients, angiographic assessment of patency was studied and linked to left ventricular function and mortality. Maximum benefit was achieved in those patients who had grade 3 reperfusion and this has once more greatly promoted the open artery hypothesis. Although the importance of grade 3 reperfusion had been suggested in the TEAM Study of anistreplase, these present data give major credence to these observations.

FTT

The Fibrinolytic Therapy Trialist (FTT) Collaborative Group[45] performed a systematic overview of the effects of thrombolytic therapy in death and major morbidity in various patient categories, with a meta-analysis of the major trials in which >1000 patients were randomised. This included: GISSI, ISAM, AIMS, ISIS-2, ASSET, USIM, ISIS-3, EMERAS and

LATE. This meta-analysis demonstrated the wide range of patients who benefit from thrombolytic therapy and it may be that some do not receive this in clinical practice. The analysis also categorised the early excess in deaths and strokes associated with fibrinolytic therapy. The greatest reduction in mortality occurs in those patients presenting with ST elevation, particularly those with anterior infarcts, although benefits are also seen in those with inferior infarction and those with left bundle branch block pattern. There is little evidence of benefit in patients presenting with ST depression and if the ECG is normal, there is a high risk/benefit ratio.

Time between symptom onset and symptoms

Benefit in some of the early thrombolytic trials was shown in patients treated up to 24 hours later. Recent studies, however, have thrown some doubt on this and suggested a narrower effective time band. The use of TPA was assessed in 5711 patients entered into the LATE Study[46] who had ECG changes but presented at more than six hours following onset of symptoms. In those treated at between seven and 12 hours, there was a significant reduction in mortality and a further analysis suggested that if patients presented later than 12 hours but had typical ECG changes and a typical history, advantage was maintained. In the EMERAS Study,[47] assessing streptokinase versus placebo, similar results were obtained but no benefit was shown in the group treated at between 13 and 24 hours.

Early therapy is most efficient and each hour lost prior to treatment is associated with a reduced benefit of 1·6–2 patients/1000. There is continued doubt concerning the benefits to patients presenting beyond 12 hours after onset of symptoms, even after the results of the ISIS-2, EMERAS and LATE studies. It appears there may be a continued benefit between 13 and 18 hours, but the numbers in general are small for such a subdivision. The FTT review suggests that late treatment may be associated with a higher mortality on days 0–1 and therefore emphasises the early hazard of thrombolytic therapy. In the elderly, there is an early excess of deaths but the subsequent improvement in mortality is similar to younger age groups. In patients with cardiac failure or cardiogenic shock, alternative reperfusion strategies have been advocated. This study suggests the greatest benefit of thrombolysis occurs in patients with hypotension and tachycardia, but once more the numbers are relatively small. The early hazard associated with fibrinolytic therapy appears related to the development of electromechanical dissociation or cardiac rupture.

Adjunctive heparin

There was a higher incidence of bleeds associated with heparin therapy – 655 (10·6%) versus 364 (5·9%) – in GISSI-2, but there was a reduction in pulmonary and systemic thromboembolism.[42] There was no difference in major bleeds with respect to thrombolytic agent (30 versus 35) but those patients treated with heparin had a higher incidence (44 versus 21). In the International Study Group subcutaneous heparin was used because it was practicable, safe and effective.[43] There was a lower in-hospital mortality observed when subcutaneous heparin was used compared with SK alone, but it was associated with the highest incidence of major bleeds. The use of subcutaneous heparin has been questioned as the regimen does not fully anticoagulate. It is proposed that in ISIS-3 an improved level of reperfusion would have been achieved if full anticoagulation had been given and the anticoagulant response serially measured.

Magnesium following myocardial infarction

Diverse beneficial effects of magnesium post-MI were suggested by several experimental studies. Acute administration doubling the physiological plasma level (0·7–0·95 mmol/L) causes endothelium dependent vasodilation mediated in part by prostacyclin. It also inhibits vascular smooth muscle cell contraction[48] and its withdrawal potentiates vasoconstriction reponses to a number of agonists including angiotensin 2 and noradrenaline.

Observations of early mortality following successful coronary artery reperfusion suggest that reperfusion damage may occur. Studies in experimental myocardial ischaemia suggest that magnesium protects myocardial contractile function against injury and that stunning is associated with an uncontrolled rise in intracellular calcium and depletion of high energy phosphates which is modified by magnesium therapy.

Magnesium has an electrophysiological action by slowing conduction through the AV node, with prolongation of the A-H interval, inhibiting the slow calcium current mediating conduction through the upper AV node. Sinus node function and QT interval duration remain unchanged.[49] Magnesium is effective in terminating multifocal atrial tachycardia and is highly effective in terminating torsade de pointes. This action appears independent of the initiating cause and does not seem to be mediated by correction of underlying magnesium depletion.[50] In models of the long QT syndrome, the amplitude of after potentials is reduced. Patients with low magnesium concentrations who have had acute myocardial infarction are more commonly prone to ventricular arrhythmias. In acutely ischaemic myocardium magnesium automatically impartially depolarises cells and inhibits the calcium current. Moreover, in some animal experiments, the concentration of magnesium shown to be efficacious is unobtainable in man and there are marked species variations. An antiplatelet effect is also evident with inhibition of platelet function by stimulating release of prostacyclin from human vascular endothelium.[51]

Prior to 1990 there were several small studies of IV magnesium in

31

patients with suspected acute myocardial infarction. There were seven randomised trials involving 1301 patients, with treatment being commenced within 12 hours of onset of chest pain, with the only exclusion criterion being a high degree of AV block and elevated serum creatinine. Magnesium sulphate was used in five studies and magnesium chloride in the remaining two studies. The total dose administered was 30–90 mmol, the duration of the infusion was 24–48 hours and there was a variable follow-up. The reduction in mortality was significant (25 of 657 versus 53 of 644 controls, 3·85% versus 8·2%). The one-year mortality was recorded in the study of Rasmussen.[52] The reduction in mortality occurred early and there was no further divergence in the first year. There was a reduction in ventricular arrhythmias in the magnesium treated group, compared to controls. An overview suggested a reduction in mortality and arrhythmias, but reservations have been expressed concerning the relatively small numbers studied, the different infusion regimen used and the small numbers of deaths in control and study groups. A positive bias in the reporting of such studies has also been suggested.

The LIMIT-2 Study[53, 54] examined the effects of magnesium infusion on the 28-day mortality in patients who had suspected acute myocardial infarction. An IV regimen of magnesium sulphate or placebo was introduced in 2316 subjects. Twenty-eight day mortality was 10·3% versus 7·8%, i.e. a 16% reduction for those patients treated with IV magnesium. There was also benefit shown in the incidence of congestive cardiac failure (clinical 11·2% versus 14·9%, p = 0·009; radiological 17·2% versus 22%, p = 0·004). The follow-up data confirmed reduction in mortality from ischaemic heart disease by 21% (5–35%, p = 0·01). All-cause mortality was reduced by 16% (2–29%, p = 0·03).

In contrast, in the ISIS-4 Study,[55] IV magnesium showed no beneficial effect, in fact a slight excess mortality was evident. This may reflect the late introduction of therapy as the lytic phase was complete before trial randomisation, whereas the LIMIT Study was in keeping with the previous study design, with early pre-reperfusion therapy.

The mechanism of any benefit of magnesium treatment is unclear. The reduction in afterload in the LIMIT Study was minor and no apparent antiarrhythmic effect was noted. The lack of interaction with aspirin appears to exclude an effect on platelets and the lack of interaction with previous diuretic therapy suggests that significant pretherapy depletion was not a factor.

Adjunctive therapy after myocardial infarction

Oral anticoagulants

In 1980 (prethrombolytic era) the Sixty Plus Reinfarction Study examined patients who had received anticoagulants for a mean of six years post-myocardial infarction. They were randomised to continued anticoagulants or placebo and there was an increase in cardiovascular complications after withdrawal.[56] The Norwegian (WARIS) Study[57] found a substantial reduction in mortality (24%), recurrent myocardial infarction (34%), and reduced stroke (55%). The ASPECT Study[58] was a randomised placebo-controlled double blind multicentre trial in 3404 hospital survivors of myocardial infarction, randomly assigned to anticoagulation or placebo therapy within six weeks of discharge from hospital (2·8–4·8 times INR). In this patient group only 25% received thrombolytic therapy and 51% were receiving β-blockade. This was a mortality reduction of 10%, a significant reduction in the risk of recurrent myocardial infarction (114 versus 242) and reduction in the risk of first cerebrovascular event (37 versus 62). However, major bleeding was commoner in the anticoagulant group (73 versus 19) with intracranial bleeding being more common (17 versus 2). Sixty-two percent of the patients were controlled within the target range of INR with 29% below and 9% above. However, after three years about half of the patients had discontinued therapy.

Several studies have compared antiplatelet with anticoagulant strategy. In the German–Austrian Trial[59] patients with MI were randomised to aspirin, placebo or anticoagulants with follow-up over a two-year period. There was a non-significant reduction in all-cause mortality of 26%, compared with a coronary death reduction of 46·3% with anticoagulants. In the EPSIM Trial[60] patients were randomised to aspirin or oral anticoagulants with a mean follow-up of 29 months. Mortality was 11·1% in those treated with aspirin versus 10·3% with anticoagulants. Conversely, in the APRICOT Study, aspirin was shown to be superior to warfarin in terms of both the angiographic and clinical outcome when oral warfarin was added following intravenous heparin.[61]

The results of two trials are awaited – the CARS Trial with patients randomised to 160 mg aspirin daily versus aspirin 80 mg plus 3 mg of warfarin daily or aspirin 80 mg and 1 mg daily, and the CHAMP Study of 160 mg aspirin versus aspirin 80 mg plus warfarin with an INR of 1·5–2·5.

β-Blockers in acute myocardial infarction

During the 1970s and 1980s β-adrenoreceptor antagonist drugs (β-blockers) established their efficacy and safety in the management of ischaemic heart disease. All β-blockers act as competitive antagonists at β-adrenoreceptors which are widely distributed through the body; β1-adrenoreceptors are found mainly in the heart and β2 are located in other tissues including the lungs, peripheral blood vessels, and skeletal muscles. Some β-blockers preferentially and predominantly antagonise β1-receptor mediated effects, but none of the agents demonstrates absolute selectivity. Some agents have partial agonist activity (PAA) or intrinsic

33

sympathomimetic activity (ISA). Under basal conditions they act as mild agonists on the β-adrenoreceptor, but in the presence of enhanced adrenergic tone, the β-blocking activity predominates. In practice, the main effect is on resting heart rate. Early studies to salvage myocardium included the use of β-blocking compounds. Their beneficial haemodynamic changes included reduction of heart rate, contractility and wall stress, associated with a reduction in systolic blood pressure, both at rest and under catecholamine stress.

Beneficial electrophysiological changes occur, with resulting anti-arrhythmic properties. Experimental studies suggest that β-blockers reduce myocardial infarct size and, by reducing myocardial wall stress, may reduce the incidence of early cardiac rupture. β-Blockers elevate the threshold for ventricular fibrillation in animal experiments and also reduce the incidence of complex ventricular arrhythmias in clinical studies.[62] By the above action, they would be expected to reduce the mortality following myocardial infarction and reduce cardiac rupture, reinfarct and the incidence of ventricular fibrillation.

Clinical studies have examined the immediate and late effects of the introduction of β-blockers and the later studies examined β-blockade in conjunction with thrombolysis.

In the ISIS-1 Study[63] vascular deaths were reduced by 15% during the week of treatment (3·9% in β-blocker versus 4·6% in control group, $p < 0·05$). Further pooled data suggested a reduction in deaths by 13% (95% CI 2–25%) in the first week and the benefits were maintained for the first year of follow-up.

The long term use of β-blockers has been evaluated in many studies, but with variable times of introduction and duration of treatment. The mortality is significantly reduced by β-blockade (7·6% versus 9·4% amongst controls) with a 22% reduction (95% CI −16–30%).[64]

Detailed analysis of the results based on subgroups including divisions for age, sex, site of myocardial infarction, and risk category failed to show specific preference, but absolute benefit was greater for the group with poor rather than good prognosis in the MIAMI Trial.[65]

The TIMI Phase 2 Trial examined β-blockade in the thrombolytic era.[66, 67] A subgroup of 1390 patients were randomly assigned to treatment with metoprolol given IV immediately followed by oral therapy or oral metoprolol commenced at day 6. The total mortality at hospital discharge and at day 42 showed no difference, but there was a significant reduction in non-fatal infarction and recurrent ischaemic episodes in the early β-blocking treated group (123 versus 178, $p < 0·005$). The results were extended to a total of 1424 patients and a subset analysis undertaken, those patients who were defined as having low risk appearing to benefit in terms of mortality (no deaths at six weeks in immediate β-blocking group versus seven deaths in the deferred group). The overall view of the investigators, however, was that early treatment, although associated with reduced myocardial ischaemia and reinfarction in the first week, showed no benefit over late therapy in improving left ventricular function or in reducing mortality.

As favourable effects have been reported with the use of atenolol,[63] metoprolol,[65] timolol,[68] propranolol,[69] and alprenolol[70] and there is an absence of studies showing favourable effects with agents with intrinsic sympathomimetic activity, then these latter agents should be avoided.

Starting treatment early with IV β-blockade and continuing with oral therapy for up to 1–2 years appears the best clinical strategy.

Calcium channel blockers

Calcium channel blockers have been shown in animal models to preserve left ventricular function by reducing myocardial necrosis after experimental coronary artery occlusion. These effects occur by several mechanisms including a reduction in left ventricular contraction, a reduction in afterload leading to reducing oxygen consumption and by increasing coronary blood flow, due to coronary vasodilation and the reduction of myocardial cell damage by decreasing intracellular calcium overload during

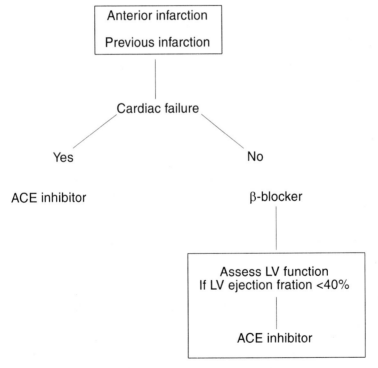

Fig 2.2   Long term management.

ischaemia.[71]

The major subclasses of calcium channel blockers are presented by nifedipine, diltiazem and verapamil. Nifedipine has peripheral vasodilating action which may be associated with tachycardia. Verapamil has a significant electrophysiological effect, as well as a negative inotropic action. Diltiazem has intermediate effects.

Held et al.[72] reviewed the actions of calcium channel blockers in acute myocardial infarctions. The overview of 16 trials strongly suggested that the currently available calcium channel blockers are unlikely to reduce the rate of infarct development, infarct size, rate of reinfarction or mortality and the negative results of clinical studies of unstable angina refute the suggestion that preischaemia (infarction) administration is necessary. The Multicentre Diltiazem Post-Infarction Trial claimed significant bidirectional interaction,[73] a favourable but non-significant beneficial trend in those without pulmonary congestion, but significant adverse effects in those with pulmonary congestion. In the SPRINT-1 Trial[74] nifedipine treatment was introduced at 7–20 days in a dose of some 30 mg/day. The results were negative, but criticism was made concerning the late introduction of therapy at a fairly low dose. The SPRINT-2 Study[75] was designed in which nifedipine 60 mg/day was administered early (within 48 hours) to 1006 patients in the course of myocardial infarction. During the first six days, however, active treatment was associated with an increased mortality (6·8% versus 5·5%). During the six months follow-up of 826 patients who continued to receive therapy, there was no difference in mortality nor in the rates of non-fatal myocardial infarction and unstable angina.

Recent meta-analysis of the treatment of patients with acute myocardial infarction with calcium channel blockers interpreted the results as showing a dose related increase in hospital mortality in studies in which > 80 mg of nifedipine was used.[76] Although this data interpretation has been challenged, it seems appropriate to avoid high dose therapy with short acting dihydropyridines.[77, 78] No trials of sustained release preparations of nifedipine have been reported. In the MDPIT and the DAVIT-2[79] Trial, subgroup analysis suggested a reduction in mortality in patients free from cardiac failure. In patients with ongoing ischaemia and contraindications to β-blockade, the cautious introduction of verapamil or diltiazem may be indicated in the absence of cardiac failure.

Nitrate therapy

The use of nitrates as adjunctive therapy to relieve ischaemic chest pain has been discussed above. Early studies have confirmed a reduction in left ventricular dilation following infarction with intravenous nitrates using an infusion regimen designed to reduce systemic pressure and avoid the development of tolerance.[80, 81] In general, although early advantage may be obtained, the use of nitrates has been superseded by the use of the angiotensin converting enzyme inhibitors.

In the GISSI-3 Study[82] IV nitrates were used for the first 24 hours followed by transdermal GTN 10 mg daily. This systematic administration of transdermal GTN did not show any independent effect, while the survival curve showed a small but non-significant benefit. It should be noted that of the 9442 patients assigned to the control group, 5392 (57·1%) received some kind of nitrate therapy with 1071 continuing treatment for longer than five days. In the GISSI-3 pilot study it was shown that there was no effect on systolic blood pressure after 24 hours of therapy, suggesting developing tolerance. There appeared to be some additive effect of GTN and lisinopril on both mortality and the combined endpoint results. In the ISIS-4 Study, no benefit was shown from early treatment with slow release isosorbide mononitrate (Imdur). To avoid tolerance, this drug was given in a once-a-day therapy, but would therefore not have sustained haemodynamic effects.

Angiotensin converting enzyme inhibitors

This group of drugs, which have been shown to favourably influence symptomatic heart failure and mortality in long term studies of patients with heart failure, have now also been shown to be of benefit in defined patients post-MI. This benefit is seen in LV function, further cardiac events and total mortality.

LV Remodelling

Infarct size is determined by the size of arterial occlusion, the presence of previous myocardial infarction and of developed collaterals. Progressive left ventricular dilation may be observed during the early period following acute myocardial infarction.[83] This consists of expansion of the infarct segment within the first few days which extends over weeks to months after the onset of infarction.[84]

Ventricular remodelling describes a series of morphological changes leading to dilation and systolic dysfunction. In the remodelling process, myocyte hypertrophy is associated with side-to-side slippage of myocytes in the non-infarct zone, leading to increased cardiac volume while the thickness of the ventricular wall is maintained or reduced. With time, increased wall stress induces the development of eccentric ventricular hypertrophy, with further growth of cardiac myocytes and progressive myocardial fibrosis and rearrangement of the extracellular matrix architecture.

Segmental dilation is common in large transmural infarctions, particularly of the anteroapical surface which has the greatest curvature which thins and elongates.[85] Rearrangement of the myofibrils across the ventricular wall and eccentric secondary compensatory hypertrophy can occur in the non-infarcted zone, leading to significant remodelling. Coronary reperfusion reduces the degree of left ventricular dilation. This occurs whether successful reperfusion is achieved early or late.

A preclinical phase of left ventricular dysfunction may occur in which subjects are asymptomatic but continued increased wall stress and afterload may lead to increased infarct expansion.[86] Although some pharmacological methods have been shown to be effective in salvaging myocardium in animal models, such as the administration of steroids and non-steroidal anti-inflammatory drugs, when translated into the clinical trials they have led to the development of thinner scar formation and enhanced expansion with resultant slowing of the healing process.

Diuretics have been used extensively in the treatment of acute cardiac failure and their efficacy is well established. Serial measurements of left ventricular function, however, show continued deterioration in left ventricular contraction, with resulting dilation in patients with asymptomatic left ventricular dysfunction postinfarct.[86] The neurohumeral responses secondary to diuretic administration may lead to activation of the renin angiotensin system, with resulting increased afterload.

Acute myocardial infarction, with its impact on left ventricular function, leads to activation of various neuroendocrine systems. It has long been recognised that there is enhanced sympathetic activity following an acute myocardial infarction early in its course.[87, 88] The degree of elevation reflects the degree of cardiac damage and its resulting haemodynamic consequences. Very marked increases in catecholamine levels occur in the presence of pulmonary oedema and shock and may predispose to serious ventricular arrhythmias. Local sympathetic overactivity may occur with exocytolic release of noradrenaline from cardiac sympathetic nerve terminals. This may lead to very high local levels in myocardium and may even result in localised necrosis.[89] Deleterious effects of sympathetic drive include oxygen-wasting tachycardia, increased peripheral resistance and possible induction of tachyarrhythmias. The renin angiotensin system is activated and myocardium sensitised by increased angiotensin 2 receptors in the infarct zone. Angiotensin 2 may increase myocardial contractility, thus stimulating myocardial growth, and induce fibroblast proliferation and therefore contribute to myocardial hypertrophy and fibrosis during the ventricular remodelling process.[90] The use of ACE inhibitors may have a localised role as well as a general effect on haemodynamic changes.

The use of ACE inhibitors early in acute myocardial infarction has shown reduction in early dilation of the infarct segment in both experimental models and clinical infarction.[84] In asymptomatic patients with documented left ventricular dysfunction,[86] reduced dilation was shown using ACE inhibitors compared to treatment with placebo or diuretics. There was a significant improvement in end systolic and end diastolic volumes and ejection fraction seen at one year.

Following these initial promising observations, ACE inhibitors have been widely applied in the treatment of patients with acute myocardial infarction. Studies have been performed using two major strategies: a low risk approach which involved the early application of ACE inhibitors to patients at a variable time following myocardial infarction or to all patients early in their clinical course, regardless of presence of left ventricular dysfunction. The alternative approach has been to identify those patients with clinical evidence of left ventricular failure or with measured left ventricular dysfunction, using objective radionuclide or echocardiographic assessments of left ventricular function.

In the SMILE Study[91] 1500 patients with myocardial infarction who were ineligible for thrombolytic therapy were randomised, introducing ACE inhibition using zofenopril at 24 hours and continuing treatment for one year. This study showed a reduced risk of new cardiac events (22%) and a significant reduction in the development of heart failure (49%).

The CONSENSUS 2 Study[92] was conducted in 103 Scandinavian centres to examine the effects on mortality of the ACE inhibitor enalapril introduced within 24 hours of the onset of acute myocardial infarction defined with typical ECG changes and enzyme elevation. Treatment was introduced using an intravenous infusion of 1 mg enalapril over two hours or placebo, followed by oral therapy at six hours. The dose schedule increased daily from 5 mg to 20 mg, but was modified according to the precipitation of hypotensive episodes. The primary endpoint was death within six months, with secondary endpoints of death at one month, cause of death reinfarction, worsening heart failure requiring a change in treatment or hospitalisation and progressive heart failure. Ten thousand three hundred and eighty-seven patients were screened with 41% excluded. Nine thousand and ninety were randomised, the mean age of entry was 66 years with 73% males, 24% had previous infarct and 6% had heart failure prior to trial entry. Eighteen percent developed heart failure with the index infarction. Fifty-seven percent received thrombolytic therapy. Patients were followed up for a minimum of 41–280 days, with 598 deaths in total – 286 placebo and 312 enalapril (9·4% versus 10·2%, p = 0·26). The increased mortality appeared to be secondary to progressive heart failure.

Adverse events were also more frequent in patients receiving enalapril than placebo. This study was disappointing despite the observation that 82% of the patients were able to take the top dose of enalapril (20 mg) and it was discontinued prematurely in view of the early results. After the results of subsequent trials, critical re-evaluation of this study has occurred. The entry criteria did not require the presence of left ventricular dysfunction and it was suggested that very early administration of the ACE inhibitor may have inhibited beneficial compensatory changes of cellular proliferation during early healing. An early hypotensive effect may have adversely affected perfusion and it may be that the treatment should have been longer than the six months observed, as in other studies benefit has only been evident after longer term follow-up.

The SAVE Study (1992)[93] examined the effects of captopril on morbidity and mortality in 2231 patients with left ventricular dysfunction following myocardial infarction. Entry was of either sex surviving for three days with a radionuclide ejection fraction of <40%, although patients were excluded if there was a requirement to treat cardiac failure. If patients had evidence of recurrent ischaemia, angiography was indicated and revascularisation undertaken during the hospital admission. Patients were treated using 6·25 mg of captopril, followed by 12·5 mg, increasing to 25 mg tid by time of discharge and the maximum 25 mg tid during the follow-up. Thirty-three percent of the population received thrombolytic therapy, 60% had coronary angiography and 25% had revascularisation. The endpoints studied were death from all causes, death from cardiovascular causes and death plus a further reduction in ejection fraction of 9% units. Other endpoints included new onset of congestive cardiac failure and occurrence of non-fatal infarction. Hospitalisation for treatment of CCF was also noted. Of 503 deaths, 275 of 1116 (25%) occurred with placebo and 228 of 1115 (20%) occurred with captopril. There was a 19% reduction (95% CI 3–32%, p = 0·019). Eighty-four deaths were of cardiovascular origin. There was a 21% reduction in death or major CV events with captopril, range 5–35%, p < 0·014. The reduction in deaths appeared to be due to a reduction in progressive heart failure. There was a 37% reduction in development of CCF with captopril (95% CI 20–50%, p < 0·001). There was a reduced need for hospitalisation. An unexpected result showed a significant reduction in recurrent acute myocardial infarction with 170 associated with placebo and 133 with captopril (25% reduction in risk, 95% CI 5–40%, p = 0·015). Eighty percent of patients maintained the target dose of captopril and there was a small excess of dizziness, taste alteration and cough.

The summary confirmed the hypothesis that therapies which attenuate progression of LV dysfunction should be beneficial and that the attenuation of ventricular modelling should affect mortality. This may be due to the benefits of inhibiting the deleterious effects of neurohumeral activation. The anti-ischaemic mechanism may be secondary to alteration in plasma renin activity or to alteration in baseline fibrinolysis, both of which are independent markers for the risk of myocardial infarction. The benefits shown in the SAVE Study were observed in patients who received standard additional therapy, including thrombolytic therapy (33%), β-blockade (36%), and aspirin (59%).

The TRACE Study randomised 1749 patients who had a myocardial infarction with a significant wall motion abnormality to treatment with trandolopril or placebo. The drugs were introduced between three and seven days following infarction with a median of some four days. The follow-up was a minimum of 24 months. There was an 18% reduction in mortality.[94]

The AIRE Study (1993)[95] was a multicentre, multinational, double blind, randomised, placebo controlled study enrolling patients with definite myocardial infarction and clinical evidence of cardiac failure as defined by LV failure on chest X-ray or on clinical grounds, including the findings of bilateral crepitations to one third of the chest, presence of a third heart sound or persistent tachycardia. Patients with severe heart failure were excluded. Two thousand and six patients were randomised between days 3–10 to ramipril 2·5 mg bd or placebo, then 5 mg bd after 48 hours. The primary endpoint of the study was all-cause mortality, while the secondary endpoint included the time to the first secondary event, defined as death, progression to severe cardiac failure, reinfarction or stroke. Of a total of 52,019 screened patients, 2006 were randomised, 23% had previous myocardial infarction and 8·2% previous heart failure. The mean time to randomisation was 5·4 days, with a minimum follow-up of six months, with a mean follow-up of 15 months. Fifty-eight percent of patients received thrombolytic therapy. The results showed an early separation between active and placebo therapies in all-cause mortality with an early and continued divergence. There was a 17% mortality in the ramipril group versus 23% in the placebo group (27% reduction, 95% CI 11–40%, $p = 0·002$). There was a 19% reduction in secondary endpoints of reinfarction or development of severe resistant cardiac failure (95% CI 5–31%, $p = 0·008$). Three hundred and fifty-two patients were prematurely withdrawn from ramipril therapy and 318 in the placebo group; 126 were intolerant to ramipril with 68 intolerant to placebo. Significantly fewer[58] developed severe cardiac failure with ramipril than with placebo.[92] Of those randomised to ramipril, 9% could not maintain the therapy and 14% were on 2·5 mg twice daily, therefore 23% could not tolerate the peak dose.

A comparison of the SAVE and AIRE studies highlights the differences in clinical practice between the UK and the US, as many in the SAVE Study had early angiography and intervention (60% angiography, 25% intervention). The AIRE study is of major importance as only simple clinical tests were used prior to entry and although some patients with asymptomatic left ventricular dysfunction were not treated, a high risk group of patients was identified as shown by the early evidence for reduction in mortality. There was a trend to reduction in incidence of myocardial infarction, but there also appeared to be a possible small increase in the number of strokes. Forty percent of the patients had no diuretics at the time of randomisation and it was felt that the action of ramipril was complementary to the action of β-blockade.

In the GISSI-3 Study[82] 19,394 patients were randomised from 200 CCUs in Italy within 24 hours of the onset of symptoms. They received oral lisinopril 5 mg then 10 mg daily, nitrates intravenously, then transdermal 10 mg GTN daily or no treatment for six weeks. Complete clinical data has been reported from 18,895 patients. After six weeks of therapy, the mortality overall was 6·7%. Those patients treated with lisinopril showed a statistically significant reduction in mortality compared with placebo (odds ratio 10·88, 95% CI 0·79–0·99) and there was a reduced incidence of death and development of severe left ventricular dysfunction. There was no significant difference shown between the nitrate and placebo groups. The combination of lisinopril and nitrates was found to significantly reduce mortality, compared to placebo or to either treatment given individually. The GISSI Study was an open label study and only 49% of patients were titrated up to the target dose of lisinopril. One thousand two hundred and fifty-six of the 9460 patients allocated to placebo had an ACE inhibitor given on clinical grounds and 10·4% had this therapy for more than five days. This suggests that the potential beneficial results of lisinopril may have been greater than demonstrated in this study. There was no difference in the reinfarction rates between the placebo and lisinopril groups.

The ISIS-4[55] Collaborative Group assessed the separate and combined effects on vascular mortality of adding nitrates, captopril and IV magnesium in patients with definite or suspected acute myocardial infarction; 70% received standard thrombolysis therapy and 94% had antiplatelet therapy.

Neither oral mononitrates (30–60 mg) nor intravenous magnesium (8 mmol bolus followed by 72 mmol infusion), begun with two hours of the start of thrombolysis on half the patients and within six hours of thrombolysis in 75%, influenced mortality. Captopril was given immediately after the early lytic phase of thrombolysis, beginning with 6·25 mg and titrated up to 50 mg twice daily. There was a significant reduction in five-week mortality (absolute reduction by 4·9/1000 deaths) in treated patients. There appeared also to be even more benefit in patients with previous myocardial infarction or heart failure. The benefit of active treatment was sustained for 12 months. Although there was an increase in documented hypotensive episodes, captopril treatment did appear safe with no excess of early deaths (day 0–1).

The Chinese Study[96] of the early mortality and complications with captopril has been reported, using 12·5 mg tid within 36 hours of onset of acute myocardial infarction in patients with suspected or confirmed infarct. An interim analysis of data from 11,345 has suggested a positive trend, reducing mortality at four weeks. Full reporting of the trial is awaited.

Primary angioplasty

A series of randomised studies in the late 1980s demonstrated that as an adjunct to thrombolysis, there was no advantage to immediate angioplasty over deferred investigation and treatment.[97–99] In the TAMI study 386 patients were enrolled and underwent angiography 90 minutes after administration of TPA.[97] This demonstrated infarct related vessel patency in 288 patients (75%). Of these 197 patients were randomised to either undergo immediate angioplasty (99 patients) or to have further intervention deferred for 7 days (98 patients). This study compared two groups both of whom underwent angioplasty following TPA, the comparison being of the timing of the angioplasty. There was no significant difference in outcome between the patient groups in terms of in-hospital mortality, regional wall motion abnormalities or re-occlusion. A similar sized study examined the effect of angioplasty as immediate adjunctive therapy after thrombolysis compared with continued conservative management.[99] Randomisation to the invasive treatment limb (183 patients) was followed in 180 patients by angiography, and angioplasty was attempted in 168 patients. A further 184 patients were investigated invasively only if clinically indicated. There was a higher 14 day mortality rate (7% versus 3%) in those allocated the interventional therapy, and also more recurrent ischaemia in the first 24 hours (17% versus 3%) when compared with conservatively managed patients. Bleeding complications were also greater in those assigned to angiography and angioplasty. There has been no evidence of benefit from adjuvant angioplasty.

More recently comparisons have been made between primary angioplasty and thrombolysis as the sole treatment for an acute myocardial infarction.[100-102] Improvements in patency rates of the infarct associated artery, left ventricular function and subsequent acute coronary events were observed after angioplasty. In the PAMI study there was a significant reduction in the combined endpoint of death and non-fatal infarct and also a reduction in stroke when angioplasty was compared with thrombolysis.

In contrast, an observational study based in Seattle compared patients assigned to either treatment on the basis of local clinical practice only.[103] This large non-randomised study appeared to compare patients with similar profile, though there was an excess of patients who had had previous bypass grafting or a history of GI bleed in those treated by immediate angioplasty. There were no significant outcome benefits between the two treatments assigned on this basis. A non-randomised observational study has many confounding variables, but equally the efforts expanded on a randomised clinical trial may not reflect a scenario applicable in practice. An additional consideration must be the recent reports of high rates of restenosis after immediate angioplasty for acute MI (47% at one year).[104]

Where facilities are available primary angioplasty may have some advantages in general, but specifically is a useful option for patients with contraindications to thrombolysis. Interestingly, this means the elderly may have most to gain from an aggressive interventional approach. The results of immediate angioplasty for infarction in 55 octogenarians were surprisingly good.[105] Technical success in 96% and a 60 day mortality of 16% in this high risk group would seem to compare favourably with thrombolysis results in these patients who are most vulnerable to cerebral haemorrhage and stroke.

Summary

If multiple variations and therapies need to be given to the peri-infarct patient, simple regimes are required to ensure that the majority of patients receive optimal treatment. Early diagnosis of myocardial infarction should lead to early aspirin and thrombolysis. The majority of the current evidence cannot differentiate between thrombolytic agents in terms of outcome. Only GUSTO II, demonstrated an advantage for TPA. Other comparative studies and meta analyses have not demonstrated benefits for TPA over streptokinase. The regime used to administer TPA in GUSTO II may have been a major factor in the results. GUSTO suggests a particular advantage for accelerated TPA in anterior myocardial infarction, presenting within 6 hours, in younger patients (<75 years). In older patients the increased risk of stroke counteracted the cardiac benefits. Anistreplase may be useful in remote areas (hence its choice in the Grampian Highlands-based GREAT study) as it can be given as a single bolus before a long journey to a distant hospital is undertaken.

β-Blocker treatment (a class effect by all accounts) should be begun early by IV injection then oral administration in patients in whom frank heart failure, bradycardias or coexisting pulmonary disease does not contra-indicate it.

The large ISIS 4 study did not demonstrate any benefit from intravenous magnesium, though the administration in that trial was generally late. This perhaps illustrates the increasing complex management of the acute infarct. Few centres would advocate magnesium therapy at present, except perhaps where early administration to patients with a contraindication to thrombolysis is possible.

The advantages of ACE inhibitor therapy post-myocardial infarction are also a class effect and there will be little to choose between agents. The ISIS 4 results support early oral administration (of captopril) but other large studies have shown benefit even with the later introduction of the ACE inhibitor. Adverse effects of early IV administration of enalapril in the Consensus 2 study has discouraged many from immediate IV ACE inhibitor therapy. Benefits appear to be greater when patients are selected by clinical or simple investigational evidence of a substantial myocardial infarction and/or heart failure, and the benefits persist over a prolonged follow-up period. A simple regime may be the oral administration of an ACE inhibitor on the day following admission, to those with clinical indications or a "large" Q-wave myocardial infarction by whatever criteria. A review, possibly with echocardiography at six weeks may indicate those with a good LV in whom the advantages of continued treatment are low and in whom the costly ACE inhibitor could be discontinued. In those who have evidence of heart failure or signs of left ventricular dysfunction (ejection fraction less than 40%) then ACE inhibitor therapy should be continued indefinitely.

Adjuvant angioplasty is of no advantage and the role of primary angioplasty is not yet fully defined. It is in any case largely academic at this time. The majority of hospitals which receive myocardial infarction patients have no facilities for such intervention. The major goal remains early recanalisation by whatever means.

1 Pell S, Fayerweather W. Trends in the incidence of myocardial infarction and in associated mortality and morbidity in a large employed population. *N Engl J Med* 1985; **312**: 1005.
2 National Heart Attack Alert Programme Co-ordination Committee. 60 mins to treatment working group. Emergency department: rapid identification and treatment of patients with acute myocardial infarction. *Ann Emerg Med* 1994; **23**: 311.
3 Herlitz J, Elmfeldt D, Hjalmarson A *et al.* Effect of metoprolol on direct signs of the size and severity of acute myocardial infarction. *Am J Cardiol* 1983; **51**: 1282–88.
4 Alderman EL, Barry WH, Graham AF *et al.* Haemodynamic effects of morphine and pentazocine differ in cardiac patients. *N Engl J Med* 1972; **287**: 623–7.
5 Kerr F, Donald KW. Analgesia in myocardial infarction. *Br Heart J* 1974; **36**: 117–21.
6 Seminkovich CF, Jasse AS. Adverse effects due to morphine sulphate. Challenge to previous clinical doctrine. *Am J Med* 1985; **79**: 325–30.
7 Neilsen JR, Pedersen KE, Dahlstrom CG *et al.* Analgesic treatment in acute myocardial infarction. A controlled clinical comparison of morphine, nicomorphine and pethidine. *Acta Med Scand* 1984; **215**: 349–54.
8 Come PC, Pitt B. Nitroglycerine induced severe hypotension and bradycardia in patients with acute myocardial infarction. *Circulation* 1976; **34**: 624.
9 Kinch JW, Ryan TJ. Right ventricular infarction. *N Engl J Med* 1994; **330**: 1211.
10 Chamberlain D. Betablockers and calcium antagonists. In: Julian D, Braunwald, E. eds. *Management of acute myocardial infarction.* London: W.B. Saunders, 1994.
11 Madias JE, Hood WB Jnr. Reduction of precordial ST segment elevation in patients with anterior myocardial infarction by oxygen breathing. *Circulation* 1976; **53**: 198.
12 Antman EM, Berkin JA. Declining incidence of ventricular fibrillation in myocardial infarction. Implications for the use of lidocaine. *Circulation* 1992; **84**: 764.
13 Hine LK, Laird N, Hewitt P. Meta-analytic evidence against prophylactic use of lidocaine in acute myocardial infarction. *Arch Intern Med* 1989; **149**: 2694.
14 Lynch M, Littler WA, Pentecost BL, Stockley RA. Immunoglobulin response to intravenous streptokinase in acute myocardial infarction. *Br Heart J* 1990; **66**: 139–42.
15 Elliot J, Cross D, Cederholm-Williams S, White H. High streptokinase times 4 years after administration of intravenous streptokinase. New Zealand Cardiac Society Meeting, August 1991.
16 Fears R, Hearn J, Standring R *et al.* Lack of influence of pretreatment antistreptokinase antibody on efficacy in a multicentre patency comparison of i.v. streptokinase and anistreplase in acute myocardial infarction. *Am Heart J* 1992; **124**: 305.
17 *British National Formulary* 1997; 33:2:10:111.
18 Neuhof H, Hey D, Glaser E, Wolf H, Lasch HG. Haemodynamic reactions induced by streptokinase therapy in patients with acute myocardial infarction. *Eur J Intensive Care Med* 1975; **6**: 27–30.
19 Smith RAG, Dupe RJ, English PD, Green J. Fibrinolysis with acyl enzymes: a new approach to thrombolytic therapy. *Nature* 1981; **290**: 505–8.
20 Ferres H. Pre-clinical pharmacological evaluation of anysolated plasminogen streptoki- nase activator complex. *Drugs* 1987; **33**(Suppl 3): 33–50.
21 GREAT Group. Feasibility, safety and efficacy of domiciliary thrombolysis by general practitioners: Grampian Region Early Anistreplase Trial. *Br Med J* 1992; **305**: 548.

22 Van de Werf F, Ludbrook PA, Bergman SR. Coronary thrombolysis with tissue type plasminogen activator in patients with evolving myocardial infarction. *N Engl J Med* 1984; **310**: 609.

23 Garabedian HD, Gold HK, Leinbach RC. Comparative properties of two clinical preparations of recombinant human tissue type plasminogen activator inpatients with acute myocardial infarction. *J Am Coll Cardiol* 1987; **9**: 599.

24 Gold HK, Leinbach RC, Garabedian HD *et al.* Acute coronary reocclusion after thrombolysis with recombinant human tissue type plasminogen activator: prevention by a maintenance infusion. *Circulation* 1986; **73**: 347.

25 The GUSTO Angiographic Investigators. The comparative effects of tissue plasminogen activator, streptokinase, or both on coronary artery patency, ventricular function and survival after acute myocardial infarction. *N Engl J Med* 1993; **329**: 1615.

26 Tennant SN, Dickson J, Venable TC *et al.* Intracoronary thrombolysis in patients with acute myocardial infarction. Comparison of the efficacy of urokinase with streptokinase. *Circulation* 1984; **69**: 756.

27 Fletcher AP, Alkajaersig N, Smyniotis FE. The treatment of patients suffering from early myocardial infarction with massive and prolonged streptokinase therapy. *Trans Assoc Am Phys* 1958; **71**: 287.

28 Neuhaus KL, Tebbe U, Sauer G, Kostering H, Kreuzer H. High dose intravenous streptokinase infusion in acute myocardial infarction. *Eur Heart J* 1981; **2**: 144.

29 Collen D. Coronary thrombolysis: streptokinase or recombinant tissue type plasminogen activator? *Ann Intern Med* 1990; **112**: 529–38.

30 Hogg KJ, Hornung RS, Howie CA, Hockings N, Dunn FG, Hillis WS. Electrocardiographic prediction of coronary artery patency after thrombolytic treatment in acute myocardial infarction: use of the ST segment as a non-invasive marker. *Br Heart J* 1988; **60**: 275–80.

31 Hogg KJ, Lees KR, Hornung RS, Howie CA, Dunn FG, Hillis WS. Electrocardiographic evidence of myocardial infarction. *Br Heart J* 1989; **61**: 489–95.

32 Schroder R, Neuhaus KL, Leizorovicz A. A prospective placebo-controlled double-blind multi-centre trial of intravenous streptokinase in acute myocardial infarction (ISAM): longterm mortality and morbidity. *J Am Coll Cardiol* 1987; **9**: 197.

33 Lenderik T, Simoons ML, Van Es G-A. Benefits of thrombolytic therapy sustained throughout 5 years and related to TIMI perfusion grade 3, but not grade 2 flow discharge. *Circulation* 1995; **92**: 1110.

34 Yusuf S, Collins R, Peto R *et al.* Intravenous and intracoronary fibrinolytic therapy in acute myocardial infarction: overview of results on mortality, reinfarction and side-effects from 33 randomised controlled trials. *Eur Heart J* 1985; **6**: 556–85.

35 GISSI. Effectiveness of intravenous thrombolytic treatment in acute myocardial infarction. *Lancet* 1986; **i**: 397–401.

36 GISSI. Long-term effects of intravenous thrombolysis in acute myocardial infarction: final report of the GISSI Study. *Lancet* 1978; **ii**: 871–4.

37 ISIS 2. International Study of Infarct Survival. Intravenous streptokinase given within 0–4 hours of onset of myocardial infarction reduced mortality in ISIS-2. *Lancet* 1987; **i**:500.

38 AIMS Trial Study Group. Effect of intravenous APSAC on mortality after acute myocardial infarction: preliminary report of a placebo-controlled clinical trial. *Lancet* 1988; **i**: 545.

39 AIMS Trial Study Group. Long-term effects of intravenous anistreplase in acute myocardial infarction. Final report of the AIMS Study. *Lancet* 1990; **325**: 427–32.

40 Van de Werf F, Arnold AER and the European Cooperative Study Group for Recombinant Tissue-type Plasminogen Activator (r-tPA). Intravenous tissue plasminogen activator and size of infarct, left ventricular function and survival in acute myocardial infarction. *Br Med J* 1988; **297**: 1374–8.

41 Wilcox RG, von der Lippe G, Olsson CG, Jensen G, Skene AM, Hampton JR for the ASSET Study Group. Trial of tissue plasminogen activator for mortality reduction in acute myocardial infarction. Anglo-Scandinavia Study of Early Thrombolysis (ASSET). *Lancet* 1988; **ii**: 525–30.

42 GISSI-2 Study Group. GISSI-2: a factorial randomised trial of alteplase versus

streptokinase and heparin versus no heparin among 12,490 patients with acute myocardial infarction. *Lancet* 1990; **336**: 65–71.

43 The International Study Group. In-hospital mortality and clinical course of 20,891 patients with suspected acute myocardial infarction randomised between alteplase and streptokinase with or without heparin. *Lancet* 1990; **336**: 71–5.

44 ISIS-3 (Third International Study of Infarct Survival) Collaborative Study Group. ISIS-3: a randomised comparison of streptokinase vs tissue plasminogen activator vs anistreplase and of aspirin plus heparin vs aspirin alone among 41,299 cases of suspected acute myocardial infarction. *Lancet* 1992; **339**: 753–70.

45 Fibrinolytic Therapy Trialists (FTT Collaborative Group). Indications for fibrinolytic therapy and suspected acute myocardial infarction: collaborated overview of early mortality and major morbidity results from all randomised trials in more than 1000 patients. *Lancet* 1994; **343**: 311–22.

46 LATE Study Group. Late assessment of thrombolytic efficacy (LATE) study with alteplase 6–24 hours after onset of acute myocardial infarction. *Lancet* 1993; **342**: 759–66.

47 EMERAS Collaborative Group. Randomised trial of late thrombolysis in patients with suspected acute myocardial infarction. *Lancet* 1993; **342**: 767–72.

48 Altura BM, Altura BT, Carella A, Gebrewold A, Murakawa T, Nishio A. Mg^{2+}–Ca^{2+} interaction in contractility of vascular smooth muscle: Mg^{2+} versus organic calcium channel blockers on myogenic tone and agonist-induced responsiveness of blood vessels. *Can J Physiol Pharmac* 1987; **65**: 729–45.

49 Rasmussen HS, Thomsen PEB. The electrophysiological effects of intravenous magnesium on human sinus mode, atrioventricular node, atrium and ventricle. *Clin Cardiol* 1989; **12**: 85–90.

50 Tzivoni D, Banai S, Schuger C *et al.* Treatment of torsade de pointes with magnesium sulphate. *Circulation* 1988; **77**: 392–7.

51 Briel RC, Lippert TH, Zahradnik HP. Veranderungen von Blutgerinnung. Thrombozytenfunktion und vaskularer Prostazyklinsynthese durch Magnesium-sulfat. *Gerburtsh U Fraun heilk* 1987; **47**: 332–6.

52 Rasmussen HS, Gronbaek M, Cintin C, Balslov S, Norregard P, McNair P. One-year death rate in 270 patients with suspected acute myocardial infarction initially treated with intravenous magnesium or placebo. *Clin Cardiol* 1988; **11**: 377–81.

53 Woods KL, Fletcher S, Roffe C, Haider Y. Intravenous magnesium sulphate in suspected acute myocardial infarction: results of the second Leicester Intravenous Magnesium Intervention Trial (LIMIT-2). *Lancet* 1992; **339**; 1553–8.

54 Woods KL, Fletcher S. Long-term outcome after intravenous magnesium sulphate in suspected acute myocardial infarction: the second Leicester Intravenous Magnesium Intervention Trial (LIMIT-2). *Lancet* 1994; **343**: 816–19.

55 ISIS-4 (Collaborative Group). ISIS-4: a randomised factorial trial assessing early oral captopril, oral mononitrate and intravenous magnesium sulphate in 58,050 patients with suspected acute myocardial infarction. *Lancet* 1995; **345**: 669.

56 The Sixty Plus Reinfarction Study Research Group. A double-blind trial to assess long-term oral anticoagulant treatment in elderly patients after myocardial infarction. *Lancet* 1980; **ii**: 989–93.

57 Smith P, Arnesen H, Holme I. The effect of warfarin on mortality and reinfarction after myocardial infarction. *N Engl J Med* 1990; **323**: 147–52.

58 Anticoagulants in the Secondary Prevention of Events in Coronary Thrombosis (ASPECT) Research Group. Effect of long-term oral anticoagulant treatment on mortality and cardiovascular morbidity after myocardial infarction. *Lancet* 1994; **343**: 499–503.

59 Breddin K, Loew D, Lechner K *et al.* The German-Austrian aspirin trial: a comparison of acetyl salicylic acid, placebo and phenprocoumon in secondary prevention of myocardial infarction. *Circulation* 1980; **62** (Suppl V): V-63–V-72.

60 The EPSIM Research Group. A controlled comparison of aspirin and oral anticoagulants in prevention of death after myocardial infarction. *N Engl J Med* 1982; **307**: 701–8.

61 Meijer A, Verheugt FWA, Weter CJPJ *et al.* Aspirin versus cumadin in the prevention of reocclusion and recurrent ischaemia after successful thrombolysis, a prospective placebo

angiographic study. *Circulation* 1993; **87**: 1524–30.

62 Rossi PRF, Yusuf S, Ramsdale D *et al.* Reduction of ventricular arrhythmias by early intravenous atenolol in suspected acute myocardial infarction. *Br Med J* 1983; **286**: 506–10.

63 ISIS-1 Collaborative Group. A randomised trial of intravenous atenolol among 16,027 cases of suspected acute myocardial infarction. *Lancet* 1986; **ii**: 57–66.

64 Yusuf S, Wittes J, Friedman L. Overview of results of randomised clinical trials in heart disease. I. Treatments following myocardial infarction. *JAMA* 1988; **260**: 2088–93.

65 The MIAMI Trial Research Group. Metoprolol in acute myocardial infarction (MIAMI): a randomised placebo-controlled international trial. *Eur Heart J* 1985; **6**: 199–226.

66 The TIMI Study Group. Comparison of invasive and conservative strategies after treatment with intravenous tissue plasminogen activator in acute myocardial infarction: results of the Thrombolysis in Myocardial Infarction (TIMI) phase 2 trials. *N Engl J Med* 1989; **320**: 618–27.

67 Roberts R, Rogers WJ, Mueller HS *et al.* Immediate versus deferred betablockade following thrombolytic therapy in patients with acute myocardial infarction: results of the Thrombolysis in Myocardial Infarction (TIMI) 2-B study. *Circulation* 1981; **83**: 422–37.

68 The Norwegian Multi-study Group. Timolol induced reduction in mortality and reinfarction in patients surviving acute myocardial infarction. *N Engl J Med* 1981; **304**: 801.

69 Betablocker Pooling Project Research Group. The Betablocker Pooling Project (BBPP): subgroup findings from randomised trials in post-infarction patients. *Eur Heart J* 1988; **9**: 8.

70 Yusuf S, Peto R, Lewis J. Betablockage during and after myocardial infarction. An overview of the randomised trials. *Prog Cardiovasc Disease* 1985; **27**: 335.

71 Kloner RA, Braunwald E. Effects of calcium antagonists on infarcting myocardium. *Am J Cardiol* 1987; **59**: 84B–94B.

72 Held PH, Yusuf S, Furberg CD. Calcium channel blockers in acute myocardial infarction and unstable angina: an overview. *Br Med J* 1989; **299**: 1187–92.

73 Multicenter Diltiazem Postinfarction Trial Research Group. The effect of diltiazem on mortality and reinfarction after myocardial infarction. *N Engl J Med* 1988; **319**: 385–92.

74 The Israeli SPRINT Study Group. Secondary Prevention Reinfarction Israel Nifedipine Trial (SPRINT). A randomised intervention trial of nifedipine in patients with acute myocardial infarction. *Eur Heart J* 1988; **9**: 354–64.

75 Goldbourt U, Behar S, Reicher-Reiss H, Zion M, Mandelzweig L, Kaplinsky E, for the SPRINT Study Group. The Secondary Prevention Reinfarction Israel Nifedipine Trial 2 Study. Early administration of nifedipine in suspected acute myocardial infarction. *Arch Intern Med* 1993; **153**: 345–53.

76 Furberg CD, Psaty BM, Meyer JV. Nifedipine: dose-related increase in mortality in patients with coronary heart disease. *Circulation* 1995; **92**: 1236.

77 Yusuf S. Calcium antagonists in coronary artery disease and hypertension: time for re-evaluation. *Circulation* 1995; **92**: 1079.

78 Opie LH, Messerli RH. Nifedipine and mortality: grave defects on the dossier. *Circulation* 1995; **92**: 1068.

79 The Danish Study Group on Verapamil and Myocardial Infarction. The effects of verapamil on mortality and major events after acute infarction (The Danish Verapamil Infarction Trial 2 – DAVIT 2). *Am J Cardiol* 1990; **66**: 779.

80 Bussmann WD, Passec D, Seidel W. Reduction of CK and CKMB indexes of infarct size by intravenous nitroglycerine. *Circulation* 1981; **63**: 615.

81 Jugdutt BI, Warnica JW. Intravenous nitroglycerine therapy to limit myocardial infarct size. Expansion, and complications: effect of timing, dosage and infarct location. *Circulation* 1988; **78**: 906.

82 Gruppo Italiana per lo Studio della Sprawivenza nell'infarto Miocardico (GISSI-3). GISSI-3 effects on lisinopril and transdermal glyceryl trinitrate singly and together on 6 week mortality and ventricular function after acute myocardial infarction. *Lancet* 1994; **343**: 1115–22.

83 Ito H, Hisahiro Y, Tomooka T *et al.* Incidence and time course of left ventricular dilation in the early convalescent stage of reperfused anterior wall acute myocardial infarction. *Am*

J Cardiol 1994; **73**: 539–43.

84 Pfeffer M, Braunwald E. Ventricular remodelling after myocardial infarction. Experimental observations and clinical implications. *Circulation* 1990; **81**: 1161–72.

85 Eaton LW, Weiss JL, Bulkley BH, Garrison JB, Weisfelds ML. Regional cardiac dilatation after acute myocardial infarction. Recognition by two-dimensional echocardiography. *N Engl J Med* 1979; **300**: 57–62.

86 Sharpe N, Murphy J, Smith H, Hannan S. Preventative treatment of asymptomatic left ventricular dysfunction following myocardial infarction. *Eur Heart J* 1990; **11**(Suppl B): 147–56.

87 McAlpine HM, Morton JJ, Leckie B, Rumley A, Gille G, Dargie J. Neuroendocrine activation after acute myocardial infarction. *Br Heart J* 1988; **60**: 117–24.

88 Rouleau JL, de Champlain J, Klein M *et al.* Activation of neurohormonal systems in post-infarction left ventricular dysfunction. *J Am Coll Cardiol* 1993; **22**: 390–8.

89 Schomig A. Catecholamines in myocardial infarction. *Circulation* 1990; **82**(Suppl 2): 13–22.

90 Lindpaintner K, Niedermaier N, Drexler H, Ganten D. Left ventricular remodelling after myocardial infarction: does the cardiac renin-angiotensin system play a role? *J Cardiovasc Pharmacol* 1992; **20**(Suppl): S41–7.

91 Ambrosini E, Borghi C, Magnani B. The effect of angiotensin converting enzyme inhibitor zofenopril on mortality and morbidity after anterior myocardial infarction. *N Engl J Med* 1995; **332**: 80–5.

92 Swedberg K, Held P, Kjekshus J. Effects of early administration of enalapril on mortality in patients with acute myocardial infarction: results of the Co-operative North Scandinavian Enalapril Survival Study 2 (Consensus 2). *N Engl J Med* 1992; **327**: 678.

93 Pfeffer MA, Braunwald E, Moye LA *et al.* on behalf of the SAVE Investigators. Effect of captopril on mortality and morbidity in patients with left ventricular dysfunction after myocardial infarction. Results of the Survival and Ventricular Enlargement Trial. *N Engl J Med* 1992; **327**: 669–77.

94 Kober L, Torp-Pedersen C, Carlsen JE. A clinical trial of the angiotensin converting enzyme inhibitor trandolapril in patients with left ventricular dysfunction after myocardial infarction. *N Engl J Med* 1995; **333**: 1670.

95 The Acute Infarction Ramipril Efficacy (AIRE) Study Investigators. Effect of ramipril on mortality and morbidity of survivors of acute myocardial infarction with clinical evidence of heart failure. *Lancet* 1993; **342**: 821–8.

96 Chinese Cardiac Study Collaborative Group. Oral captopril versus placebo among 13,634 patients with suspected myocardial infarction: interim report from the Chinese Cardiac Society (CCS-I). *Lancet* 1995; **345**: 686.

97 Topol EJ, Califf RM, George BS *et al.* for the Thrombolysis and Angioplasty in Myocardial Infarction Study Group. A randomized trial of immediate versus delayed elective angioplasty after intravenous tissue plasminogen activator in acute myocardial infarction. *N Engl J Med* 1987; **317**: 581–8.

98 Guerci AD, Gerstenblith G, Brinker JA *et al.* A randomized trial of intravenous tissue plasminogen activator for acute myocardial infarction with subsequent randomization to elective coronary angioplasty. *N Engl J Med* 1987; **317**: 1613–18.

99 Simoons ML, Arnold AER, Betriu A *et al.* for the European Co-operative Study Group for Recombinant Tissue-type Plasminogen Activator. Thrombolysis with tissue plasminogen activator in acute myocardial infarction; no additional benefit from immediate percutaneous coronary angioplasty. *Lancet* 1988; **i**: 197–202.

100 Grines CL, Browne KF, Marco J *et al.* for the Primary Angioplasty in Myocardial Infarction Study Group. A comparison of immediate angioplasty with thrombolytic therapy for acute myocardial infarction. *N Engl J Med* 1993; **328**: 673–9.

101 Zijlstra F, Jan de Boer M, Hoorntje JCA, Reiffers S, Rieber JHC, Suryapranata H. A comparison of immediate coronary angioplasty with intravenous streptokinase in acute myocardial infarction. *N Engl J Med* 1993; **328**: 680–4.

102 Gibbons RJ, Holmes DR, Reeder GS, Bailet KR, Hopfenspringer MR, Gersh BJ for the Mayo Coronary Care Unit and Cardiac Catheterisation Laboratory Groups. Immediate angioplasty compared with the administration of a thrombolytic agent followed by conservative treatment for myocardial infarction. *N Engl J Med* 1993; **328**: 685–91.

103 Every NR, Parsons LS, Hlatky M, Martin JS, Weaver WD for the Myocardial Infarction Triage and Intervention Investigators. A comparison of thrombolytic therapy with primary coronary angioplasty for acute myocardial infarction. *N Engl J Med* 1996; **335**: 1253–60.

104 Nakagawa Y, Iwasaki Y, Kimura T *et al.* Serial angiographic follow-up after successful angioplasty for acute myocardial infarction. *Am J Cardiol* 1996; **78**: 980–4.

105 Laster SB, Rutherford BD, Giogi LV *et al.* Results of direct percutaneous transluminal coronary angioplasty in octogenarians. *Am J Cardiol* 1996; **77**: 10–13.

3: Antiplatelet drugs

JM RITTER

Introduction

Platelets are key elements in the processes of haemostasis and thrombosis. Arterial thrombosis is the leading cause of death and morbidity in industrialised countries and drugs that interfere with platelet function ("antiplatelet drugs") are proving of great value in its treatment and prevention. As would be anticipated, these drugs can cause haemorrhage but by interfering selectively with various aspects of platelet function, this is much less of a problem than is caused by thrombocytopaenia. There are many links between platelet activation and the coagulation cascade (Figure 3.1) so it is not surprising that anticoagulants can also have beneficial effects in prevention of coronary artery disease or that antiplatelet drugs such as aspirin have some effect on venous thrombosis. Indeed, the interrelatedness of these systems leads to some semantic problems: for instance, thrombin, which is the pivotal factor in coagulation, also acts on specific receptors on platelets so there is a sense in which anticoagulants that inhibit thrombin are also antiplatelet drugs. This chapter briefly describes processes involved in platelet activation and function followed by a description of antiplatelet drugs in clinical use and finally a short discussion of potential future antiplatelet strategies and some recommendations for use of antiplatelet drugs.

Platelet function

Platelets are activated by agonists (for example, thrombin, adenosine diphosphate, 5-hydroxytryptamine, thromboxane A_2, platelet activating factor) acting on specific surface receptors or by contact with foreign substances including collagen and other subendothelial components.[1,2] Circulating von Willebrand factor, synthesised by endothelial cells, combines with glycoprotein Ib receptors on the platelet surface, linking platelets with subendothelial molecules and leading to the formation of an adherent platelet monolayer covering areas of vascular injury. Activated platelets change shape and their contained granules become centralised and granule contents are secreted into a cannalicular system that communicates with

51

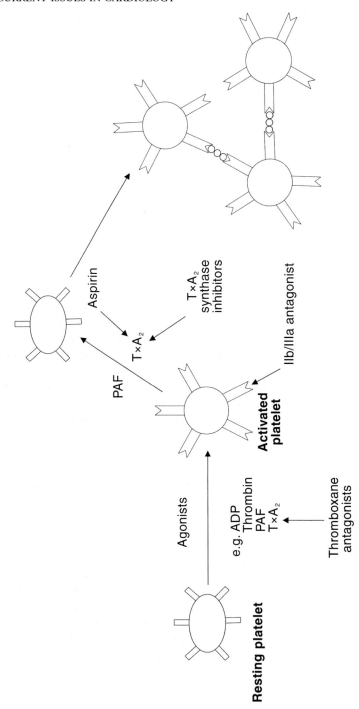

Fig 3.1   Platelet activation and aggregation.

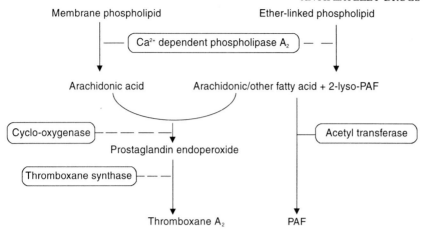

Fig 3.2   Biosynthesis of thromboxane A_2 and of platelet activating factor (PAF). Enzymes are outlined.

the exterior. Granule contents include several agonists (for example, adenosine diphosphate, 5-hydroxytryptamine) in addition to coagulation factors (fibrinogen, Va) and growth factors (platelet derived growth factor, transforming growth factor β). In addition to secretion of preformed agonists, lipid derived mediators including thromboxane A_2 and platelet activating factor are formed *de novo* (Figure 3.2). Receptors for these various agonists are linked via the inositol signalling pathway to increased cytoplasmic Ca^{2+} and membrane diacylglycerol.[3,4] Platelet activation therefore results in a complex series of events including the appearance of negatively charged phospholipid moieties (e.g. phosphatidyl serine) and of glycoprotein IIb/IIIa receptors on the outer membrane surface. These respectively promote coagulation (by binding Ca^{2+} and factors Va, IXa, VIIa and Xa) and cause aggregation. Aggregation entails attachments of platelets to one another via fibrinogen which links activated glycoprotein IIb/IIIa receptors on adjacent platelets. As further platelets are activated, the aggregate propagates as white thrombus that can occlude a vessel or break off and embolise downstream.

Platelets are inactive in healthy individuals under physiological conditions. They do not adhere to healthy endothelium. This lines the vasculature and acts as a container that preserves the circulating blood in its fluid state. Endothelium possesses a complex array of antithrombotic mechanisms. Endothelial cells synthesise several mediators[5] that inhibit platelet function, including prostacyclin and endothelium derived relaxing factor, now known to be identical with nitric oxide[6] or closely related to it. Prostacyclin is synthesised at sites of vascular trauma and acts on specific receptors on the platelet surface membrane that are linked via a stimulatory G-protein to

53

adenylyl cyclase.[7] The resulting increase in cyclic adenosine monophosphate causes phosphorylation of specific proteins and inhibition of all of the pathways leading to aggregation while having little effect on adhesion to foreign surfaces.[8] Unlike prostacyclin, nitric oxide is synthesised continuously in the endothelium of human resistance arteries *in vivo*. It diffuses into platelets and activates soluble cytoplasmic guanylyl cyclase (by combining with a haem moiety) thereby increasing cytoplasmic cyclic guanosine monophosphate.[9] This phosphorylates cytoplasmic proteins, altering their function and inhibiting the increase in cytoplasmic Ca^{2+} caused by agonists. NO potently inhibits both aggregation and adhesion *in vitro*.[10] Whether endogenous nitric oxide has antiplatelet activity *in vivo* is less certain, however, since it is avidly bound by the abundant haemoglobin in red cells.

Antiplatelet drugs in clinical use

Rather few antiplatelet drugs are used clinically and of these, aspirin is overwhelmingly the most important. Sulphinpyrazone is the only other cyclo-oxygenase inhibitor for which there is some evidence of clinical efficacy as an antiplatelet drug, but it is now seldom used for its antiplatelet effects. Dipyridamole has effects on platelet function but its place in therapeutics remains unclear despite many years of clinical use. Ticlopidine is effective but has distinct toxicities. It is used in North America but is not as yet licensed in the United Kingdom. Epoprostenol must be given intravenously. It has distinct but limited clinical indications. Abciximab is a monoclonal antibody directed against glycoprotein IIb/IIIa receptors. It is used by some experts as a single administration as an adjunct to heparin and aspirin in high risk patients undergoing coronary angioplasty. Finally, various drugs that are used primarily because of other pharmacological actions also have effects on platelets. These include β-adrenoreceptor antagonists, Ca^{2+} channel antagonists and nitrovasodilators. The concentrations of these drugs that influence platelet function are generally too high for it to be likely that their antiplatelet actions contribute to their therapeutic effects, although it is possible that conversion of nitrovasodilators to NO by vascular smooth muscle could contribute to antiplatelet effects *in vivo*.[11]

Aspirin

Aspirin reduces vascular deaths by approximately 25% in patients with established coronary or cerebrovascular disease.[12, 13] It reduces fatal events in patients with acute myocardial infarction by approximately 21%, a similar magnitude of effect to that of streptokinase, with which it is additive (Figure 3.3).[14] It reduces the risk of myocardial infarction in patients with unstable angina (by approximately 50%)[15-18] and in patients who have

54

recovered from myocardial infarction (by approximately 30%)[19] and in apparently healthy middle aged men.[20] It is not, however, recommended generally as prophylaxis in asymptomatic men, because in this setting its benefits are probably outweighed by adverse effects.[21] It also reduces the risk of acute reocclusion following angioplasty or bypass grafting.[22, 23] Aspirin reduces the risk of stroke in patients with transient cerebral

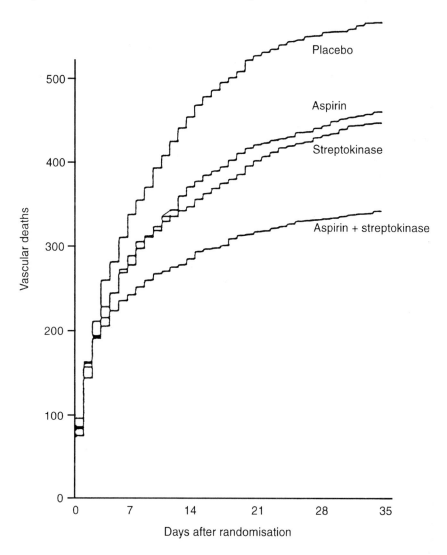

Fig 3.3   Cumulative vascular mortality following diagnosis of myocardial infarction in patients allocated streptokinase, aspirin, streptokinase and aspirin or placebo in the ISIS-2 trial (redrawn from[12]).

ischaemic attacks by approximately 10%.[24] It reduces the risk of thromboembolism in patients with atrial fibrillation[25] but is less effective than warfarin for this indication. Low dose (60 or 75 mg/day) aspirin may be justified in pregnant women who are especially liable to early onset severe pre-eclampsia, for which indication it is started early in the second trimester. Routine prophylactic or therapeutic aspirin for all pregnant women at increased risk of pre-eclampsia or intrauterine growth retardation is, however, not justified.[26, 27]

The mechanism of the antithrombotic action of aspirin is mainly or exclusively through inhibition of thromboxane A_2 biosynthesis in platelets. It irreversibly inhibits cyclo-oxygenase-1 (COX-1) by acetylation of serine 530, thereby preventing access of substrate (arachidonic acid) to the active site by steric hindrance. Thromboxane A_2 is the main cyclo-oxygenase product of activated platelets and acts as a positive feedback, recruiting more platelets to sites of platelet activation. Although non-steroidal anti-inflammatory drugs such as ibuprofen and indomethacin also inhibit cyclo-oxygenase, they are much less effective than aspirin at inhibiting platelet thromboxane A_2 biosynthesis, possibly because, unlike aspirin, they are reversible inhibitors of the enzyme. It should not therefore be assumed that patients receiving such drugs for another indication are thereby necessarily receiving adequate antiplatelet therapy. In this regard, the uricosuric drug and cyclo-oxygenase inhibitor sulphinpyrazone appears to be a special case. There is some evidence of clinical efficacy of sulphinpyrazone following myocardial infarction (albeit much debated)[28–32a] and it causes only partial and reversible inhibition of cyclo-oxygenase via a slowly formed sulphide metabolite. However, it has additional actions on platelets that distinguish it from other cyclo-oxygenase inhibitors, including inhibition of platelet activation factor induced aggregation and normalisation of shortened platelet survival in various clinical situations.

Numerous different actions of aspirin have been described *in vitro*. These include effects on thrombolysis, on membrane fluidity, on the formation of lipid bodies in leucocytes from which eicosanoids may be released, and from COX-2 in leucocytes. In contrast to COX-1, aspirin interaction with the COX-2 active site results in formation of 15-*R*-HETE with unknown consequences. Aspirin may also alter inflammatory processes by inhibiting the mobilisation of nuclear factor-*k*B (NF*k*B). These additional actions of aspirin have been discussed in a recent editorial[32b] which points out that although these mechanisms are intriguing, their clinical importance remains to be established. They raise the possibility of improved dose regimens of aspirin aimed at augmenting the already impressive effects of low dose (60–160 mg/day) aspirin in the treatment of cardiovascular disease.

Aspirin is rapidly absorbed from the gastrointestinal tract and rapidly deacetylated to yield salicylate which has anti-inflammatory but little if any antiplatelet activity at ordinary doses.[33, 34] There has been considerable interest in the possibility that very low doses of aspirin (40 mg per day or less) may selectively inhibit platelet thromboxane A_2 biosynthesis without reducing prostacyclin biosynthesis in blood vessels.[35] This strategy has yet to be shown to result in increased antithrombotic efficacy and it is possible that it will not produce uniformly satisfactory inhibition of platelet thromboxane A_2 biosynthesis in all patients, especially those with severe atheromatous disease.

A simpler approach to achieving selectivity is to use a substantial dose interval between larger doses of aspirin that reliably cause essentially complete inhibition of platelet thromboxane A_2 biosynthesis. Within limits, the longer the dose interval the greater the specificity for platelet thromboxane A_2 biosynthesis, because platelets do not possess nuclei and can not resynthesise cyclo-oxygenase after inhibition by aspirin, whereas in human endothelium cyclo-oxygenase appears to be completely resynthesised within approximately six hours (Figure 3.4).[34, 36] Appreciable recovery of platelet thromboxane A_2 biosynthesis occurs only after 48 hours,[37] and then continues over the time span with which new platelets enter the circulation from megakaryocytes (complete in 7–10 days). Consequently, if aspirin is given once every 24 or 48 hours, platelet thromboxane A_2 biosynthesis is essentially completely inhibited throughout the entire dose interval, whereas endothelial prostacyclin biosynthesis is inhibited on average only one quarter or one eighth of the dose interval. Aspirin was given in a dose of 150 mg every 24 hours in the ISIS-2 trial[12] and a dose of 320 mg every 48 hours in the American Physicians Trial.[18] In one positive study of unstable coronary disease the dose was 75 mg daily.[14]

Dose related adverse effects consequent on the pharmacological effect of aspirin on cyclo-oxygenase are common; approximately 25% of British physicians were intolerant of it in a trial that required regular prolonged daily use.[38] Furthermore, although available over the counter for nearly a century, some of the adverse effects of aspirin are serious. The commonest severe effect is upper gastrointestinal haemorrhage and the commonest symptom dyspepsia. These are related to inhibition of prostaglandin E_2 biosynthesis in the stomach.[39] Prostaglandin E_2 is the main cyclo-oxygenase product of this organ and has a number of effects that help protect it from ulceration, including mucus secretion, inhibition of acid secretion, vasodilation of vessels in the submucosa that carry away hydrogen ions that have diffused back through the mucosal barrier, and possibly a cytoprotective effect on mucosal cells themselves. Inhibition of prostaglandin E_2 biosynthesis consequently predisposes to ulceration. Should an ulcer occur during aspirin treatment, bleeding is likely to be increased because of inhibition of platelet thromboxane biosynthesis. Active ulcer disease contraindicates the use of aspirin and a past history of ulcer disease also argues against its use, although if the indication is strong enough, the risk

57

may be judged clinically acceptable. In such cases coincident treatment with an H_2 antagonist such as cimetidine or with a stable prostaglandin E_1 analogue (misoprostol) may be useful. Constipation is less well recognised as an unwanted effect of aspirin than are upper gastrointestinal symptoms but is not uncommon.[38] It may also relate to inhibition of prostaglandin E_2 biosynthesis since this prostaglandin increases gastrointestinal mobility, reduces absorption of water, and causes secretory diarrhoea when administered therapeutically.

Some patients with asthma (especially those with a history of nasal polyps) are sensitive to aspirin.[40] The mechanism is not fully established, although this adverse effect appears likely to be due to cyclo-oxygenase inhibition rather than to an idiosyncrasy, since individuals who are aspirin sensitive are also sensitive to other structurally unrelated cyclo-oxygenase

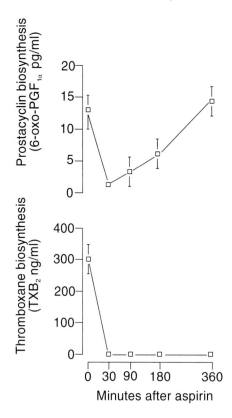

Fig 3.4   Recovery of prostanoid biosynthesis after a single dose of aspirin in healthy men. Thromboxane biosynthesis by platelets is profoundly inhibited and inhibition persists. Prostacyclin biosynthesis (in response to pulsed intravenous infusions of bradykinin) is also profoundly inhibited, but recovers within six hours (redrawn from[36]).

inhibitors (for example, indomethacin and piroxicam). It is possible that it is caused by a disturbance in the usual balance between cyclo-oxygenase and lipoxygenase products in the lung. In contrast, symptoms of salicylism are unrelated to cyclo-oxygenase inhibition. These occur only in overdose or when aspirin is used for high dose anti-inflammatory indications and not with therapeutic regimens used to inhibit platelet function.

Epoprostenol (prostacyclin)

Epoprostenol is the approved drug name of synthetic prostacyclin, the principal endogenous prostaglandin of mammalian large and medium sized arteries.[7] It is used in the preparation of washed platelet concentrates. Epoprostenol relaxes pulmonary as well as systemic vascular smooth muscle and this underlies its use in patients with primary pulmonary hypertension who are, however, also at risk of thromboembolic disease. It has been administered chronically to such patients for periods of months and even years while awaiting heart–lung transplantation.[41] Epoprostenol inhibits platelet activation during haemodialysis. It can be used with heparin, but is also effective when used as sole anticoagulant in this setting and is therefore particularly useful for haemodialysis in patients in whom heparin is contraindicated.[42, 43] It has also been used in other kinds of extracorporeal circuit (for example, during cardiopulmonary bypass and during charcoal column haemoperfusion). Epoprostenol has been used with apparent benefit in patients with acute retinal vessel thrombosis and with critical limb ischaemia.[44] It is also used in patients with platelet consumption due to multiple organ failure,[45] especially those with meningococcal sepsis. Rigorous proof of efficacy is difficult to provide in such settings.

Epoprostenol is dissolved immediately before use in alkaline buffer and is infused intravenously (or, in the case of haemodialysis, into the arterial limb supplying the dialyser). The starting dose is 2 ng/kg body weight/minute. This can be increased in stepwise increments of 2 ng/kg/min if necessary to as much as 16 ng/kg/min, with frequent monitoring of blood pressure and heart rate during dose titration. A modest reduction in diastolic pressure with an increase in systolic pressure and reflex tachycardia is the expected and desired haemodynamic effect. Occasionally, a vagal syndrome super-venes; if bradycardia occurs, the infusion should be temporarily discontinued and the patient's legs elevated if there is hypotension. Other adverse effects include flushing, headache, nausea, abdominal discomfort, diarrhoea and uterine cramps but these effects are usually mild and much less pronounced than with E-series prostaglandins. Crushing chest pain is, rarely, experienced by individuals without evidence of ischaemic heart disease and jaw ache is common during chronic administration.[41] These effects usually resolve within minutes of stopping or reducing the infusion. Bleeding complications, which were anticipated, have in fact been rare, perhaps because although prostacyclin is very potent at inhibiting platelet aggregation, it is much less effective at inhibiting platelet adhesion.[8] Consequently, the haemostatic function of platelets is little influenced by prostacyclin despite its antithrombotic action. Stable analogues such as carbacyclin and iloprost have been developed but not yet marketed in the UK. The half life of prostacyclin in the circulation is approximately three minutes so steady state is achieved rapidly and dose increments can be made safely every 8–12 minutes. Prostacyclin hydrolyses spontaneously to an inactive product (6-oxo-prostaglandin $F_{1\alpha}$) which is excreted in urine both unchanged and as further metabolites, of which the major one is 2,3 dinor-6-oxo-prostaglandin $F_{1\alpha}$.[46] Measurements of these products are used to quantify endogenous prostacyclin biosynthesis in kidney and systemic circulations respectively.[47]

Ticlopidine

Ticlopidine does not inhibit cyclo-oxygenase and its mechanism is entirely different from that of aspirin. It is an inactive prodrug that is converted in the liver to unstable biologically active metabolites that have not been characterised. It is inactive when added to platelet-rich plasma *in vitro*, but when platelet-rich plasma is prepared from a subject who has ingested the drug, aggregation to a wide variety of agonists including adenosine diphosphate (ADP) is inhibited. This wide spectrum of activity is explained by inhibition of fibrinogen binding to activated glycoprotein IIb/IIIa. Ticlopidine also reduces fibrinogen concentrations by about 10% during chronic treatment, although the importance of this is unknown. It is used in North America as prophylaxis against stroke or myocardial infarction in patients at high risk, in peripheral arterial disease, diabetic microangiopathy, and to reduce platelet activation in extracorporeal circulations. It reduces the risk of recurrence in patients who have recovered from ischaemic stroke and even appears rather more effective than aspirin (650 mg bd) for this indication.[48, 49] It also reduces the risk of stroke and myocardial infarction in patients with intermittent claudication.[50] In patients with unstable angina, addition of ticlopidine to β-blockers, nitrates and Ca^{2+} channel antagonists resulted in approximately a 50% reduction in myocardial infarction,[51] which is similar to the effect of aspirin. Ticlopidine reduces the rate of progression of microaneurysms in patients with diabetes mellitus about three-fold, but the clinical importance of this is unknown.[52a] The usual dose is 250 mg twice daily. Adverse events are common and can be severe. Neutropenia occurs in some 2·4% of patients, usually in the first 12 weeks, and is severe in 0·8%. Thrombocytopenia and pancytopenia have also been described but are less common. Cholestatic jaundice has occurred in the first few months of treatment and is reversible on stopping the drug. Gastrointestinal symptoms are common (around 40%) and include nausea, anorexia, vomiting, epigastric pain, and diarrhoea. These usually occur early and may resolve despite continued treatment or not recur on reinstituting treatment. Rashes occur. Plasma lipid concentrations increase by about 10% during chronic treatment. All subfractions are affected so the LDL/HDL ratio is unchanged. As compared with conventional anticoagulant therapy (intra-venous heparin, an oral anticoagulant and aspirin) combined antiplatelet therapy with ticlopidine plus aspirin was found to reduce cardiac events and haemorrhagic and vascular complications after placement of coronary artery stents.[52b]

Clopidogrel

Clopidogrel is structurally related to ticlopidine. Like ticlopidine it inhibits ADP induced platelet aggregation and possibly also has actions on the glycoprotein IIb/IIIa receptor. It has been compared (in a dose of 75 mg/day) with aspirin (325 mg/day) in patients at risk of ischaemic events.[52c] Clopidogrel was found to be marginally more effective (relative risk reduction 8·7% in favour of clopidogrel) than this relatively large dose of aspirin at reducing the risk of a composite outcome cluster of ischaemic stroke, myocardial infarction or vascular death. The safety profile was similar for clopidogrel and aspirin. The precise place of clopidogrel in therapeutics remains to be established.

Dipyridamole

Dipyridamole was introduced as a vasodilator but is now promoted, often in combination with aspirin, for its effects on platelet function. There is no doubt that dipyridamole influences platelet function *in vitro* and *ex vivo* but the mechanism of these effects as well as of its vasodilator action is incompletely understood. The mechanism probably involves inhibition of phosphodiesterase with consequent reduced breakdown of cyclic adenosine and guanosine monophosphates. Dipyridamole also inhibits adenosine uptake with consequent enhancement of the actions of this mediator on platelets and vascular smooth muscle. (Adenosine acts on receptors that are linked via a stimulatory G-protein to adenylyl cyclase and so inhibits platelet aggregation.)

Clinical trials have not supported any additional benefit over that of aspirin alone in the prevention of stroke or myocardial infarction.[53-57] The combination of aspirin with dipyridamole is effective in reducing the incidence of graft occlusion following coronary artery bypass grafting but has not been directly compared with aspirin alone. Addition of dipyr-idamole to warfarin in patients with prosthetic heart valves apparently reduced the risk of thromboembolism in one study[58a], but the incidence of such events in the group treated with anticoagulation alone was unusually high, casting doubt on this conclusion. Clinical use at present is therefore limited mainly to its intravenous use as a diagnostic agent in dipyridamole/

61

thallium scanning in patients for whom a stress test is indicated but who are unable to exercise. Intravenous dipyridamole acts as a pharmacological stress and enables areas of reversible cardiac hypoperfusion to be identified in such individuals.

Platelet glycoprotein IIb/IIIa receptor antagonists

A hybrid murine/human monoclonal antibody (abciximab) directed against the glycoprotein IIb/IIIa receptor inhibits fibrinogen binding and prevents platelet aggregation (see above). Abciximab was found to reduce immediate acute myocardial infarction and the need for subsequent revascularisation in a group of high risk patients undergoing coronary angioplasty at the expense of a higher rate of bleeding events.[58b] Other potentially useful inhibitors have been derived from viper venom (e.g. trigramin) although their peptide structure makes them potentially antigenic. Other peptides have been based on the Arg-Gly-Asp (RGD) sequence common to ligands for IIb/IIIa receptors. While linear peptides on this template are unstable, cyclic peptides are stable. Further modifications (e.g. amidino or benzamidino derivatives) improve resistance to enzymic breakdown further. Several new drugs based on this concept (e.g. lamifiban, tirofiban) are currently in investigational use in humans. The potential of this class of drugs to cause immune thrombocytopenia is being closely monitored.

Potential future antiplatelet strategies

From the above it will be appreciated that there is excellent evidence that aspirin is of value in the treatment and prevention of arterial thrombotic disease, but that the magnitude of its effect is modest (approximately 10–50% reductions in event rates in various settings) and it is not tolerated by a substantial minority (approximately 25% during prolonged use). Other antiplatelet drugs either lack convincing evidence of clinical efficacy (dipyridamole) or are associated with serious adverse effects (ticlopidine) or are inconvenient to administer (epoprostenol).

What are the prospects for improved efficacy and/or reduced adverse event rates? One strategy ripe for exploration by clinical trial is the combination of aspirin with drugs used to treat other specific risk factors for vascular disease – hyperlipidaemia, hypertension, and diabetes in particular. The outcome of such trials is far from a foregone conclusion and at present physicians treating patients with these disorders lack the information needed to make firm recommendations.

A second strategy being evaluated is the combination of aspirin with anticoagulant therapy. By inhibiting platelet function and coagulation cascades simultaneously the hope is for improved antithrombotic efficacy without unacceptable bleeding. The results of a recent study of patients following heart valve replacement are encouraging in this regard; the patients were all treated with warfarin and randomly allocated to placebo or aspirin 100 mg daily in addition. There was some increase in bleeding in the aspirin group but this was more than offset by a considerable benefit in terms of reduced mortality, especially from vascular causes.[59]

A third strategy is to explore drugs whose pharmacology suggests that they may have advantages over aspirin. Of these, thromboxane A_2 receptor antagonists, thromboxane synthase inhibitors and drugs with combined synthase inhibitor/receptor antagonist actions offer potential therapeutic advantages over aspirin, although their clinical development has been slow.

Thromboxane receptor antagonists

Thromboxane receptor antagonists provide the possibility of blocking the actions of thromboxane A_2 without reducing prostaglandin biosynthesis. Whether preserves prostacyclin biosynthesis is likely to improve efficacy is uncertain, however. In view of the fairly high selectivity for platelet thromboxane A_2 biosynthesis of intermittent low dose aspirin, it seems unlikely that such drugs will have markedly greater efficacy than aspirin on this account. Preservation of gastric prostaglandin E_2 biosynthesis means, however, that thromboxane receptor antagonists will lack the adverse effects of aspirin on the stomach that are caused by inhibition of prostaglandin E_2 and this could be of great value to patients who cannot tolerate aspirin because of gastrointestinal side effects. Potent and long acting drugs of this variety have been used in humans[60, 61] but have not undergone comparative clinical trials with aspirin.

Thromboxane synthase inhibitors

Thromboxane synthase inhibitors block thromboxane A_2 biosynthesis without reducing prostaglandin formation. Unlike thromboxane receptor antagonists, they actually increase prostacyclin biosynthesis,[62] probably as a result of diversion of endoperoxide intermediates from platelets to the walls of blood vessels. This is potentially important, because prostacyclin inhibits all pathways of platelet aggregation, not only the thromboxane pathway. Thromboxane synthase inhibitors could therefore have greater efficacy than intermittent low dose aspirin. Early thromboxane synthase inhibitors had unfavourable pharmacokinetic properties, however, and lack the potency of aspirin in inhibiting thromboxane biosynthesis.[62] Furthermore, thromboxane synthase inhibitors have only small and variable effects on platelet aggregation. This has been attributed to accumulation of endoperoxides, since prostaglandin H_2 is itself an agonist on thromboxane receptors. If such accumulation occurs during platelet activation *in vivo* it could offset the antiplatelet effects of thromboxane synthase inhibition. A means of circumventing this is to use thromboxane synthase inhibitors and thromboxane receptor antagonists in combination, the thromboxane receptor antagonist preventing actions of any accumulated endoperoxide on thromboxane receptors.[63] Ridogrel is a potent and long lasting thromboxane synthase inhibitor that also has moderate thromboxane receptor antagonist activity.[64] It profoundly reduces thromboxane biosynthesis and moderately increases prostacyclin biosynthesis[65a] but has as yet to be compared with aspirin in clinical trials.

Drugs that inhibit adenosine diphosphate, thrombin and 5-hydroxytryptamine receptors are also in development. It is hard to assess their potential compared with aspirin in the setting of our limited understanding of the roles of specific platelet agonists in different clinical situations.

A rational regime for the use of antiplatelet drugs

Healthy individuals who are asymptomatic and without recognised coronary, cerebral or peripheral vascular disease should not receive prophylactic aspirin. Patients who have known stable coronary (e.g. angina or previous MI) or cerebrovascular disease (transient ischaemic attack or previous non-haemorrhagic stroke) should receive aspirin (75–160 mg/day). The treatment of patients with unstable angina should include aspirin. Aspirin is given in acute MI and continued indefinitely. It is often stopped perioperatively in patients undergoing bypass surgery but should be restarted soon thereafter.

The use of antiplatelet therapy as adjuvant treatment for surgical or coronary interventions is dealt with in Chapter 10.

It has been claimed that higher doses of aspirin (650–1300 mg/day) are more effective than lower doses in preventing stroke, but the evidence for this is not convincing.[65b] While the optimum dosing regimen remains disputed, we favour the lowest dose demonstrated to be effective, namely 75 mg/day, especially in patients who give a history of aspirin intolerance. If aspirin intolerance is problematic, it can be coadministered with an H_2 blocker (e.g. ranitidine).

1 Weiss HJ. *Platelets: pathophysiology and antiplatelet drug therapy.* New York: Alan R Liss, 1982.
2 Longenecker GL. *The platelets: physiology and pharmacology.* Orlando: Academic Press, 1985.
3 Rink TJ, Sanchez A, Hallam TJ. Diacylglycerol and phorbol ester stimulate secretion without raising cytoplasmic free calcium in human platelets. *Nature* 1983; **305**: 317–19.
4 Hallam TJ, Sanchez A, Rink TJ. Stimulus-response coupling in human platelets. Changes evoked by platelet-activating factor in cytoplasmic free calcium monitored with the fluorescent calcium indicator quin2. *Biochem J* 1984; **218**: 819–27.
5 Vane JR, Ångård EE, Botting RM. Regulatory functions of the vascular endothelium. *N Engl J Med* 1990; **323**: 27–35.
6 Palmer RMJ, Ferrige AG, Moncada S. Nitric oxide release accounts for the biological activity of endothelium-derived relaxing factor. *Nature* 1987; **327**: 524–6.
7 Moncada S, Vane JR. Arachidonic acid metabolites and the interactions between platelets and blood vessel walls. *N Engl J Med* 1979; **300**: 1142–7.
8 Higgs EA, Moncada S, Vane JR, Caen JP, Michel H, Tobelem G. Effect of prostacyclin

(PGI$_2$) on platelet adhesion to rabbit arterial subendothelium. *Prostaglandins* 1978; **16**: 17–22.

9 Moncada S, Palmer RMJ, Higgs EA. Nitric oxide: physiology, pathophysiology and pharmacology. *Pharmacol Rev* 1991; **43**: 109–42.

10 Radomski MW, Palmer RMJ, Moncada S. The role of nitric oxide and cGMP in platelet adhesion to vascular endothelium. *Biochem Biophys Res Comm* 1987; **148**: 1482–9.

11 Benjamin N, Dutton JAE, Ritter JM. Human vascular smooth muscle cells inhibit platelet aggregation when incubated with glyceryl trinitrate: evidence for generation of nitric oxide. *Br J Pharmacol* 1991; **102**: 847–50.

12 Antiplatelet Trialists' Collaboration. Collaborative overview of randomised trials of antiplatelet therapy, I: prevention of death, myocardial infarction and stroke by prolonged antiplatelet therapy in various categories of patients. *Br Med J* 1994; **308**: 81–106.

13 Antiplatelet Trialists' Collaboration. Secondary prevention of vascular disease by prolonged antiplatelet therapy. *Br Med J* 1988; **296**: 320–31.

14 ISIS-2 (Second International Study of Infarct Survival) Collaborative Group. Randomised trial of intravenous streptokinase, oral aspirin, both, or neither among 17,187 cases of suspected acute myocardial infarction: ISIS-2. *Lancet* 1988; **ii**: 349–60.

15 Lewis HD Jr, Davis JW, Archibald DG. Protective effects of aspirin against acute myocardial infarction and death in men with unstable angina: results of a Veterans' Administration cooperative study. *N Engl J Med* 1983; **309**: 396–403.

16 The RISK Group. Risk of myocardial infarction and death during treatment with low dose aspirin and intravenous heparin in men with unstable coronary artery disease. *Lancet* 1990; **336**: 827–30.

17 Cairns JA, Gent M, Singer J. Aspirin, sulphinpyrazone or both in unstable angina: results of a Canadian multicentre trial. *N Engl J Med* 1985; **313**: 1369–75.

18 Théroux P, Quimet H, McCans J. Aspirin, heparin or both to treat unstable angina. *N Engl J Med* 1988; **319**: 1105–11.

19 Antiplatelet Trialists' Collaboration. Secondary prevention of vascular disease by prolonged antiplatelet treatment. *Br Med J* 1988; **296**: 320–31.

20 Steering Committee of the Physicians' Health Study Research Group. Final report on the aspirin component of the ongoing physicians' health study. *N Engl J Med* 1989; **321**: 129–35.

21 Willard JE, Langar A, Hillis LD. Current concepts: the use of aspirin in ischaemic heart disease. *N Engl J Med* 1992; **327**: 175–81.

22 Barnathan ES, Schwartz JS, Taylor L. Aspirin and dipyridamole in the prevention of acute coronary thrombosis complicating coronary angioplasty. *Circulation* 1987; **76**: 125–34.

23 Goldmann S, Copeland J, Moritz T. Saphenous vein graft patency one year after coronary artery bypass surgery and effects of antiplatelet therapy: results of a Veterans' Administration Cooperative Study. *Circulation* 1989; **80**: 1190–7.

24 UK-TIA Study Group. United Kingdom transient ischaemic attack (UK-TIA) aspirin trial: interim results. *Br Med J* 1988; **296**: 316–20.

25 Stroke Prevention in Atrial Fibrillation Study Group Investigators. Preliminary report of the stroke prevention in atrial fibrillation study. *N Engl J Med* 1990; **322**: 863–8.

26 Italian Study of Aspirin in Pregnancy. Low-dose aspirin in prevention and treatment of intrauterine growth retardation and pregnancy-induced hypertension. *Lancet* 1993; **341**: 396–400.

27 Collaborative Low-dose Aspirin Study in Pregnancy. Collaborative Group. CLASP: a randomised trial of low-dose aspirin for the prevention and treatment of pre-eclampsia among 9,364 pregnant women. *Lancet* 1994; **343**: 619–29.

28 The Anturane Reinfarction Trial Research Group. Sulfinpyrazone in the prevention of cardiac death after myocardial infarction: the Anturane Reinfarction Trial. *N Engl J Med* 1978; **298**: 289–95.

29 The Anturane Reinfarction Trial Research Group. Sulfinpyrazone in the prevention of sudden death after myocardial infarction. *N Engl J Med* 1980; **302**: 250–6.

30 Temple R, Pledger GW. The FDA's critique of the Anturane Reinfarction Trial. *N Engl J Med* 1980; **303**: 1488–92.

31 The Anturane Reinfarction Trial Policy Committee. The Anturane Reinfarction Trial: reevaluation of outcome. *N Engl J Med* 1982; **306**: 1005–8.

32a Anon. Sulphinpyrazone in post-myocardial infarction: report from the Anturane Reinfarction Italian Study. *Lancet* 1982; **i**: 237–42.

32b Rocca B, FitzGerald GA. Simply read: erythrocytes modulate platelet function. Should we rethink the way we give aspirin? *Circulation* 1997; **95**: 11–13.

33 Rosenkranz B, Fischer C, Meese CO, Frölich JC. Effects of salicylic and acetylsalicylic acid alone and in combination on platelet aggregation and prostanoid synthesis in man. *Br J Clin Pharmacol* 1986; **21**: 309–17.

34 Ritter JM, Cockcroft JR, Doktor HS, Beecham J, Barrow SE. Differential effect of aspirin on thromboxane and prostaglandin biosynthesis in man. *Br J Clin Pharmacol* 1989; **28**: 573–9.

35 Patrono C. Aspirin and human platelets: from clinical trials to acetylation of cyclo-oxygenase and back. *Trends Pharmacol Sci* 1989; **10**: 453–8.

36 Heavey DJ, Barrow SE, Hickling NE, Ritter JM. Aspirin causes short-lived inhibition of bradykinin-stimulated prostacyclin production in man. *Nature* 1985; **318**: 186–8.

37 Patrono C, Ciabattoni G, Pinca E, Pugliese F. Low dose aspirin and inhibition of thromboxane B_2 production in healthy subjects. *Thromb Res* 1980; **17**: 317–27.

38 Peto R, Gray R, Collins R *et al.* Randomised trial of prophylactic daily aspirin in British male doctors. *Br Med J* 1988; **296**: 313–16.

39 Whittle BJR. The mechanisms of gastric damage by non-steroid anti-inflammatory drugs. In: Cohen M. ed. *Biochemical protection with prostaglandins.* Boca Raton: CRC Press, 1986.

40 Barnes PJ, Thomson NC. Drug induced asthma. In: Barnes PJ, Rodger IW, Thomson, NC, eds. *Asthma: Basic mechanisms and clinical management,* 2nd edn. London: Academic Press, 1992, Ch. 30.

41 Butt AY, Higenbottam TW, Wallwork J. Prostaglandins and primary pulmonary hyper-tension. In: Vane J, O'Grady J. eds. *Therapeutic applications of prostaglandins.* London: Edward Arnold, 1993.

42 Rylance PB, Gordge MP, Keogh AM, Parsons V, Weston MJ. Epoprostenol during haemodialysis. *Lancet* 1984; **ii**: 744–5.

43 Zusman RM, Ruben RH, Cato AE, Cochetto DM, Crow JM, Tolkoff-Ruben N. Haemodialysis using prostacyclin instead of heparin as the sole antithrombotic agent. *N Engl J Med* 1981; **304**: 934–9.

44 Belch JJF, McKay A, McArdle V. Epoprostenol (prostacyclin) and severe arterial disease; a double blind trial. *Lancet* 1983; **i**: 315–17.

45 Bihari D, Smithies M, Gimson A, Jinker J. The effects of vasodilation with prostacyclin on oxygen delivery and uptake in critically ill patients. *N Engl J Med* 1987; **317**: 397–403.

46 Rosenkranz B, Fischer C, Weimer KE, Frölich JC. Metabolism of prostacyclin and 6-keto-prostaglandin F_{1a} in man. *J Biol Chem* 1980; **255**: 10194–8.

47 FitzGerald GA, Pedersen A, Patrono C. Analysis of prostacyclin and thromboxane biosynthesis in cardiovascular disease. *Circulation* 1983; **67**: 1174–7.

48 Gent M, Blakely JA, Easton JD and the CATS Group. The Canadian-American ticlopidine study (CATS) in thromboembolic stroke. *Lancet* 1989; **i**: 1215–20.

49 Hass WK, Easton JD, Adams HP *et al.* A randomised trial comparing ticlopidine hydrochloride with aspirin for the prevention of stroke in high risk patients. *N Engl J Med* 1989; **321**: 501–7.

50 Janzon L, Bergquist D, Boberg J *et al.* Prevention of myocardial infarction and stroke in patients with intermittent claudication: effects of ticlopidine. Results from STIMS, the Swedish ticlopidine study. *J Int Med* 1990; **227**: 301–8.

51 Balsano F, Rizzon P, Violi F, Scrutinio D, Cimmineielo C and the STAI Group. Antiplatelet treatment with ticlopidine in unstable angina: a controlled multicentre clinical trial. *Circulation* 1990; **82**: 17–26.

52a The TIMAD Study Group. Ticlopidine treatment reduces the progression of non-proliferative diabetic retinopathy. *Arch Ophthalmol* 1990; **108**: 1577–83.

52b Schomig A, Neumann FJ, Kastrati A *et al.* A randomised comparison of antiplatelet and anticoagulant therapy after the placement of coronary artery stents. *N Engl J Med* 1996; **334**: 1084–9.

52c CAPRIE Steering Committee. A randomised, blinded, trial of clopidogrel versus aspirin in patients at risk of ischaemic events (CAPRIE). *Lancet* 1996; **348**: 1329–39.

53 FitzGerald GA. Dipyridamole. *N Engl J Med* 1987; **316**: 1247–57.

54 The Persantin-Aspirin Reinfarction Study Research Group. Persantin and aspirin in coronary heart disease. *Circulation* 1980; **62**: 449–61.

55 Cheesebro JH, Clements IP, Fuster V. A platelet inhibitor drug trial in coronary artery bypass operations. *N Engl J Med* 1982; **307**: 73–8.

56 Bousser MG, Eschwege E, Haguenau M. AICLA controlled trial of aspirin and dipyridamole in the secondary prevention of atherothrombotic cerebral ischaemia. *Stroke* 1983; **14**: 5–14.

57 American-Canadian Cooperative Study Group. Persantine aspirin trial in cerebral ischaemia Part II. End point results. *Stroke* 1985; **16**: 406–15.

58a Sullivan JM, Harker DE, Gorlin R. Pharmacologic control of thromboembolic complications of cardiac valve replacement. *N Engl J Med* 1971; **284**: 1391–4.

58b EPIC Investigators. Use of a monoclonal antibody directed against the platelet glycoprotein IIb/IIIa receptor in high-risk coronary angioplasty. *N Engl J Med* 1994; **330**: 956–61.

59 Turpie AGG, Gent M, Laupacis A *et al*. A comparison of aspirin with placebo in patients treated with warfarin after heart-valve replacement. *N Engl J Med* 1993; **329**: 524–9.

60 Le Breton GC, Venton DK, Enke SE, Haluschka PV. 13-aza-prostanoic acid: a specific antagonist of the human blood platelet thromboxane/endoperoxide receptor. *Proc Nat Acad Sci USA* 1979; **76**: 4097–101.

61 Ritter JM, Benjamin N, Doktor HS *et al*. Effects of a selective thromboxane receptor antagonist (GR32191B) and of glyceryl trinitrate on bleeding time in man. *Br J Clin Pharmacol* 1990; **29**: 431–6.

62 FitzGerald GA, Brash A, Oates JA, Pedersen AK. Endogenous prostacyclin biosynthesis and platelet function during selective inhibition of thromboxane synthase in man. *J Clin Invest* 1983; **72**: 1336–43.

63 Gresel P, Arnout J, Deckmyn H, Huybrechts E, Peiters G, Vermylen J. Role of proaggregatory and antiaggregatory prostaglandins in hemostasis: studies with combined thromboxane synthase inhibition and thromboxane receptor antagonism. *J Clin Invest* 1987; **80**: 1435–45.

64 De Clerck F, Beetens J, van de Water A, Vercammen E, Janssen PAJ. R68070: thromboxane A_2 synthetase inhibition and thromboxane A_2/prostaglandin endoperoxide receptor blockade combined in one molecule. *Thromb Haemostas* 1989; **61**: 35–42.

65a Ritter JM, Barrow SE, Doktor HS *et al*. Thromboxane A_2 receptor antagonism and synthase inhibition in essential hypertension. *Hypertension* 1993; **22**: 197–203.

65b Patrono C, Roth GJ. Aspirin in ischemic cerebrovascular disease: how strong is the case for a different dosing regimen? *Stroke* 1996; **27**: 756–60.

4: Anticoagulation and heart disease

SMC HARDMAN AND MR COWIE

Although a common complication of cardiac disease, thromboembolism can have devastating consequences for the patient whilst leaving the physician with a sense of frustration that the embolism, which so often lodges in the cerebral circulation, might have been prevented. Anticoagulants such as warfarin have long been used to prevent thromboembolism and are largely effective in this respect. Since the main side effect is haemorrhage, which can be fatal, the decision to prescribe an anticoagulant to prevent thromboemboli should ideally be based upon a considered assessment of a particular patient's risk without treatment and the likely benefit and side effects of the proposed level of anticoagulation. Unfortunately the literature on the use of warfarin is unable to provide guidance for many patient groups. Much of the published work involves small patient populations, non-comparable assessment of the level of anticoagulation and inadequate documentation of the achieved levels. Reported series are often incomplete retrospective analyses or prospective studies with widely varying rigour and duration of follow-up. The literature on the risks of haemorrhage associated with anticoagulation is subject to similar criticisms.

This chapter will discuss the use of warfarin in a number of clinical situations and, within the limitations of the literature, provide practical guidelines including, where appropriate, algorithms. These have been inserted at the end of the relevant sections rather than at the end of the chapter but this should not detract from the strong unifying theme stressed throughout the chapter, namely risk stratification for individual patients. The use of antiplatelet agents is discussed extensively in Chapter 3.

Anticoagulation control

In clinical practice the dose of warfarin is titrated against the induced coagulation defect assessed by a biological assay, the prothrombin time (which represents the clotting time of a recalcified tissue thromboplastin). However, the prothrombin ratio, of treated against untreated control, varies markedly depending upon the thromboplastin source. Although in the UK these inconsistencies have for some years been minimised through national quality control (using a UK reference thromboplastin source) this has not applied to laboratories elsewhere. Widespread acceptance of the international normalised ratio (INR) now makes it more possible to compare the reported levels of anticoagulation. This measure, introduced by the World Health Organisation in 1983,[1-3] is based upon quantifying the responsiveness of various thromboplastin agents against a reference preparation but was only recently adopted in the USA. Much of the existing literature is based on estimated INR values which are not equivalent to values derived using a reference source of thromboplastin.

In the UK anticoagulation is predominantly monitored by anticoagulant clinics where decisions on warfarin dosing may be entirely physician based or computer assisted,[4] with resulting variations in achieved levels of anticoagulation. A similar approach is found in other European countries[5] but in North America greater variations in monitoring patterns are found.[6] Reported series suggest patients may be inadequately anticoagulated for significant periods of time,[7,8] which in some studies appear to correlate with significant morbidity. Inadequate warfarin dosing occurs more often in the more intense target range (e.g. 3·0–4·5) when this is physician determined than when a computer based system is used.[9] Computer assisted dosing algorithms can be designed to weight dosing recommendations towards the midpoint of a target range rather than assuming that levels at either end of a range are equally acceptable. This might facilitate the practice of a target INR level within an accepted INR range, as recently advocated by the European Atrial Fibrillation Trial Study Group[10] and supported by others.[6]

Historically, the recommended intensities of anticoagulation have been broadly divided into low (INR 2·0–3·0) and high (INR 3·0–4·5) intensity ranges. Actual INR levels below 2·0 are associated with increased thromboembolic events and those above 5·0 with increased bleeding complications.[5,10] In our own recommendations (see final algorithms, p. 85) we advocate three target levels of anticoagulation (2·5, 3·0, 3·8) corresponding to low, medium or high intensity warfarin with acceptable levels for those patients ranging from 2·0 to 3·0, 2·5 to 3·5, and 3·0 to 4·5 respectively. Medium intensity anticoagulation may offer a compromise between the high intensity anticoagulation which the patient's thromboembolic risks may advocate and a lower level of anticoagulation on the basis of their increased bleeding risk. For such patients this intermediate level of anticoagulation should avoid the risks associated with INRs below 2·0 or above 5·0 which seem to be inevitable for at least some of the time with target ranges of 2·0–3·0 and 3·0–4·5 respectively.

69

Bleeding risks with warfarin

The risk of warfarin related bleeding is highest at the start of therapy with the risk during the first month of treatment being 10 times the risk at 12 months.[11] Patients with cerebrovascular, renal, cardiac and hepatic disease are at increased risk of bleeding. A history of previous gastrointestinal bleeding, but not a history of peptic ulceration alone, is also associated with a significant increased risk of bleeding,[12-14] as is severe anaemia.[15] The commonest sites of anticoagulant related bleeding include the gastro-intestinal tract, the urinary tract, the soft tissues, and the oropharynx. Intracranial bleeding is relatively rare, accounting for about 2% of anticoagulant related bleeding, but is the commonest cause of fatal bleeding. Atrial fibrillation may also be a risk factor for anticoagulant related bleeding[14, 16] although the results of recent trials suggest the benefits outweigh the risks.[17-23] The issue of whether age itself is associated with increased risk of bleeding remains unresolved[24] and controversial.[11] It is well established, however, that the risk of anticoagulant related bleeding is closely related to the anticoagulant level:[11, 25-28] the higher the INR, the greater the risk of bleeding. The recent trials of anticoagulation in non-rheumatic atrial fibrillation also emphasise another aspect of anticoagulant related bleeding, namely that the incidence can be reduced with diligent clinical follow-up.[17-23] These trials reported an incidence of major bleeding events of 1·3% in patients taking warfarin compared with 1% in controls, whereas an incidence of 3% was reported in an overview of 25 studies of patients given anticoagulation in routine practice.[11]

Non-rheumatic atrial fibrillation

Although a common cardiac arrhythmia, atrial fibrillation is not benign and is the commonest cause of cardiogenic stroke.[29] The prevalence of atrial fibrillation varies enormously from one population to another; within the general community the best currently available estimates suggest a prevalence of 0·5% for those aged 50–59 years but this increases with age and dramatically in the years beyond 70 (Figure 4.1). In the presence of cardiac failure, hypertension, and rheumatic heart disease, the prevalence is much higher. As many as 25% of patients presenting with an acute stroke will be in atrial fibrillation.[31, 32] Although this association between atrial fibrillation and stroke can largely be explained by the propensity for thrombus to form within the fibrillating atria and subsequently to embolise, a small but significant proportion of the strokes are not due to cardiogenic embolus: atrial fibrillation can also be a marker for coexistent cerebro-vascular disease.

It does not follow, however, that all patients with atrial fibrillation will benefit from formal anticoagulation and the decision to treat an individual patient with warfarin should be based upon convincing evidence that their

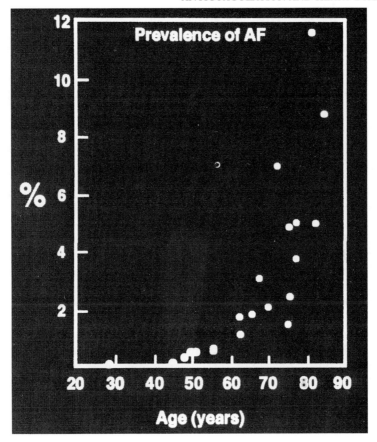

Fig 4.1   The prevalence of atrial fibrillation as a percentage of the population as a function of age. (Reproduced with permission after Wheeldon[30])

risk of a thromboembolic event is greater than their risk of a significant bleed. The age of the patient appears, either directly or indirectly, to be an important determinant of events. For patients with lone atrial fibrillation (no evidence of any concurrent heart disease) aged less than 60, the risk of a serious bleed is of the order of 1·3% or above (see below), and greater than that of a thromboembolic event which is of the order of 0·55%.[33] The difficulty in identifying individual patients in whom the potential benefits of treatment with warfarin outweigh potential risks may be one factor contributing to the continued reluctance of physicians, including cardiologists, to initiate this treatment.[34–36] The recent publication of the randomised trials for primary prevention in patients with non-rheumatic atrial fibrillation[17–22] and one which specifically addresses secondary prevention[23] clarifies some of these issues but raises others. The consensus

71

from these trials is that warfarin therapy is effective prophylaxis for thromboembolic events but its use is generally associated with an increase in haemorrhagic events.[30,37] An appreciation of the limitations of these anticoagulant trials is a prerequisite for the safe and effective prevention of stroke in non-rheumatic atrial fibrillation and the development of further trials to clarify remaining contentions. Wheeldon's review provides useful insights into these trials.[30]

The patient populations under investigation in these trials varied enormously (making direct comparisons difficult), with the only consistent theme being that only a minority of potentially eligible patients were randomised with a nadir of 3·4% in the Stroke Prevention in Atrial Fibrillation Study (SPAF 1).[20] To extrapolate data from such highly selected patients to a hospital based population is arguably hazardous and to the general community potentially more so.[38] Five of the trials were terminated early on "ethical" grounds when interim analyses revealed a significant benefit from anticoagulation whilst the Canadian Atrial Fibrillation Anticoagulation Trial was terminated because of the results of other trials.[19]

The classification of endpoints in the various trials differed but if reported events are reclassified then the overall risk of stroke was 4·32% per annum in the control group as compared with 1·3% per annum in those treated with warfarin, which represents a 60% reduction in the incidence of stroke for primary prevention (personal communication MS Leaning, MR Cowie, DLH Patterson, Report 304 for the Clinical Operational Research Unit, University College London). This would mean treating 1000 patients with warfarin over 12 months to prevent 30 strokes. The overall incidence of haemorrhagic events for the control group was 0·93% as against 1·3% for those receiving warfarin. A similar relative risk reduction for secondary prevention translates into prevention of 80 strokes per year for every 1000 patients treated.[23]

Notwithstanding the limitations of the atrial fibrillation trials, the best data currently available for risk stratification probably come from the Stroke Prevention in Atrial Fibrillation Trial where multivariate analysis was used to determine the clinical and echocardiographic variables most predictive of risk of thromboembolism in the 568 patients randomised.[39,40] A history of recent congestive cardiac failure (i.e. within the last three months), a history of treated or untreated hypertension and previous thromboembolism were each significantly and independently associated with substantial risk of thromboembolism. As Table 4.1 shows, the more clinical risk factors found in a patient, the greater their risk of stroke.

The same applied to the presence of a large left atrium or global left ventricular dysfunction and the effect of including these echocardiographic variables was to reclassify as high risk some of the patients who clinically would have been considered low risk (Table 4.2). This argues in favour of

Table 4.1   Risk stratification for thromboembolic events by clinical assessment in patients with non-rheumatic AF

Score*	0	1	2+
Number	241	259	68
% thromboembolic events (per annum)	2·5%	7·2%	17·6%

Thromboembolic event rate by clinical score for patients with non-rheumatic AF aged over 60. Data from SPAF[38] n = 568
* Scoring one point each for a history of hypertension (both treated and untreated), congestive cardiac failure within the previous three months and previous thromboembolism. n = 568.

echocardiographic assessment of any patient with atrial fibrillation. From this analysis patients without any of these clinical or echocardiographic criteria probably do not warrant anticoagulation but in the presence of one or more there will be a likely benefit from warfarin (where there is no increased risks of bleeding). This argument becomes more powerful where more risk factors for thromboemboli are present. These observations are also supported by reanalysis of pooled data from the major studies of anticoagulation in atrial fibrillation.[41]

The potential benefits of warfarin increase with age above 60. However, with increasing age there may be an increasing tendency to the complications of anticoagulation including problems related to disturbances of balance and mobility, as well as cerebral haemorrhage.[22] Although the exact numbers of patients included in the trials aged 75–80 and over 80 remain unpublished it is clear that the numbers of patients randomised to receive warfarin over the age of 75 were small and above 80 probably negligible. Whilst on this basis it may be hard to justify the initiation of warfarin for patients aged 80 or over, those patients in whom anticoagulant therapy has been well tolerated (following appropriate decision making at a younger age) should not be deprived of this treatment simply because they enter their ninth decade. Anticoagulation should be withdrawn if significant new complications develop or become likely.

Table 4.2   Risk stratification for thromboembolic events by combined clinical and echocardiographic assessment in patients with non-rheumatic AF

Score*	0	1–2	3+
Number	147	336	78
% thromboembolic events (per annum)	1·0%	6·0%	18·6%

Thromboembolic event rate by combined clinical and echocardiographic score for patients with non-rheumatic AF aged over 60.
Data from SPAF[38, 39] n = 561
* Scoring one point for a history of hypertension (both treated and untreated), congestive cardiac failure within the previous three months, and previous thromboembolism, global left ventricular dysfunction, and LA size >2·5 cm²/m² body surface area.
NB: The effect of adding the echocardiographic score allows reclassification of patients who clinically appear at low risk.

73

The trials of anticoagulation in atrial fibrillation give no reliable guidance on the level of anticoagulation. They were predominantly monitored using prothrombin ratios and different thromboplastin sources and even if the translated INR ranges are accepted, these vary considerably between trials. We suggest an attempt is made to grade the patients using the criteria discussed above and that patients with numerous risk factors are given more intense levels of anticoagulation than those with fewer risk factors where an INR range of 2–3 is generally recommended.

The hypothesis that the combination of fixed dose, low intensity warfarin combined with aspirin might confer similar benefit to higher dose warfarin but with fewer side effects was not proven when these two treatment strategies were compared in a group of 1000 patients with non-rheumatic AF at high risk of thromboemboli.[42] The randomised trial was terminated early, after just over one year of follow-up, because of the discrepancy between the benefit of anticoagulation with warfarin, in a target range of 2·0–3·0, and a relative lack of benefit in those receiving aspirin with fixed dose, low intensity warfarin designed to maintain an INR range of 1·2–1·5. However, not only was the combination therapy less effective in preventing systemic embolism but interestingly it failed to confer any benefit over conventional warfarin treatment in terms of major bleeding.

Aspirin treatment is often recommended for elderly patients with non-rheumatic atrial fibrillation on the basis that it will confer protection against thromboembolic events but whilst the likely risks may be less than those of warfarin, so are the likely benefits, on the basis of the trials which have compared these different treatment strategies.[17, 22, 23] When considering treatment with aspirin as alternative to warfarin it is pertinent to remember that there is no evidence of its efficacy in doses of less than 325 mg daily for primary prevention.[17, 22]

Paroxysmal atrial fibrillation

Paroxysmal atrial fibrillation is usually considered to carry a lesser risk of thromboembolism than chronic atrial fibrillation.[43–47] The recent trials of anticoagulation in non-rheumatic atrial fibrillation were inconsistent in their inclusion of these patients and individually provide no additional insights, though subsequent reanalysis of pooled data[41] supports the contention that patients with paroxysmal and chronic (or sustained) atrial fibrillation share a similar risk of stroke.[48–50] Paroxysmal atrial fibrillation covers a wide spectrum of disease severity with the duration and frequency of attacks varying markedly both between and within individuals. As episodes become more frequent and of longer duration, the risks may approximate to those of chronic atrial fibrillation with factors such as associated cardiac pathology and left ventricular function further modifying these risks and these patients should be anticoagulated accordingly.

1. Assess

> **Thromboembolic risk, increased with:**
> Previous thromboemboli
> Recent congestive cardiac failure
> Hypertension (treated or untreated)
>
> Left atrium >2·5 cm²/m² body surface area
> Global left ventricular dysfunction

2. Assess

> **Anticoagulant related bleeding risk, increased with:**
> Serious co-morbid disease including anaemia,
>   cerebrovascular, renal, cardiac and hepatic disease
> Previous gastrointestinal bleed
> Erratic and excessive alcohol abuse
> Immobility
> Modified by quality of clinical and anticoagulant monitoring

> 3. Does the thromboembolic risk outweigh the bleeding risk?
>   (NB: Patient may have informed "preferences" for potential complication)

YES
Anticoagulate

Minimum target INR of 2·5 (range 2·0 to 3·0) but consider higher level where high thromboembolic risk

NO
Aspirin 300 mg per day (unless clear contraindication)

Other categories of non-rheumatic atrial fibrillation

Lone AF under 60 years of age: Aspirin if well tolerated; no indication for long term anticoagulation.

Paroxysmal AF: Overall may be lower risk group but not true for all individuals. Anticoagulation justified when risk factors (as above) are present (which include age over 60) and where attacks are frequent and prolonged.

Chronic AF in patients over 80 years of age: If warfarin has previously been well tolerated up to this age it should not be stopped but no hard evidence in favour of initiation in this group (yet). Where warfarin prescribed target INR should be 2·5 and when aspirin is prescribed the dose should be 300 mg.

AF due to acute thyrotoxicosis: Should be fully anticoagulated. This should be maintained until sinus rhythm has been present for 2–3 months in a euthyroid patient. (Many revert spontaneously to sinus rhythm within 8–12 weeks of being euthyroid: the remainder are susceptible to DC cardioversion.)

Fig 4.2   Long term anticoagulation of patients with non-rheumatic AF aged 60 to late 70s.

Cardioversion of atrial fibrillation and anticoagulation

Direct current (DC) shock has been used to restore sinus rhythm since the early 1960s.[51] The return to sinus rhythm can give profound symptomatic benefit, may reduce the long term incidence of thromboemboli (although this has never been proven) and may even prevent a chronic cardiomyopathy.[52-54]. However, an increased incidence of embolic events (0·8–5·6%) has consistently been reported in the weeks following cardioversion[51, 55-58] even though sinus rhythm is maintained. For many years the working assumption had been that emboli following cardioversion were due to pre-existing atrial thrombi which were dislodged with the restoration of effective atrial contraction. The practice of anticoagulation for 3–4 weeks prior to cardioversion was based on an assumption that this would abolish and/or stabilise atrial clot and thereby reduce the embolic risk. This has not been assessed on a prospective randomised basis although there is circumstantial evidence to suggest that the embolic rates may be reduced from 5–7% to 1·6% with this sort of strategy.[51, 55-58]

The advent of transoesophageal echocardiography has improved the sensitivity and specificity with which the left atrium, including the left atrial appendage, can be examined for the presence of clot[59, 60] and additionally allows functional assessment of the left atrial appendage,[61, 62] providing new insights into the mechanisms of thromboemboli complicating cardioversion. Using this technique persistent thrombus has been reported in some patients despite anticoagulation for the standard four weeks,[63] five weeks[64, 65] and even 12 weeks.[65] Both spontaneous[67] and DC cardioversion[68] of atrial fibrillation are associated with evidence of impaired left atrial and left atrial appendage function postcardioversion. Their recovery appears to be related to the duration of atrial fibrillation at the time of cardioversion and returns to normal within 24 hours in patients who cardiovert within a few days of onset of atrial fibrillation[69] but in patients with atrial fibrillation of longer duration, recovery of atrial function is slower and may continue for up to 12 weeks (depending upon the preceding duration of atrial fibrillation).

Transoesophageal echocardiography has demonstrated the development of new clot as a result of DC cardioversion[65, 70] and spontaneous contrast in the left atrium (which is associated with thrombus formation)[66, 71] following both DC cardioversion[72] and spontaneous reversion to sinus rhythm.[67] Furthermore, patients who have undergone cardioversion without anticoagulation, after left atrial and left atrial appendage clot have been excluded by transoesophageal echocardiography, have subsequently developed thromboemboli.[70] The suggestion that following cardioversion the "stunned atrium" is the source of stasis with thrombus formation and subsequent embolisation when effective atrial contraction returns[72] seems plausible and emphasises the need for anticoagulation at the time of cardioversion and subsequently.

It has long been argued that recent onset atrial fibrillation (less than two or three days duration) can be safely cardioverted without anticoagulation but the basis for these recommendations is entirely empirical[73] and is increasingly questioned.[74] A recent study from Stoddard et al.[75] provides further support for our view that this approach is not without hazard; of 143 patients with atrial fibrillation of less than three days duration, left atrial appendage thrombus was found in 20 using transoesophageal echocardiography. Moreover, the same study identified left atrial thrombus with a similar frequency in the patients with atrial fibrillation of recent onset (<three days duration) and thromboemboli as in patients with more chronic atrial fibrillation and thromboemboli.

Since early cardioversion appears to offer an increased likelihood of successful cardioversion[76-79] and sustained sinus rhythm[80] a strong case can be made for initiating anticoagulation in patients who present within the first few days of onset of atrial fibrillation and using transoesophageal echocardiography to screen those who fail to revert spontaneously or to cardiovert chemically. In the absence of thrombus DC cardioversion can be undertaken provided there is full anticoagulation which should be maintained for 48 hours thereafter. Patients with thrombus would undergo a period of prolonged anticoagulation with warfarin before reassessment for cardioversion with repeat transoesophageal echocardiography. Where transoesophageal echocardiography is not available patients should undergo a transthoracic study but could be discharged home on a combination of warfarin and antiarrhythmics designed to control ventricular rate and restore sinus rhythm. Elective DC cardioversion can then be arranged for those who remain in atrial fibrillation at the end of four weeks. These recommendations are not advocated for patients with previous thromboemboli or rheumatic mitral valve disease.

The use of transoesophageal echocardiography to reduce the requirement for precardioversion anticoagulation has similarly been proposed for atrial fibrillation which has been present for longer periods.[64, 81, 82] Preliminary studies[64, 66, 83] and a completed prospective study of over 200 patients in whom atrial fibrillation has been present for more than two days[84] suggest it may be safe to use transoesophageal echocardiography to identify patients who have no left atrial thrombus and then proceed to cardioversion as soon as they are anticoagulated (with heparin or warfarin). Anticoagulation is maintained for the usual four weeks or more following cardioversion. Patients with detectable thrombus would undergo a conventional period of anticoagulation with warfarin and a repeat transoesophageal study before reconsideration for cardioversion.[81] A larger series of over 7000 patients randomised to compare such transoesophageal guided DC cardioversion with the conventional approach has completed the pilot phase[85] and is now underway. It has been suggested that the projected savings of reduced

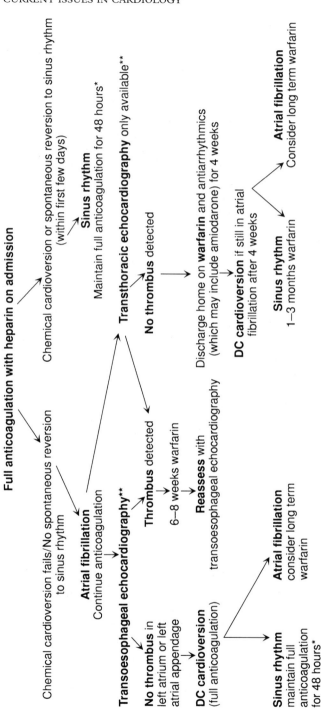

Fig 4.3   Anticoagulation for cardioversion of AF of <3 days duration (without previous thromboembolism).

anticoagulation and morbidity would meet the increased costs of trans-oesophageal echocardiography if the postcardioversion embolic rate was reduced from 1·6% (and above) to 0·9% or less[86] but this needs formal evaluation. This would have important implications for cardiological practice in the UK where, although transoesophageal echocardiography is increasingly available, echocardiography is more usually limited to the transthoracic approach. The latter remains an important investigation for patients presenting with atrial fibrillation and should be undertaken before cardioversion. Transthoracic echocardiography will usefully identify thrombus in certain patients and document previously undiagnosed cardiac disease in others. In all patients an assessment of left atrial and ventricular size and of left ventricular function will be important in weighing the requirements for long term anticoagulation where cardioversion is unsuccessful (or not undertaken). Nonetheless, transthoracic echocardiography is not recommended as an alternative to precardioversion anticoagulation and neither transthoracic nor transoesophageal echocardiography precludes the need for anticoagulation at the time of and for a period after cardioversion.[74, 87]

The duration of anticoagulation postcardioversion has traditionally been limited to the period during which the patient has been assumed to be at increased risk relating to that single rhythm change (as discussed above): usually from one to three months. However, significant numbers will relapse into atrial fibrillation over the next year. If instead of discontinuing warfarin at 1–3 months anticoagulation were maintained for 12 months, this would protect the patient from any associated thromboembolic risk and allow an aggressive approach of immediate repeat cardioversion. This strategy is likely to minimise the electrical instability of the atrium which follows any relapse into atrial fibrillation[80] and may result in a higher incidence of long term sustained sinus rhythm. This approach may not be suitable for all patients but should certainly be considered for those patients in whom the side effects of atrial fibrillation are unacceptable and for those in whom chronic atrial fibrillation would justify long term anticoagulation.

Atrial flutter

It is often suggested that atrial flutter does not carry the same thromboembolic risk at the time of cardioversion. We have been unable to find any convincing data to support this suggestion or justify the associated practice of cardioversion without anticoagulation. We are, however, aware of a number of cases, not reported perhaps for obvious reasons, of patients in whom atrial flutter has been cardioverted without anticoagulation and who have subsequently developed systemic emboli. The issue is complex because atrial flutter is an unstable rhythm and may degenerate into atrial fibrillation in some patients; in others, Holter recording often demonstrates

Full anticoagulation

↓

Transthoracic echocardiography*
(to exclude undiagnosed cardiac pathology, to identify thrombus, to determine left atrial and
left ventricular size and to assess left ventricular function)**

If **thrombus** identified   If **no thrombus** identified
6–8 weeks of anticoagulation   4 weeks anticoagulation

↓   ↓

Transoesophageal echocardiography **DC cardioversion** (fully anticoagulated)
To ensure left atrial and left appendage
thrombus does not preclude   **Atrial fibrillation** **Sinus rhythm**
cardioversion   Consider long term Continue warfarin for 1–3
                                 anticoagulation   months but consider
                                                    anticoagulation for 12
                                                        months (see text)

* NB: Initial results suggest that where available, transoesophageal echocardiography can be used to guide cardioversion, obviating the need for prolonged anticoagulation precardioversion. Pending further studies the following algorithm may be appropriate in selected cases where reducing either the overall duration of anticoagulation or delay before cardioversion is deemed of paramount importance. These patients will require full anticoagulation at the time of cardioversion and following cardioversion as elsewhere.

** If mitral stenosis is found cardioversion should only be undertaken after a transoesophageal study in consultation with a cardiologist since cardioversion may not be appropriate. Long term warfarin is required.

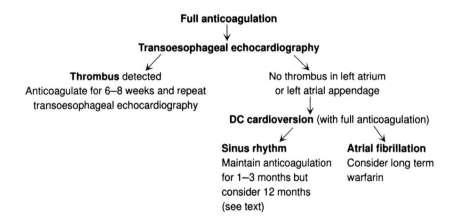

Fig 4.4 Anticoagulation for cardioversion of AF of >3 days duration (without previous thromboembolism).

alternation between atrial fibrillation and atrial flutter. Bikkina and coworkers[88] have recently reported a prevalence of intra-atrial thrombus of 21% in a group of 24 unselected hospital patients found to be in atrial flutter of unknown duration as compared with a 3% prevalence rate in a control group of patients in sinus rhythm undergoing transoesophageal echocardiography within the same hospital. Furthermore, evidence is emerging of atrial standstill immediately postcardioversion in some patients with atrial flutter.[89] On current evidence we therefore recommend that patients with atrial flutter should be anticoagulated, prior to and following cardioversion, in the same way as patients with atrial fibrillation.

Rheumatic valve disease and anticoagulation

Patients with atrial fibrillation and rheumatic valve disease have an increased risk of thromboembolism compared with patients in sinus rhythm and require long term anticoagulation. This includes patients with rheumatic valvular heart disease and paroxysmal, as opposed to chronic, atrial fibrillation. In the presence of mitral (or tricuspid) stenosis and sinus rhythm, indications for anticoagulation include an enlarged atrium, the presence of atrial clot or evidence of previous thromboembolism, more than mild stenosis and arguably the presence of spontaneous contrast within the atrium (detected by transoesophageal echocardiography). These patients should also be referred for formal cardiological opinion because of the importance of ensuring optimal timing of intervention.

Long term anticoagulation following myocardial infarction

Thrombosis on a substrate of plaque fissure in the coronary arteries is the usual precipitant of acute myocardial infarction with the interruption of myocardial flow resulting in tissue necrosis. Thrombolytic agents (such as streptokinase or tissue plasminogen activator) act to dissolve the occluding thrombus and thereby abort the infarction. However, even after dissolution of the thrombus, the fissured plaque remains a potent stimulus for rethrombosis and antiplatelet agents (such as aspirin) and anticoagulants have an important role in preventing rethrombosis and so reinfarction in the acute phase. This is discussed in Chapters 2 and 3.

Longer term anticoagulation following myocardial infarction has attracted considerable interest over the last 30 years. Most of the early trials were undertaken when patients were maintained on strict bed rest for many weeks with the consequent increased risk of deep venous thrombosis and pulmonary embolism and they reported only limited series of patients who were seldom randomised. Although an overview of several of the larger, more recent and better designed studies suggested a 22% reduction in mortality after myocardial infarction in patients taking warfarin compared to those who were not,[90] most of the trials included in this meta-analysis predated the use of thrombolytic agents.

One of the most recent studies of oral anticoagulation following myocardial infarction is the ASPECT study.[91] This provided evidence of a reduction in the number of reinfarctions and cerebrovascular events in a large group of patients postinfarction randomised to warfarin (target INR of 2·8–4·8) compared with placebo, following discharge from hospital. In absolute terms, for every 1000 patient-years of anticoagulation there were 28 fewer first reinfarctions and five fewer cerebrovascular events at the expense of ten additional "major" haemorrhages. Interestingly, this benefit was not significantly different in any subgroup, including those thrombolysed as against those who did not receive thrombolysis.[92] This degree of benefit (which comes at not inconsiderable cost and inconvenience to the patient and the health service) has not been high enough to persuade most units in the UK to adopt a policy of long term anticoagulation postmyocardial infarction. The same study reported a 10% reduction in mortality but this reduction failed to achieve statistical significance.

Whether or not aspirin confers any additional benefit if combined with oral anticoagulation has yet to be established but until the report of the CARS (Coumarin Aspirin Reinfarction Study), which was designed to establish this, is available, it is usual practice to stop aspirin if warfarin is to be given because of the increased risk of haemorrhage.

Long term anticoagulation following myocardial infarction should be considered in patients at especially high risk of thromboembolism postinfarction: those who are immobile or with severe heart failure, left ventricular thrombosis or aneurysm and those with a past history of deep venous thrombosis or pulmonary embolism. Left ventricular mural thrombus may form in up to 40% of patients with an acute anterior myocardial infarction and usually within the first 48 hours. The risk of embolism is not clear but has been as high as 40% in some series and can be reduced by anticoagulation.[93] The risk of mural thrombus forming can be reduced with high dose heparin (12,500 units bd subcutaneously).[94] It would seem sensible to consider anticoagulation (initially with heparin and thereafter with warfarin) in all patients with extensive anterior myocardial infarction and especially where this is complicated by heart failure or by aneurysm formation. If at the end of three months (the highest risk period for thromboembolism postinfarction) echocardiography fails to demonstrate persistent thrombus, severe anterior akinesia or ventricular aneurysm, consideration should be given to discontinuing anticoagulation.

Anticoagulation and heart failure

Thromboembolism is not uncommon in heart failure, with reported rates varying from 2·5% per annum in patients with symptoms on mild to moderate exertion[95] to 20% in hospital based patients with dilated cardiomyopathy,[96] although subclinical thromboemboli may be more common.[97] Retrospective analyses of the role of anticoagulation (or antiplatelet agents) in reducing either mortality or thromboembolism in patients with heart failure have produced conflicting results. Several studies which may answer these questions are actively recruiting, including the WASH Study in the UK (aspirin versus warfarin versus placebo). Until these trials report, anticoagulation should be considered at least in those patients with high risk of embolism (which includes patients with atrial fibrillation, left ventricular thrombus and previous thromboembolism). Less stable patients with cardiac failure (who are likely to be at increased risk) will require especially careful monitoring of their anticoagulation because varying hepatic congestion will alter their warfarin requirements and anticoagulant control.

Anticoagulation of prosthetic heart valves

A diseased valve can be replaced with either a mechanical valve (ball, tilting disc or bileaflet) or a tissue valve (homograft or xenograft). The major advantage of mechanical prostheses over tissue valves is their longevity but they do require lifelong anticoagulation to prevent valve thrombosis and thromboembolism. Although valve thrombosis is often grouped together with thromboembolism as a single entity[98] the mechanisms appear largely distinct. In disc and bileaflet valves there appears to be no definite relation between valve thrombosis and embolism,[99] although in caged ball valves where the apex of the cage, the area most vulnerable to clot formation, is repeatedly struck by the ball, recurrent embolism can portend valve thrombosis.[100-102]

The risk of systemic embolism appears to be largely unrelated to the type or position of valve prosthesis but instead reflects patient related risk factors including cardiac failure, atrial fibrillation, previous embolism, hypertension, smoking, and left atrial size.[103-106] Embolic rates taken from the larger series reported since 1985 and restricted to those trials with more rigorous statistical analyses show greater variation between one series and another than between the different valve types[104] which include caged ball, tilting disc, and bileaflet valves. The potential benefit of tissue valves is the avoidance of anticoagulation because they are less likely to thrombose. But even these patients will require anticoagulation if other risk factors for embolism are present either at the time of implantation or on subsequent follow-up.

In contrast certain valves are especially vulnerable to thrombosis and this complication reflects prosthesis type and position, surgical technique and adequate anticoagulation. Valves with the highest risk of thrombosis include the Bjork–Shiley (but not the Monostrut valve) and St Jude valves in the mitral position whilst the Medtronic Hall prosthesis appears to have a low thrombosis rate.[106]

Whilst there is convincing circumstantial evidence that warfarin produces a marked reduction in thrombosis and thromboembolic events with mechanical valve prostheses,[107, 108] the recommended levels of anticoagulation for mechanical valves are often arbitrary. They are based on inadequate scientific data and reflect established clinical practice which has tended to ascribe all the risks to a particular prosthesis and its position.

The need for anticoagulation and its intensity should be dictated by the thrombogenicity of a particular prosthesis and the individual patient's risk factors for embolic events, which must be balanced against an assessment of their bleeding risk with anticoagulation (factors which should all contribute to the surgeon's choice of prosthesis). Patients with prosthetic valves at high risk of thrombosis with numerous risk factors for thromboembolism or with a history of previous thromboembolism require a more intense level of anticoagulation than patients with less thrombogenic valves and no risk factors for thromboemboli. There is continuing controversy over the ideal target levels for anticoagulation.[5, 6] Current guidelines issued by the British Society of Haematology recommended the INR be maintained between 3·0 and 4·5 in patients with mechanical valves[109] and until recently this policy was also that of the American College of Physicians.[110] Although this remains the policy of many anticoagulant clinics in the UK considerable differences are found between centres.[111] Important influences in final anticoagulant levels include the varying recommendations from cardiac surgeons and other clinicians and the character of the local anticoagulant clinic.

A recent study from The Netherlands suggests optimal anticoagulation lies within an actual INR range of 2·5–4·9 achieved using a computer assisted system and a target INR range of 3·0–4·0.[5] In contrast, the most recent American guidelines now suggest a lower level of anticoagulation for mechanical valves with a target INR range of 2·5–3·5[110] with this policy modification heavily influenced by only two studies,[105, 112] neither of which compared the newly advocated level of anticoagulation with those previously recommended.

The risk of embolism is relatively high soon after operation but falls to a more stable long term risk over subsequent months,[106, 111, 113] so that a more aggressive approach to anticoagulation can be justified in the early postoperative months. These increased risks in the early postoperative period may reflect the difficulties of achieving adequate anticoagulation in the first few postoperative days, rhythm changes over the same period and incomplete endothelialisation of raw intracardiac surfaces, sewing ring and suture knots. Bioprosthetic valves are subject to the same hazards.[113] These early risks of thromboemboli do appear to be reduced by warfarin[113] so unless contraindications exist all patients should have anticoagulation

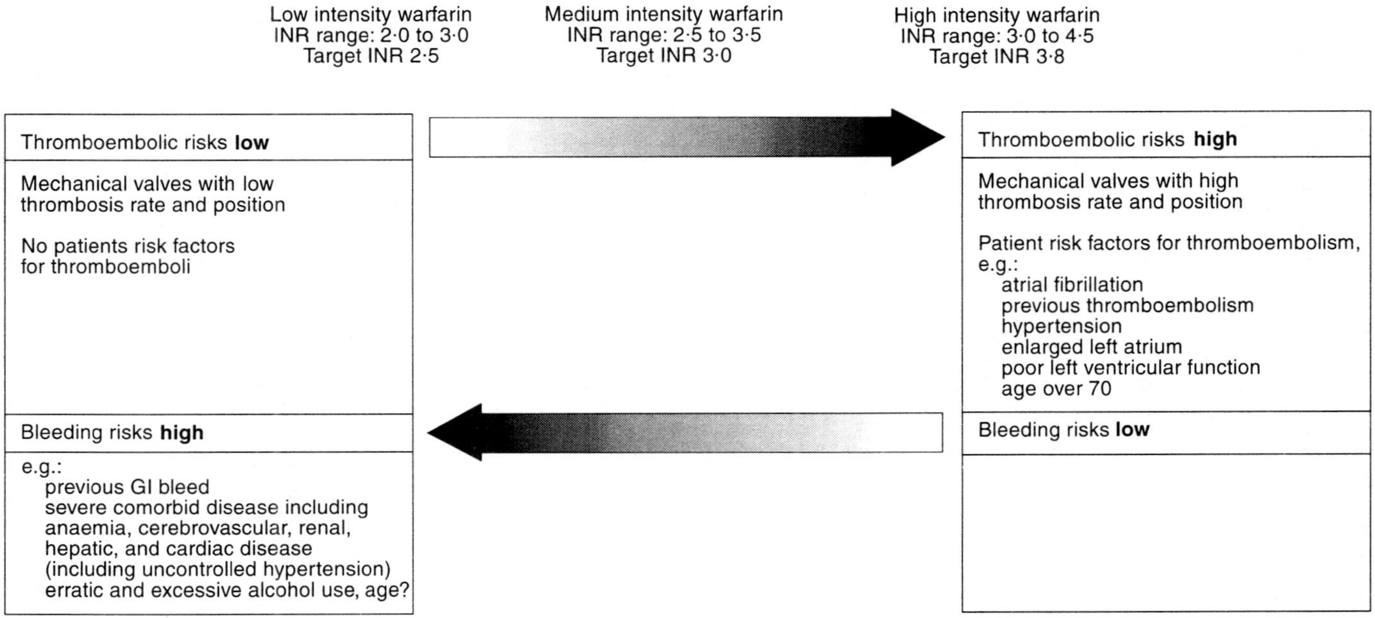

Low intensity warfarin
INR range: 2·0 to 3·0
Target INR 2·5

Medium intensity warfarin
INR range: 2·5 to 3·5
Target INR 3·0

High intensity warfarin
INR range: 3·0 to 4·5
Target INR 3·8

Thromboembolic risks **high**

Mechanical valves with high thrombosis rate and position

Patient risk factors for thromboembolism, e.g.:
atrial fibrillation
previous thromboembolism
hypertension
enlarged left atrium
poor left ventricular function
age over 70

Bleeding risks **low**

Thromboembolic risks **low**

Mechanical valves with low thrombosis rate and position

No patients risk factors for thromboemboli

Bleeding risks **high**

e.g.:
previous GI bleed
severe comorbid disease including anaemia, cerebrovascular, renal, hepatic, and cardiac disease (including uncontrolled hypertension) erratic and excessive alcohol use, age?

The bleeding risk is reduced as the INR level falls and as the anticoagulant monitoring and clinical care improves.

NB: Following surgery even patients with bioprostheses should receive three months anticoagulation unless strong contraindications exist. Anticoagulation beyond this period is unusual because bioprostheses are now usually restricted to those patients in whom the long term risks of bleeding are unacceptably high with formal anticoagulation.

Fig 4.5   Long term anticoagulation of patients with prosthetic heart valves.

85

initiated as early as possible in the immediate postoperative period and maintained for three months. At the end of this period the indications for and risks of anticoagulation in each individual should be formally reviewed. In patients with bioprosthetic valves anticoagulation beyond three months is only indicated where the patient has specific risk factors for thromboemboli (which outweigh the bleeding risks) and in their absence it is normal practice to withdraw anticoagulation at this stage.

A small number of patients continue to experience emboli despite higher level warfarin treatment. In these patients the combination of higher level warfarin and low dose aspirin can be justified[114] but on current evidence there appears to be no advantage to be gained by increasing the INR to a target beyond 3·8 (range 3·0–4·5).[5] When all else fails replacement of the prosthetic valve is sometimes undertaken for recurrent thromboemboli but this should not be contemplated within the first six months.

Anticoagulation, prosthetic valves and pregnancy

Pregnancy for women with prosthetic valves remains hazardous and where appropriate, child bearing should be encouraged before valve replacement is indicated. Since this is not practicable for all young women the debate has focused on the relative merits of mechanical valves which require anticoagulation with potential risks for mother and foetus versus bioprostheses which are not as durable and which may be associated with an increased rate of deterioration during pregnancy.[115, 116] "Redo" surgery carries a much higher mortality than the first operation and this may be increased further when surgery is required during the pregnancy. In some patients the need for anticoagulation and risks of "redo" surgery may be obviated by the Ross procedure (where the diseased aortic valve is replaced with the patient's own pulmonary valve and a homograft implanted in the pulmonary position).[117–121]

Pregnancy is associated with an increased risk of thromboembolic complications[122–124] due to the hypercoagulable state[125, 126] and anti-coagulation is essential for all women with mechanical valves or bioprostheses with risk factors for thromboembolism, which include atrial fibrillation and previous thromboembolism. There is no international consensus as to the optimum approach to anticoagulation during pregnancy.[127–131] This reflects the hazards of heparin and warfarin therapy to mother and foetus, the consequences of inadequate anticoagulation control, the lack of well reported prospective trials, the small numbers and the inevitable bias of retrospective studies. The discrepancy in current recommendations from Western cardiac centres, where young women with prosthetic valves are a relative rarity, emphasises the paucity of evidence on which to base current practice.

warfarin is associated with an embryopathy[115, 132] which is thought to occur between the sixth and ninth week, resulting in foetal wastage and malformation. The reported incidence varies enormously, with Sbarouni and Oakley,[116] Chen et al.,[133] Ben Ismail et al.[134] and Pavakumar et al.[135] reporting no cases in retrospective series of 36, 22, 53, and 47 patients respectively. In contrast, the prospective cohort study of Iturbe-Alessio et al.[136] describes a 29% risk of embryopathy (10/35) and Wong et al.[137] a 67% risk (12/18) in another retrospective cohort. Cotrufo et al.[138] suggest the foetal risk of warfarin is not manifest in mothers whose requirement is less than 5 mg per day (which may reflect the stronger anticoagulant effect seen in the foetus as compared with the mother) but this observation was again based on small numbers only. Treatment with heparin between six and 12 weeks of gestation and warfarin thereafter until week 38 has been recommended in the US[128] but not in the United Kingdom where the use of warfarin until week 38 is more usually advocated.[127, 129, 130] It is generally agreed that target levels of anticoagulation should be twice the partial thromboplastin time[139] for heparin. Ginsberg argues for an INR of 3·0–4·5 in combination with aspirin from the second trimester, extrapolating from a trial which included no pregnant women.[114] Oakley also advocates anticoagulation at this level (but without the aspirin) unless the valve has a low thrombotic profile and no patient risk factors for thromboembolism, when an INR of 2·0–3·0 is suggested in keeping with current European guidelines.[140] However, whilst there is convincing evidence that this level of anticoagulation is safe in second and third generation mechanical valves with low thrombotic profiles (and no patient risk factors for thromboembolism)[106] as elsewhere there is a dearth of data to support or contend these recommendations in pregnancy.

An alternative approach has been to use heparin throughout the first 38 weeks of pregnancy although it has been suggested that this will result in a higher incidence of valve thrombosis, arterial embolism and bleeding events[116] and there is some evidence to suggest that these complications are seen more frequently even when heparin use is limited to six weeks in the first trimester.[129] Other studies of long term heparin therapy in pregnant women produced bleeding rates of 2% or less,[141, 142] but both symptomless bone loss[143, 144] and vertebral fracture[142] may complicate this treatment. Sbarouni and Oakley advocate warfarin throughout the first 38 weeks of pregnancy, arguing that subcutaneous heparin is neither safe nor effective (for the mother), though they noted a slightly improved foetal outcome in the women taking the combination of heparin in the first trimester followed by warfarin, when compared with either warfarin or heparin throughout pregnancy.[116]

There is a general consensus that warfarin at term should be avoided because of the risks of peripartum haemorrhage. warfarin should be stopped at 38 weeks and at this stage some authors advocate an elective caesarean section[130, 138] but others prefer to change to intravenous heparin until term. Wherever possible the risks and limitations of these different approaches should be discussed with future mothers prior to conception (and even valve replacement) although late presentation will preclude this approach.[145] Anticoagulation with warfarin does not induce anticoagulant defects in breast feeding infants.

Low dose molecular weight heparin is increasingly used to treat deep venous thromboses and pulmonary emboli complicating pregnancy because of its ease of administration and fewer potential side effects compared with standard heparin.[146] Low molecular weight heparin does not cross the placenta. It has, however, only been assessed to a very limited extent in pregnancy[146-148] and not at all in patients with valve prostheses.

Peroperative management of patients undergoing non-cardiac surgery on warfarin

The management of these patients is often left to the junior surgical staff who are confronted with their care at short notice even though the procedure is an elective one. This is far from ideal. Optimum management involves advance assessment of the patient and a treatment plan which reflects the individual risk of the patient. It should ensure that patients who have been asked to discontinue their anticoagulants as outpatients are not subject to last minute cancellation.

Preoperative assessment should include a decision as to whether reversal of anticoagulation is necessary for the proposed surgery, a policy which will reflect the surgical procedure and the views and skills of the surgeon. Certainly a proportion of surgery (including dental extraction) can be safely performed with the INR towards the lower end of the therapeutic range (INR 2·0) without excessive bleeding, a policy which avoids the risk of reversing anticoagulation. Those patients for whom this is not an option broadly fall into two categories: those assessed as being at high risk of developing either thrombus or emboli when anticoagulation is reversed for even short periods and those in whom this is not the case. The high risk group, which includes patients with prosthetic heart valves, should be managed so that the period without anticoagulation is minimised. Warfarin is stopped three days prior to surgery and the admission planned to coincide with an INR of 2·5 when a heparin infusion is commenced (5000 units of heparin is given as a loading dose followed by 20,000 units per 24 hours and monitoring of KPTT at four hours and at least every 24 hours· thereafter). The aim is to maintain the KPTT at between 45 to 50 seconds and heparin dose modifications should be discussed with the haematologists. The heparin should be discontinued 4–6 hours before surgery and clotting checked two hours beforehand. Intravenous heparin should be restarted about four hours after surgery (unless there are good reasons not to). The warfarin should be restarted as soon as possible in the postoperative period, usually the same evening, at the dose previously given. Heparin should be continued until the INR is greater than 2·5 (usually within 72 hours).

Patients undergoing a finite period of anticoagulation, such as treatment for a deep venous thrombosis, may benefit from deferring their surgery for that period and then having prophylactic subcutaneous heparin (5000 units eight- or 12-hourly) in the subsequent peroperative period. Lower risk patients on long term anticoagulation should stop their warfarin 3–4 days before surgery and restart as soon as possible thereafter. Subcutaneous heparin can again be given in the peroperative period.

Occasionally urgent reversal of anticoagulation with warfarin is required, either for emergency surgery or where intercurrent illness has caused marked prolongation of the INR. In this situation the clotting can be corrected using fresh frozen plasma which should be prescribed in ml according to the weight of the patient. A dose of 12–15 ml/kg is currently recommended and will correct most clotting defects. (A notable exception is patients with cirrhosis in whom clotting defects can be very difficult to correct.) Vitamin K is generally not advocated since it complicates subsequent reanticoagulation but where administered, no more than 1 mg should be given intravenously.

Despite the limitations of the literature and resulting clinical uncertainties discussed in this chapter, it is clear that the judicious use of anticoagulation is an important aspect of the management of patients with heart disease. The potential benefits of anticoagulation can be optimised by the careful assessment of the risks of thromboemboli and of haemorrhage in every individual in whom this treatment is considered. Although this approach will be time consuming the rewards for patient and clinician can be profound.

1 Shinton NK. Standardisation of oral anticoagulant therapy. *Br Med J* 1983; **287**: 1000–1.
2 Loeliger EA, Poller L, Samama M *et al.* Questions and answers on prothrombin time standardisation in oral anticoagulant control. *Thromb Haemostas* 1985; **54**: 515–17.
3 Lewis SM. Thromboplastin and oral anticoagulant control (Editorial). *Br J Haematol* 1987; **66**: 1–4.
4 Vadher BD, Patterson DLH, Leaning MS. Validation of an algorithm for oral anticoagulant dosing and appointment scheduling. *Clin Lab Haematol* 1995; **17**: 339–45.
5 Cannegieter SC, Rosendaal FR, Wintzen AR, van der Meer FJM, Vandenbroucke JP, Briet E. Optimal oral anticoagulant therapy in patients with mechanical heart valves. *N Engl J Med* 1995; **333**: 11–17.
6 Fihn SD. Aiming for safe anticoagulation (Editorial). *N Engl J Med* 1995; **333**: 54–5.
7 Duxbury B McD. Therapeutic control of anticoagulant treatment. *Br Med J* 1982; **284**: 702–4.
8 Copplestone A, Roath S. Assessment of therapeutic control of anticoagulation. *Acta Haematol* 1984; **71**: 376–80.
9 Poller L, Wright D, Rowlands M. Prospective comparative study of computer programs used for management of warfarin. *J Clin Pathol* 1993; **46**: 299–303.

10 European Atrial Fibrillation Trial Study Group. Optimal oral anticoagulant therapy in patients with non-rheumatic atrial fibrillation and recent cerebral ischemia. *N Engl J Med* 1995; **333**: 5–10.

11 Landefeld CS, Beyth RJ. Anticoagulant-related bleeding: clinical epidemiology, prediction, and prevention. *Am J Med* 1993; **95**: 315–28.

12 Peyman MA. The significance of haemorrhage during the treatment of patients with coumarin anticoagulants. *Acta Med Scand* 1958; **162** (Suppl 339): 1–62.

13 Coon WW, Willis PW III. Hemorrhagic complications of anticoagulant therapy. *Arch Intern Med* 1974; **133**: 386–92.

14 Landefeld CS, Goldman L. Major bleeding in outpatients treated with warfarin: incidence and prediction by factors known at the start of outpatient therapy. *Am J Med* 1989; **87**: 144–52.

15 Landefeld CS, McGuire E, Rosenblatt MW. A bleeding risk index for estimating the probability of major bleeding in hospitalized patients starting anticoagulant therapy. *Am J Med* 1990; **89**: 569–78.

16 Lundstrom T, Ryden L. Haemorrhagic and thromboembolic complications in patients with atrial fibrillation on anticoagulant prophylaxis. *J Int Med* 1989; **225**: 137–42.

17 Petersen P, Godfredsen J, Boysen G, Andersen ED, Andersen B. Placebo controlled, randomised trial of warfarin and aspirin for prevention of thromboembolic complications in chronic atrial fibrillation. The Copenhagen AFASAK Study. *Lancet* 1989; **i**: 175–9.

18 The Boston Area Anticoagulant Trial for Atrial Fibrillation Investigators. The effect of low dose warfarin on the risk of stroke in patients with non-rheumatic atrial fibrillation. *N Engl J Med* 1990; **323**: 1505–11.

19 Connolly SJ, Laupacis A, Gent M, Roberts RS, Cairns JA, Joyner C. Canadian Atrial Fibrillation Anticoagulation (CAFA) Study. *J Am Coll Cardiol* 1991; **18**: 349–55.

20 Stroke Prevention in Atrial Fibrillation Investigators. Stroke Prevention in Atrial Fibrillation Study – Final results. *Circulation* 1991; **84**: 527–39.

21 Ezekowitz MD, Bridgers SL, James KE *et al.* for the Veterans Affairs Stroke Prevention in Non-Rheumatic Atrial Fibrillation Investigators. warfarin in the prevention of stroke associated with non-rheumatic atrial fibrillation. *N Engl J Med* 1992; **327**: 1406–12.

22 Stroke Prevention in Atrial Fibrillation Investigators. warfarin versus aspirin for prevention of thromboembolism in atrial fibrillation: stroke prevention in atrial fibrillation II study. *Lancet* 1994; **343**: 687–91.

23 European Atrial Fibrillation Trial Study Group. Secondary prevention in non-rheumatic atrial fibrillation after transient ischaemic attack or minor stroke. *Lancet* 1993; **342**: 1255–62.

24 Scott PJW. Anticoagulant drugs in the elderly: the risks usually outweigh the benefits. *Br Med J* 1988; **297**: 1261–3.

25 Poller L. Therapeutic ranges in anticoagulant administration. *Br Med J* 1985; **290**: 1683–6.

26 Levine MN, Raskob G, Hirsh J. Hemorrhagic complications of long-term anticoagulant therapy. *Chest* 1989; **95** (Suppl): 26s–36s.

27 Van der Meer FJM, Rosendaal FR, Vandenbroucke JP, Briet E. Bleeding complications in oral anticoagulant therapy. An analysis of risk factors. *Arch Intern Med* 1993; **153**: 1557–62.

28 Hylek EM, Singer DE. Risk factors for intracranial hemorrhage in outpatients taking warfarin. *Ann Intern Med* 1994; **120**: 897–902.

29 Cerebral Embolism Task Force. Cardiogenic brain embolism. *Arch Neurol* 1986; **43**: 71–84.

30 Wheeldon NM. Atrial fibrillation and anticoagulation therapy (Review). *Eur Heart J* 1995; **16**: 302–12.

31 Friedman GD, Loveland DB, Ehrlich SP. Relationship of stroke to other cardiovascular disease. *Circulation* 1968; **38**: 533–41.

32 Terent A, Andersson B. The prognosis for patients with cerebrovascular stroke and transient ischaemic attacks. *Ups J Med Sci* 1981; **86**: 63–74.

33 Kopecky SL, Gersh BJ, McGoon MD et al. The natural history of lone atrial fibrillation. A population-based study over three decades. *N Engl J Med* 1987; **317**: 669–74.

34 Chang HG, Bell JR, Deroo DB, Kirk JW, Wasson JH. Physician variation in

anticoagulating patients with atrial fibrillation. *Arch Intern Med* 1990; **150**: 81–4.

35 Kutner M, Nixon G, Silverstone F. Physicians' attitude toward oral anticoagulants and antiplatelet agents for stroke prevention in elderly patients with atrial fibrillation. *Arch Intern Med* 1991; **151**: 1950–3.

36 Bath PMW, Prasad A, Brown MM, MacGregor GA. Survey of anticoagulants in patients with atrial fibrillation. *Br Med J* 1993; **341**: 1381–4.

37 Cleland JGF, Cowburn PJ, Falk RH. Should all patients with AF receive warfarin? Evidence from randomized clinical trials. *Eur Heart J* 1996; **17**: 674–81.

38 Sudlow CM, Rodgers H, Kenny RA, Thomson RG. Service provision and use of anticoagulants in atrial fibrillation. *Br Med J* 1995; **311**: 558–60.

39 The Stroke Prevention in Atrial Fibrillation Investigators. Predictors of thromboembolism in atrial fibrillation. I. Clinical features of patients at risk. *Ann Intern Med* 1992; **116**: 1–5.

40 The Stroke Prevention in Atrial Fibrillation Investigators. Predictors of thromboembolism in atrial fibrillation: II. Echocardiographic features of patients at risk. *Ann Intern Med* 1992; **116**: 6–12.

41 Atrial Fibrillation Investigators. Atrial Fibrillation, Aspirin, Anticoagulation Study; Boston Area Anticoagulation Trial for Atrial Fibrillation Study; Canadian Atrial Fibrillation Study; Stroke Prevention in Non-rheumatic Atrial Fibrillation Study. Risk factors for stroke and efficacy of antithrombotic therapy in atrial fibrillation. Analysis of pooled data from five randomized controlled trials. *Arch Intern Med* 1994; **154**: 1449–57.

42 Stroke Prevention in Atrial Fibrillation Investigators. Adjusted dose warfarin versus low-intensity, fixed dose warfarin plus aspirin for high-risk patients with atrial fibrillation: Stroke prevention in atrial fibrillation III randomised clinical trial. *Lancet* 1996; **348**: 633–8.

43 Takahashi N, Seki A, Imataka K, Fujii J. Clinical features of paroxysmal atrial fibrillation: an observation of 94 patients. *Jpn Heart J* 1981; **22**: 143–9.

44 Kannel WB, Abbott RD, Savage DD, McNamara PM. Coronary heart disease and atrial fibrillation: the Framingham study. *Am Heart J* 1983; **106**: 389–96.

45 Petersen P, Godtfredsen J. Embolic complications in paroxysmal atrial fibrillation. *Stroke* 1986; **17**: 622–6.

46 Weiner I, Hafner R, Nicolai M, Lyons H. Clinical and echocardiographic correlates of systemic embolization in non-rheumatic atrial fibrillation. *Am J Cardiol* 1987; **59**: 177.

47 Shimomura K, Ohe T, Uehara S, Matsuhisa M, Kamakura S, Sato I. Significance of atrial fibrillation as a precursor of embolism. *Am J Cardiol* 1989; **63**: 1405–7.

48 Roy D, Marchand E, Gagne P, Chabot M, Carter R. Usefulness of anticoagulant therapy in the prevention of embolic complications of atrial fibrillation. *Am Heart J* 1986; **112**: 1039–43.

49 Cabin HS, Clubb KS, Hall C, Perlmutter RA, Feinstein AR. Risk for systemic embolization of atrial fibrillation without mitral stenosis. *Am J Cardiol* 1990; **65**: 1112–16.

50 Moulton AW, Singer DE, Haas JS. Risk factors for stroke in patients with non-rheumatic atrial fibrillation: a case control study. *Am J Med* 1991; **91**: 156–61.

51 Lown B, Perlroth MG, Kaidbey S, Abe T, Harken DE. "Cardioversion" of atrial fibrillation: a report on the treatment of 65 episodes in 50 patients. *N Engl J Med* 1963; **269**: 325–31.

52 Peters KG, Kienzle MG. Severe cardiomyopathy due to chronic rapid atrial fibrillation: complete recovery after reversion to sinus rhythm. *Am J Med* 1988; **85**: 242–4.

53 Rodriguez LM, Smeets JLRM, Xie Bayan et al. Improvement in left ventricular function by ablation of AV nodal conduction in selected patients with lone atrial fibrillation. *Am J Cardiol* 1993; **72**: 1137–41.

54 Van Gelder IC, Crijns HJ, Blanksma PK et al. Time course of hemodynamic changes and improvement of exercise tolerance after cardioversion of chronic atrial fibrillation associated with cardiac valve disease. *Am J Cardiol* 1993; **72**: 560–6.

55 Resnekov L, McDonald L. Complications in 220 patients with cardiac dysrhythmias treated by phased direct current shock and indication for electric conversion. *Br Heart J* 1967; **29**: 926–36.

56 Bjerkelund CJ, Orning OM. The efficacy of anticoagulant therapy in preventing embolism related to DC electrical conversion of atrial fibrillation. *Am J Cardiol* 1969; **23**: 208–16.

57 Weinberg DM, Mancini GBJ. Anticoagulation for cardioversion of atrial fibrillation. *Am J Cardiol* 1989; **63**: 745–6.

58 Arnold AZ, Mich MJ, Mazurek RP, Loop FD, Trohman RG. Role of prophylactic anticoagulation for direct current cardioversion in patients with atrial fibrillation or atrial flutter. *J Am Coll Cardiol* 1992; **19**: 851–5.

59 Aschenberg W, Schluter M, Kremer P, Schroder E, Siglow V, Bleifeld W. Transoesophageal two dimensional echocardiography for the detection of left atrial appendage thrombus. *J Am Coll Cardiol* 1986; 7: 163–6.

60 Manning WJ, Weintraub RM, Waksmonski CA *et al.* Accuracy of transoesophageal echocardiography for identifying left atrial thrombi. A prospective, intraoperative study. *Ann Intern Med* 1995; **123**: 817–22.

61 Manning WJ, Leeman DE, Gotch PJ, Come PC. Pulsed Doppler evaluation of atrial mechanical function after electrical cardioversion of atrial fibrillation. *J Am Coll Cardiol* 1989; **13**: 617–23.

62 Mugge A, Kuhn H, Nikutta P, Grote J, Lopez AG, Daniel WG. Assessment of left atrial appendage function by biplane transesophageal echocardiography in patients with nonrheumatic atrial fibrillation: identification of a subgroup of patients at increased embolic risk. *J Am Coll Cardiol* 1994; **23**: 599–607.

63 Collins LJ, Silverman DI, Douglas PS, Manning WJ. Cardioversion of non-rheumatic atrial fibrillation. Reduced thromboembolic complications with 4 weeks of precardioversion anticoagulation are related to atrial thrombus resolution. *Circulation* 1995; **92**: 156–9.

64 Manning WJ, Silverman DI, Gordon SPF, Krunholtz HM, Douglas PS. Cardioversion from atrial fibrillation without prolonged anticoagulation with use of transesophageal echocardiography to exclude the presence of atrial thrombi. *N Engl J Med* 1993; **328**: 750–5.

65 Stoddard MF, Dawkins PR, Prince CR, Longlaker RA. Transesophageal echocardiographic guidance of cardioversion in patients with atrial fibrillation. *Am Heart J* 1995; **129**: 1204–15.

66 Black IW, Hopkins AP, Lee LCL, Walsh WF. Evaluation of transesophageal echocardiography before cardioversion of atrial fibrillation and flutter in non anticoagulated patients. *Am Heart J* 1993; **126**: 375–81.

67 Grimm RA, Leung DY, Black IW, Stewart WJ, Thomas JD, Klein AL. Left atrial appendage "stunning" after spontaneous conversion of atrial fibrillation demonstrated by transesophageal Doppler echocardiography. *Am Heart J* 1995; **130**: 174–6.

68 Grimm RA, Stewart WJ, Maloney JD *et al.* Impact of electrical cardioversion for atrial fibrillation on left atrial appendage function and spontaneous echo contrast: characterization by simultaneous transesophageal echocardiography. *J Am Coll Cardiol* 1993; **22**: 1359–66.

69 Manning WJ, Silverman DI, Katz SE *et al.* Impaired left atrial mechanical function after cardioversion: relation to duration of atrial fibrillation. *J Am Coll Cardiol* 1994; **23**: 1535–40.

70 Black IW, Fatkin D, Sagar KB *et al.* Exclusion of atrial thrombus by transesophageal echocardiography does not preclude embolism after cardioversion of atrial fibrillation. A multicenter study. *Circulation* 1994; **89**: 2509–13.

71 Iliceto S, Antonelli G, Sorino M, Biasco G, Rizzon P. Dynamic intracavitary left atrial echoes in mitral stenosis. *Am J Cardiol* 1985; **55**(5): 603–6.

72 Fatkin D, Kuchar DL, Thorburn CW, Fenely MP. Transesophageal echocardiography before and during direct current cardioversion of atrial fibrillation: evidence for "atrial stunning" as a mechanism of thromboembolic complications. *J Am Coll Cardiol* 1994; **23**: 307–16.

73 Yurchak PM for the Task Force Members. AHA/ACC/ACP Task Force Statement Special Report on Clinical Competence in Elective Direct Current (DC) Cardioversion. A statement from the AHA/ACC/ACP Task Force on clinical privileges in cardiology. *Circulation* 1993; **88**: 342–45.

74 Stoddard MF. Risk of thromboembolism in new onset or transient atrial fibrillation. *Progress in Cardiovascular Diseases* 1996; **39**: 69–80.

75 Stoddard MF, Dawkins PR, Prince CR, Ammash NM. Left atrial appendage thrombus is not uncommon in patients with acute atrial fibrillation and a recent embolic event: a transesophageal echocardiographic study. *J Am Coll Cardiol* 1995; **25**: 452–9.

76 Gold RL, Haffajee CI, Charos G, Sloan K, Baker S, Alpert JS. Amiodarone for refractory atrial fibrillation. *Am J Cardiol* 1986; **57**: 124–7.

77 Crijns HJGM, van Wijk LM, van Gilst WH, Kingma JH, van Gelder IC, Lie KI. Acute conversion of atrial fibrillation to sinus rhythm: clinical efficacy of flecainide acetate. Comparison of two regimens. *Eur Heart J* 1988; **9**: 634–8.

78 Van Gelder IC, Crijns HJGM, van Gilst WH, Verwer R, Lie KI. Prediction of uneventful cardioversion and maintenance of sinus rhythm from direct current electrical cardioversion of atrial fibrillation and flutter. *Am J Cardiol* 1991; **68**: 41–6.

79 Kingma JH, Suttorp MJ. Acute pharmacologic conversion of atrial fibrillation and flutter. The role of flecainide, propafenone and verapamil. *Am J Cardiol* 1992; **70**: 56A–61A.

80 Wijffels MCEF, Kirchhof JHJ, Dorland R, Allessie MA. Atrial fibrillation begets atrial fibrillation. *Circulation* 1995; **92**: 1954–68.

81 Grimm RA, Stewart WJ, Black IW, Thomas JD, Klein AL. Should all patients undergo transesophageal echocardiography before electrical cardioversion of atrial fibrillation. *J Am Coll Cardiol* 1994; **23**: 533–41.

82 Schnittger I. Value of transoesophageal echocardiography before DC cardioversion in patients with atrial fibrillation: assessment of embolic risk. *Br Heart J* 1995; **73**: 306–9.

83 Orsinelli DA, Pearson AC. Usefulness of transesophageal echocardiography to screen for left atrial appendage thrombus before elective cardioversion for atrial fibrillation. *Am J Cardiol* 1993; **72**: 1337–9.

84 Manning WJ, Silverman DI, Keighley CS, Oettgen P, Douglas PS. Transesophageal echocardiographically facilitated early cardioversion from atrial fibrillation using short-term anticoagulation: final results of a prospective 4.5 year study. *J Am Coll Cardiol* 1995; **25**: 1354–61.

85 Klein AL, Grimm RA, Black IW *et al.* Assessment of cardioversion using transesophageal echocardiography compared to conventional therapy: the ACUTE randomized pilot study (Abstract). *Circulation* 1994; **90** (Suppl 1): 1–21.

86 Klein AL, Grimm RA, Black IW *et al.* Cost effectiveness of TEE guided cardioversion with anticoagulation compared to conventional therapy in patients with atrial fibrillation. (Abstract). *J Am Coll Cardiol* 1994; **23**: 128A.

87 Manning WJ, Silverman DI. Atrial anatomy and function postcardioversion: insights from transthoracic and transesophageal echocardiography. *Progress in Cardiovascular Diseases* 1996; **39**: 33–46.

88 Bikkina M, Alpert MA, Mulekar M, Shakoor A, Massey CV, Covin FA. Prevalence of intra-atrial thrombus in patients with atrial flutter. *Am J Cardiol* 1995; **76**: 186–9.

89 Jordaens L, Missault L, Germonpre E *et al.* Delayed restoration of atrial function after conversion of atrial flutter by pacing or electrical cardioversion. *Am J Cardiol* 1993; **71**: 63–7.

90 Yusuf S, Wittes J, Friedman L. Overview of results of randomized clinical trials in heart disease. I. Treatments following myocardial infarction. *JAMA* 1988; **260**: 2088–93.

91 The ASPECT Research Group. Effect of long-term oral anticoagulant treatment on mortality and cardiovascular morbidity after myocardial infarction. *Lancet* 1994; **343**: 499–503.

92 Van Bergen PFMM, Deckers JW, Jonker JJC, van Domburg RT, Azar AJ, Hofman A. Efficacy of long-term anticoagulant treatment in subgroup of patients after myocardial infarction. *Br Heart J* 1995; **73**: 117–21.

93 Stein B, Fuster V, Halperin JL, Chesebro JH. Antithrombotic therapy in cardiac disease: an emerging approach based on pathogenesis and risk. *Circulation* 1989; **80**: 1501–13.

94 Turpie AGG. Anticoagulant therapy after acute myocardial infarction. *Am J Cardiol* 1990; **65**: 20C–23C.

95 Dunkman WB, Johnson GR, Cohn JN. Incidence of thromboembolic events in congestive heart failure: the V-HeFT study (Abstract). *Circulation* 1988; **78**: II–617.

96 Diaz RA, Obasohan A, Oakley CM. Prediction of outcome in dilated cardiomyopathy. *Br*

Heart J 1987; **58**: 393–9.

97 Schmidt R, Fazekas F, Offenbacher H, Dusleag J, Lechner H. Brain magnetic resonance imaging and neuropsychologic evaluation of patients with idiopathic dilated cardiomyopathy. *Stroke* 1991; **22**: 195–99.

98 Edmunds LH Jr, Clark RE, Cohn LH, Miller DC, Weisel RD. Guidelines for reporting morbidity and mortality after cardiac valvular operations. *J Thorac Cardiovasc Surg* 1988; **96**: 351–3.

99 Nashef SAM, Stewart M, Bain WH. Heart valve replacement: thromboembolism or thrombosis and embolism? in Bodar E. (ed.). *Surgery for heart valve disease*. London: ICR Publishers, 1990.

100 Reitz BA, Stinson EB, Griepp RB, Shumway NE. Tissue valve replacement of prosthetic heart valves for thromboembolism. *Am J Cardiol* 1978; **41**: 512–15.

101 Acar J, Enriquez-Sarano M, Farah E, Kassab R, Tubiana P, Roger V. Recurrent systemic embolic events with valve prosthesis. *Eur Heart J* 1984; **5**: (Suppl D); 33–8.

102 Acar J, Vahanian A, Dorent R *et al*. Detection of prosthetic valve thrombosis using indium platelet imaging. *Eur Heart J* 1990; **11**: 389–98.

103 Turpie AGG, Gunstensen J, Hirsch J, Nelson H, Gent M. Randomised comparison of two intensities of oral anticoagulation therapy after tissue heart valve replacement. *Lancet* 1988; **i**: 1242–5.

104 Grunkemeier GL, Rahimtoola SH. Artificial heart valves. *Ann Rev Med* 1990; **41**: 251–63.

105 Saour JN, Sieck JO, Mamo LAR, Gallus AS. Trial of different intensities of anticoagulation in patients with prosthetic heart valves. *N Engl J Med* 1990; **322**: 428–32.

106 Butchart EG, Lewis PA, Bethal JA, Breckenridge IM. Adjusting anticoagulation to prosthesis thrombogenicity and patient risk factors. Recommendations for the Medtronic Hall valve. *Circulation* 1991; **84**: III-61–III-69.

107 Stein PD, Grandison D, Tsushung AH *et al*. Therapeutic level of oral anticoagulation with warfarin in patients with mechanical prosthetic heart valves: review of literature and recommendations based on international normalised ratio. *Postgrad Med J* 1994; **70** (Suppl 1): S72–S83.

108 Cannegieter SC, Rosendaal FR, Briet E. Thromboembolic and bleeding complications in patients with mechanical heart valve prostheses. *Circulation* 1994; **89**: 635–41.

109 British Society for Haematology, British Committee for Standards in Haematology, Haemostasis and Thrombosis Task Force. Guidelines on oral anticoagulation: second edition. *J Clin Pathol* 1990; **43**: 177–83.

110 Hirsh J, Fuster V. AHA Medical/Scientific Statement. Special Report. Guide to Anticoagulant Therapy Part 2: Oral Anticoagulants. *Circulation* 1994; **89**: 1469–80.

111 Butchart EG, Lewis PA, Kulatilake ENP, Breckenridge IM. Anticoagulation variability between centres: implications for comparative prosthetic valve assessment. *Eur J Cardiothorac Surg* 1988; **2**: 72–81.

112 Altman R, Rouvier J, Garfinkel E *et al*. Comparison of two levels of anticoagulant therapy in patients with substitute heart valves. *J Thorac Cardiovasc Surg* 1991; **101**: 427–31.

113 Heras M, Chesebro JH, Fuster V *et al*. High risk of thromboemboli early after bioprosthetic cardiac valve replacement. *J Am Coll Cardiol* 1995; **25**: 1111–19.

114 Turpie AGG, Gent M, Laupacis A *et al*. A comparison of aspirin with placebo in patients treated with warfarin after heart-valve replacement. *N Engl J Med* 1993; **329**: 524–9.

115 Salazar E, Zajarias A, Guttierrez N, Iturbe I. The problem of cardiac valve prostheses: anticoagulants and pregnancy. *Circulation* 1984(Suppl. I): I-169–I-177.

116 Sbarouni E, Oakley CM. Outcome of pregnancy in women with valve prostheses. *Br Heart J* 1994; **71**: 196–201.

117 Ross DN. Observations on homograft aortic valves. *Guy's Hospital Reports* 1969; **118**: 5–11.

118 Matsuki O, Okita Y, Almeida MD *et al*. Two decades experience with aortic valve replacement with pulmonary autograft. *J Thorac Cardiovasc Surg* 1988; **95**: 705–11.

119 Elkins RC, Santangelo KL, Stelzer P, Randolph JD, Knott-Craig CJ. Pulmonary autograft replacement of the aortic valve: an evolution of technique. *J Cardiac Surg* 1992; **7**: 108–16.

120 Elkins RC, Knott-Craig CJ, Ward KE, McCue C, Lane MM. Pulmonary autograft in children: realized growth potential. *Ann Thorac Surg* 1994; **57**: 1387–93 (discussion 1393–4).

121 Westaby S. Pulmonary autograft replacement of the aortic valve (Editorial). *Br Heart J* 1995; **74**: 1–3.

122 Limet R, Grondin CM. Cardiac valve prostheses, anticoagulation and pregnancy. *Ann Thorac Surg* 1977; **23**: 337–41.

123 Bolan JC. Thromboembolic complications of pregnancy. *Clin Obstet Gynaecol* 1983; **26**: 913–22.

124 Renzulli A, De Luca L, Caruso A, Verde R, Galzerano D, Cotrufo M. Acute thrombosis of prosthetic valves: a multivariate analysis of the risk factors for a life threatening event. *Eur J Cardiothorac Surg* 1992; **6**: 412–21.

125 Todd ME, Thompson JH Jr, Bowie EJW, Owen CA. Changes in blood coagulation during pregnancy. *Mayo Clin Proc* 1965; **40**: 370–83.

126 Shaper AI. The hypercoagulable states. *Ann Intern Med* 1985; **102**: 814–28.

127 Oakley CM. Pregnancy and prosthetic valves. *Lancet* 1994; **344**: 1643–4.

128 Ginsberg JS, Barron WM. Pregnancy and prosthetic valves (Commentary). *Lancet* 1994; **344**: 1170–1.

129 Oakley CM. Anticoagulants in pregnancy (Review). *Br J Heart J* 1995; **74**: 107–11.

130 Oakley CM. Clinical perspective. Anticoagulation and pregnancy. *Eur Heart J* 1995; **16**: 1317–19.

131 Barbour LA, Pickard JP. Controversies in thromboembolic disease during pregnancy: a critical review. *Obstet Gynecol* 1995; **86**: 621–33.

132 Holzgreve W, Carey JF, Hall BD. Warfarin induced foetal abnormalities. *Lancet* 1976; **ii**: 914–15.

133 Chen WWC, Chan CS, Lee PK, Wang RYC, Wong VCW. Pregnancy in patients with prosthetic heart valves: an experience with 45 pregnancies. *Q J Med* 1982; **51**: 358–65.

134 Ben Ismail M, Abid F, Trabelsi S, Taktak M, Fekih M. Cardiac valve prostheses, anticoagulation, and pregnancy. *Br Heart J* 1986; **55**: 101–5.

135 Pavankumar P, Venugopal P, Kaul U et al. Pregnancy in patients with prosthetic cardiac valve. A 10 year experience. *Scand J Thorac Cardiovasc Surg* 1988; **22**: 19–22.

136 Iturbe-Alessio I, del Carmen Fonseca M, Mutchinik O, Santos MA, Zajarias A, Salazar E. Risks of anticoagulant therapy in pregnant women with artificial valves. *N Engl J Med* 1986; **315**: 1390–3.

137 Wong V, Cheng CH, Chan KC. Fetal and neonatal outcome of exposure to anticoagulants during pregnancy. *Am J Med Genet* 1993; **45**: 17–21.

138 Cotrufo M, de Luca TSL, Calabro R, Mastrogiovanni G, Lama D. Coumarin anticoagulation during pregnancy in patients with mechanical valve prostheses. *Eur J Cardiothorac Surg* 1991; **5**: 300–5.

139 Brill-Edwards P, Ginsberg JS, Johnston M, Hirsh J. Establishing a therapeutic range for heparin therapy. *Ann Intern Med* 1993; **119**: 104–9.

140 Ad Hoc Committee of the Working Group on Valvular Heart Disease. Guidelines for prevention of thromboembolic events in valvular heart disease. Official document of the European Society of Cardiology. *J Heart Valve Dis* 1993; **2**: 398–410.

141 Ginsberg JS, Hirsh J. Use of anticoagulants during pregnancy. *Chest* 1989; **95**: 156s–160s.

142 Dahlman TC. Osteoporotic fractures and the recurrence of thromboembolism during pregnancy and the puerperium in 184 women undergoing thromboprophylaxis with heparin. *Am J Obstet Gynecol* 1993; **168**: 1265–70.

143 Barbour LA, Kick SD, Steiner JF et al. A prospective study of heparin-induced osteoporosis in pregnancy using bone densitometry. *Am J Obstet Gynecol* 1994; **170**: 862–9.

144 Ginsberg JS, Kowalchuk G, Hirsh J et al. Heparin effect on bone density. *Thromb Haemostas* 1990; **64**: 286–9.

145 Sareli P, England MJ, Berk MR et al. Maternal and fetal sequelae of anticoagulation during pregnancy in patients with mechanical heart valve prostheses. *Am J Cardiol* 1989; **63**: 1462–5.

146 Feijgin MD, Lourwood DL. Low molecular weight heparins and their use in obstetrics

and gynecology. *Obstet Gynecol Survey* 1994; **49**: 424–31.

147 Gillis S, Shusan A, Eldor A. The use of low molecular weight heparin for prophylaxis and treatment of thromboembolism in pregnancy. *Int J Gynaecol Obstet* 1992; **39**: 297–301.

148 Sturridge F, de Swiet M, Letsky E. The use of low molecular weight heparin for thromboprophylaxis in pregnancy. *Br J Obstet Gynaecol* 1994; **101**: 69–71.

5: Treatment of hyperlipidaemia in the absence and presence of symptomatic coronary heart disease

GR THOMPSON

Before considering the treatment of hyperlipidaemia, it is appropriate first to review the evidence that lipids are indices of cardiovascular risk in subjects with as well as in those without coronary heart disease. Much of the evidence is epidemiological but this is buttressed by an increasing mass of experimental and pathological data which point to the causal role of abnormal blood lipids in promoting atherosclerosis, the process responsible for the great majority of coronary heart disease. An excellent review of this topic, especially the crucial influence of plaque cholesterol content on lesion instability and consequent clinical events, has recently been published.[1]

Cholesterol as a risk factor

Probably the most impressive epidemiological evidence for the relationship between serum cholesterol and coronary heart disease comes from the follow-up of 360,000 men aged 35–57 who were screened for possible inclusion in the Multiple Risk Factor Intervention Trial (MRFIT); the data emphasise the association between hypercholesterolaemia and premature coronary heart disease.[2] Using the age of 65 as the criterion, about 25% of coronary heart disease deaths in men are premature against less than 10% in women. Measurement of serum total cholesterol is less useful in predicting the risk of coronary heart disease in older persons, however, especially if female.[3]

The association between serum cholesterol and coronary heart disease is even stronger for those with pre-existing coronary heart disease than for asymptomatic individuals, as was shown in British civil servants by Rose *et al.*[4] Similar findings were reported by Pekkanen *et al.*[5] in 2500 men followed up for 10 years, as illustrated in Figure 5.1. It is apparent that the risk of death from coronary heart disease increases with serum cholesterol in men both without and with coronary heart disease but to a greater extent in the latter group.

Much of the association between coronary heart disease risk and total cholesterol is a reflection of the major contribution made to the latter by low density lipoprotein. This particle is known to be atherogenic, in contrast with high density lipoprotein, which seems to protect against coronary heart disease. The strong positive and negative correlations between coronary heart disease death and low and high density lipoprotein cholesterol respectively in men with pre-existing coronary heart disease are shown in Figure 5.2. Those with low density lipoprotein cholesterol >4·1 mmol/L or high density lipoprotein cholesterol <0·9 mmol/L were at greatest risk.

Total : high density lipoprotein cholesterol ratio

The opposing influences of total (or low density lipoprotein) cholesterol and high density lipoprotein cholesterol can be conveniently expressed as a ratio, as was done with men and women aged 50–90 in the Framingham Study.[6] The age adjusted incidence of coronary heart disease events

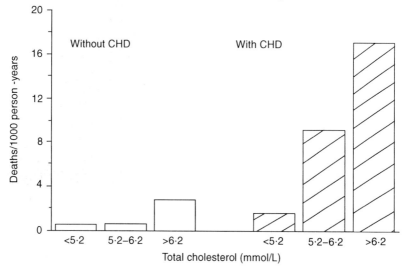

Fig 5.1 Age adjusted rates of death from coronary heart disease in 2541 men aged 40–69 without or with coronary heart disease during 10 years of follow-up (redrawn with permission from Pekkanen *et al.*, *N Engl J Med* 1990; **322**: 1700–7).

increased with increasing total:high density lipoprotein cholesterol ratios in both sexes but was higher in men than women at ratios between 3·5 and 7·4 (Figure 5.3). However, at ratios of 7·5 or greater, the risk of coronary heart disease was equally high in both sexes. Another and more recent prospective study, among male physicians, also showed a graded increase in risk of coronary heart disease according to the total:high density lipoprotein cholesterol ratio.[7] In this study, after adjusting for other variables, each unit increase in the ratio was associated with an increase in relative risk of 53%.

Triglyceride as a risk factor

A strong positive correlation exists between coronary heart disease and triglycerides, especially in case control studies. In some studies hyper-triglyceridaemia has been shown to be the commonest lipid abnormality in patients with coronary heart disease, even on multivariate analysis.[8] However, in other studies, the association is weakened or lost when other risk factors are taken into account, most notably high density lipoprotein

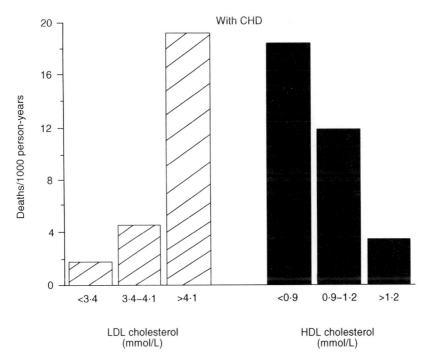

Fig 5.2 Age adjusted rates of death from coronary heart disease in 2541 men aged 40–69 with coronary heart disease in relation to low density lipoprotein and high density lipoprotein cholesterol during 10 years of follow-up (redrawn with permission from Pekkanen et al., N Engl J Med 1990; **322**: 1700–7).

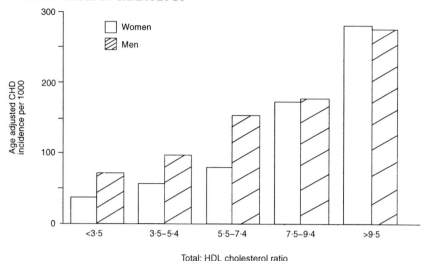

Fig 5.3 Risk of development of coronary heart disease according to total cholesterol to high density lipoprotein cholesterol ratio among men and women between the ages of 50 and 90 in Framingham (redrawn with permission from Kannel and Wilson, *Am Heart J* 1992; **124**: 768–74).

cholesterol concentration, with which triglyceride levels are inversely correlated. The strengths and weaknesses of triglycerides as a risk factor were recently considered by a panel of experts.[9] While accepting that the remnant particles of triglyceride rich lipoproteins are potentially athero-genic the panel found little evidence that reducing triglyceride levels by therapeutic means results in angiographic improvement. However, that was before the publication of the Bezafibrate Coronary Atherosclerosis Inter-vention Trial (BECAIT) which showed significant angiographic and clinical benefit in patients treated with bezafibrate for five years; this reduced triglycerides by more than 30% but had no effect on LDL cholesterol.[10] Since the drug also increased HDL cholesterol and decreased fibrinogen, it is not possible to establish with certainty that its benefits were due to its triglyceride lowering effect. However, the lack of any change in LDL is significant.

Although the significance of triglyceride measurement in isolation is debatable there is evidence that it may be discriminatory when used in conjunction with other risk factors. In the Helsinki Heart Study risk was highest in a subgroup on placebo with fasting triglycerides >2·3 mmol/L and low density lipoprotein/high density lipoprotein cholesterol ratio >5.[11] Similarly, in the Prospective Cardiovascular Münster (PROCAM) Study, the incidence of coronary artery disease in those with an identical pattern of dyslipidaemia was increased twofold.[12]

Lipoprotein(a) and coronary heart disease risk

Lipoprotein(a), usually abbreviated to Lp(a), is a low density lipoprotein-like particle with an additional protein moiety termed apo(a). Although the association between Lp(a) and coronary heart disease was first described over 20 years ago,[13] the recent discovery of close homology between apo(a) and plasminogen has markedly increased awareness of its role as a risk factor. Both prospective[14] and case control[15-19] studies have shown that a raised level of Lp(a) is correlated with coronary heart disease independently of other risk factors. A similar relationship has been demonstrated between Lp(a) and angiographically proved coronary artery disease.[20-24] Raised levels of Lp(a) may also predict the likelihood of graft stenoses after coronary artery bypass surgery[25], restenosis after angioplasty[26] and development of accelerated coronary artery disease after cardiac transplantation.[27]

Plasma levels of Lp(a) vary between individuals from undetectable to >200 mg/dL. Lp(a) is polymorphic, differences in molecular weight between the various isoforms being determined by the number of Kringle 4 repeats in apo(a). Plasma levels of Lp(a) are inversely correlated with the molecular weight of the different isoforms and in Caucasians, over 90% of interindividual variation is genetically determined.[28] The risks associated with raised levels of Lp(a) are influenced by the prevailing level of low density lipoprotein cholesterol, patients with Lp(a) levels >30 mg/dL whose low density lipoprotein cholesterol level is >4·4 mmol/L having a three- to fourfold higher odds ratio for coronary heart disease than those whose low density lipoprotein cholesterol is <4·4 mmol/L.[21]

The precise mechanism whereby elevated levels of Lp(a) increase risk of coronary heart disease remains uncertain, but *in vitro* evidence suggests that Lp(a) has both thrombogenic and antifibrinolytic potential. However, *in vivo* evidence of this is sparse, nor does Lp(a) appear to impair the action of thrombolytic agents.[29] The evidence that Lp(a) is atherogenic is stronger, in that it is demonstrable both in atheromatous plaques[30] and in coronary artery bypass grafts.[31]

Measurement of serum lipids

In the light of the evidence reviewed above, it should be apparent that measurement of serum lipids plays an important role in defining risk of development or worsening of coronary heart disease. A random assay of total cholesterol is a useful method of screening in general practice. However, when investigating individuals with coronary heart disease or a family history of coronary heart disease or hyperlipidaemia, it is preferable to take blood after an overnight fast and obtain values of total and high density lipoprotein cholesterol, together with triglyceride. To calculate low density lipoprotein cholesterol, the high density lipoprotein cholesterol and triglycerides (the latter divided by 2·2) are subtracted from total cholesterol (as long as triglycerides are less than 4·5 mmol/L). The ratio of total or low density lipoprotein cholesterol to high density lipoprotein cholesterol can then be calculated.

The importance of low density lipoprotein cholesterol levels as a determinant of therapeutic action was stressed by the National Cholesterol Education Program.[32] Similarly, measurement of high density lipoprotein cholesterol and triglycerides is increasingly regarded as essential when assessing overall risk in certain situations, specifically in individuals with coronary heart disease, familial dyslipidaemias (a term which encompasses low high density lipoprotein cholesterol as well as hyperlipidaemia) or with other risk factors such as diabetes and hypertension.[9]

The desirability of quantifying overall risk using a calculator pro-grammed with equations derived from the Framingham or PROCAM studies is discussed elsewhere.[33] Although extrapolating from population based data to individuals can be hazardous, nevertheless it is useful for both physician and patient alike to be able to quantify changes in both absolute and relative risk during the course of therapeutic measures aimed at preventing coronary heart disease.

Although the practical usefulness of measuring newer risk factors such as Lp(a) and fibrinogen remains to be established, it has been suggested that Lp(a) should be assayed in all hyperlipidaemic patients in whom drug therapy is contemplated and in those with coronary heart disease or a family history of premature coronary heart disease.[34] The detection of a raised level of Lp(a), >30–40 mg/dL, is an indication to treat vigorously other concomitant risk factors such as a raised low density lipoprotein cholesterol or lowered high density lipoprotein cholesterol. However, evidence that reduction of Lp(a) per se is beneficial is currently lacking.

Evidence that treatment is effective

The main aim of lipid lowering therapy is to reduce cardiovascular events, principally myocardial infarction, but slowing the development of symptomatic disease and reducing the requirement for revascularisation procedures are also important. A reduction in cardiac deaths and overall mortality might therefore follow. The predicted event rate (for example, cardiovascular death or non-fatal myocardial infarction) is higher for any given cholesterol level in patients with known coronary disease than in those who are asymptomatic, but clearly there is a need to know if cholesterol lowering therapies are effective and safe in both groups of patients.

Meta-analyses of primary and secondary prevention trials in the pre-statin era

Holme's meta-analysis of clinical endpoint trials of lipid lowering therapy showed a significant reduction in mortality and morbidity from coronary heart disease for both primary and secondary prevention, each 1% reduction in total cholesterol being associated with a 2·5% reduction in risk.[35] However, total mortality remained unchanged, possibly due to an increased incidence of violent or accidental deaths in treated subjects in some of the trials.[36] Alternatively, the lack of effect on total mortality may reflect the fact that none of the trials was designed to be large enough to answer this question.[37] Whether cholesterol lowering per se or the diets or drugs used to achieve this objective could have adverse effects on the psychological state of individual patients has been a subject of much speculation.[38] To date no convincing causal mechanism has been proposed nor has any dose–response relationship been documented, unlike that between cholesterol lowering and the decrease in coronary heart disease events.[36]

When separate meta-analyses of primary and secondary prevention trials are performed they show that the relative reduction in coronary heart disease events is similar but that the absolute reduction is much greater in secondary prevention trials.[39, 40] The largest meta-analysis to date is that of Law and colleagues[41] who, like Holme,[35] showed a 25% decrease in coronary heart disease mortality for every 10% reduction in serum cholesterol. The magnitude of the relative reduction in coronary heart disease was also influenced by the age of the subjects (inversely) and the duration of the reduction in serum cholesterol. These authors discounted any hazards associated with a low serum cholesterol or cholesterol lowering per se other than an increase in the risk of cerebral haemorrhage, which was confined largely to hypertensive subjects with serum cholesterol < 5 mmol/L.[42]

Lipid lowering regression trials

Between 1984 and 1994 there were a dozen randomized angiographic trials in which the effects of various forms of lipid lowering therapy on coronary artery disease were examined.[43-56] Table 5.1 lists the chief characteristics of these studies which ranged from less than 50 to over 800 subjects and lasted from one to 10 years. Most of them involved a randomised comparison of diet alone and diet combined with treatment with lipid lowering drugs. Other forms of treatment used included partial ileal bypass, exercise, and antistress measures. In the earlier trials the anion exchange resins cholestyramine and colestipol were given either alone or combined with nicotinic acid or lovastatin or both. More recent trials used monotherapy with hydroxy-methylglutaryl coenzyme A reductase inhibitors, either lovastatin or simvastatin.

The average age at entry ranged from 41 to 60, with most patients being in their 50s. Five trials were restricted to men and in the remainder, the percentage of women was usually less than 20%. Previous coronary artery bypass grafting and angioplasty were permitted in several trials; indeed,

Table 5.1 Randomised and controlled lipid lowering regression trials (from[57])

Trial (Ref)	n	Years	Treatment
NHLBI (43,44)	116	5	Cholestyramine (24 g)
CLAS I (45)	162	2	Colestipol (30 g) +
II (46)	(103)	(4)	Nicotinic acid (4 g)
POSCH (47)	838	9·7	Partial ileal bypass
FATS (48)	120	2·5	(a) Colestipol (30 g) + lovastatin (40 mg)
			(b) Colestipol (30 g) + nicotinic acid (4 g)
UCSF SCOR (49)	72	2·2	Colestipol (15–30 g) + nicotinic acid (1·5–7·5 g)
			±lovastatin (40–60 mg)
Life-Style (50)	48	1	Diet, exercise and antistress
STARS (51)	90	3·25	(a) Diet
			(b) Diet + cholestyramine (16 g)
Heidelberg (52)	113	1	Diet and exercise
MARS (53)	270	2	Diet + lovastatin (80 mg)
CCAIT (54)	331	2	Diet + lovastatin (37 mg (mean))
SCRIP (55)	300	4	Diet, exercise, and lipid lowering drugs
MAAS (56)	381	4	Diet + simvastatin (20 mg)

prior coronary artery bypass grafting was an inclusion criterion for the Cholesterol Lowering Atherosclerosis Study (CLAS). In the Multicentre Anti-Atheroma Study (MAAS) previous angioplasty was permitted but treated segments were excluded from angiographic analysis. Baseline serum concentrations of total and low density lipoprotein cholesterol were highest in the trials which involved patients with familial hypercholesterolaemia, such as the University of California, San Francisco Intervention Trial (UCSF SCOR), and lowest in those trials that used a multifactorial approach. Calculation of the weighted mean values of serum lipids showed a 31% reduction in low density lipoprotein cholesterol during the trials in treated patients (to 3·02 mmol/L) compared with those on placebo (4·36 mmol/L). This was accompanied by a 33% decrease in the frequency of progression of lesions and a doubling of the frequency of regression in treated patients on angiography (Figure 5.4). In the seven trials which used quantitative coronary angiography, the minimal lumen diameter decreased by 0·09 mm and 0·02 mm and the percent diameter stenosis increased by 2·6% and 0·69% in the placebo and treated groups respectively.[57]

Despite the quantitatively minor angiographic changes, significant reductions in coronary heart disease events occurred in treated patients in three of these trials (Program on Surgical Control of Hyperlipidemia (POSCH), Familial Atherosclerosis Treatment Study (FATS), and the St Thomas' Atherosclerosis Regression Study (STARS)). A significant correlation between angiographic change and likelihood of subsequent coronary heart disease events was evident in the POSCH trial.[58] A possible explanation is that lipid lowering therapy stabilises lesions by promoting replacement of cholesterol by collagen in atheromatous plaques.[59] Further support for the occurrence of qualitatively beneficial changes in the

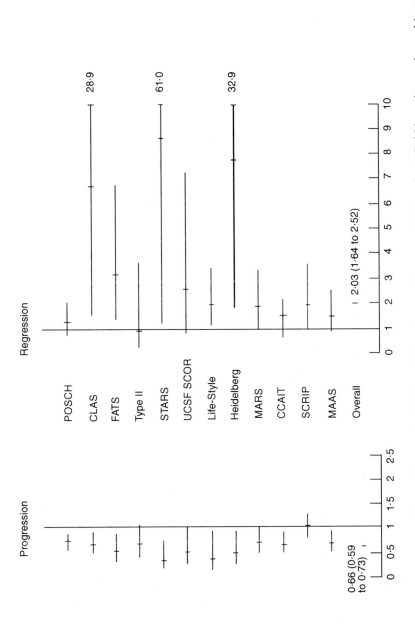

Fig 5.4 Relative risk of progression and regression (95% confidence interval) in treated subjects in 12 lipid lowering angiographic trials (reproduced with permission from Thompson, *Br Heart J* 1995; **74**: 343–7).

Table 5.2   Frequency of cardiovascular events in placebo (P) and treatment (T) groups of miscellaneous trials of statins

Trial (Ref)	Drug	Subjects	n	Duration	Events P	T	p
PLAC-I (60)	Pravastatin	CAD	408	3 months	18	7	0·014
REGRESS (61)	Pravastatin	CAD	885	2 years	93	59	0·002
ACAPS (62)	Lovastatin	Carot. IMT†	919	3 years	14	5	0·04
PLAC-II (63)	Pravastatin	CHD	151	3 years	13	5	<0·05
Multinational (64)	Pravastatin	High risk	1062	6 months	13	1	<0·001
			3425		151	77	

Carot.IMT = Carotid artery intimal-medial thickness

coronary arteries as a result of lipid lowering comes from a miscellaneous group of trials,[60–64] each of which involved the use of a statin and all of which showed a significant decrease in cardiovascular events (Table 5.2).

Recent evidence from prevention trials using a statin

The first primary prevention trial to use a statin, the West of Scotland Coronary Prevention Study (WOSCOPS), involved randomising 6595 asymptomatic men aged 45–64, with a serum total cholesterol >6·5 mmol/L and low density lipoprotein cholesterol 4·5–6 mmol/L, to pravastatin 40 mg daily or placebo for an average duration of 4·9 years.[65] Pravastatin decreased serum total and low density lipoprotein cholesterol by 20% and 26% respectively. This was accompanied by a highly significant 31% reduction in non-fatal myocardial infarction plus coronary heart disease deaths ($p < 0.001$) and a 37% reduction in the need for revascularisation procedures ($p < 0.01$). The 22% reduction in total mortality was not significant ($p = 0.051$) but there was no increase in non-cardiovascular deaths in pravastatin treated subjects. A subsequent subgroup analysis suggested that hypercholesterolaemic men who were smokers or had minor ECG abnormalities were at highest risk.[66]

The Scandinavian Simvastatin Survival Study (4S) provided the first unequivocal proof that effective treatment of hypercholesterolaemia reduces total mortality in patients with pre-existing coronary heart disease.[67] A total of 4444 patients aged 35–70 with angina or previous myocardial infarction, plus serum cholesterol of 5·5–8·09 mmol/L, were randomised to receive simvastatin (20–40 mg/day) or placebo. More than 80% of patients were men and a similar proportion had a previous myocardial infarction; less than 10%, however, had undergone myocardial revascularisation.

Simvastatin lowered total cholesterol by 25% from 6·8 mmol/L, low density lipoprotein cholesterol by 35% from 4·9 mmol/L and triglyceride by 10% from 1·5 mmol/L. High density lipoprotein cholesterol was increased by 8% from 1·2 mmol/L.

Median duration of treatment was 5·4 years, after which the trial was terminated on account of a 30% reduction in overall mortality (p = 0·0003). This was entirely the result of a 42% reduction in mortality from coronary heart disease (p = 0·00001); there were no changes in non-cardiovascular causes of death, including cancer and trauma.

In addition to its effects on mortality, simvastatin significantly reduced the occurrence of major coronary events (p = 0·00001) and the need for revascularisation procedures (p < 0·00001). The study investigators calculated that for coronary heart disease patients with total cholesterol 5·5–8·0 mmol/L, simvastatin 20–40 mg/day for six years would prevent four of every nine deaths, seven of 21 non-fatal myocardial infarctions and avert the need for six of 19 revascularisation procedures. In addition, simvastatin significantly reduced the number of cerebrovascular events without any increase in cerebral haemorrhage, even though 26% of the patients had hypertension.

The Cholesterol and Recurrent Events Trial (CARE), another secondary prevention study, involved men and women aged 24–75 with previous myocardial infarction and serum cholesterol < 6·2 mmol/L, who were randomly allocated to receive placebo or pravastatin 40 mg daily for five years.[68] Pravastatin lowered LDL cholesterol by 28%, which resulted in 24% fewer coronary deaths and non-fatal myocardial infarcts than occurred in the placebo group and a 27% decrease in the need for CABG and PTCA. Although total mortality was not significantly reduced, the findings suggested that pravastatin is effective in the secondary prevention of CHD even when cholesterol levels are 'normal', excepting those whose baseline LDL cholesterol was < 3·2 mmol/L.

These three trials provide striking evidence of the safety and effectiveness of low density lipoprotein reduction by pravastatin and simvastatin in the primary and secondary prevention of coronary heart disease over a wide range of cholesterol levels.

Current guidelines for strategies to treat dyslipidaemia

Various sets of guidelines have been proposed for the treatment of dyslipidaemia in the primary and secondary prevention of coronary heart disease. The first of these, which emanated from the National Cholesterol Education Program in 1988, stressed the importance of the low density lipoprotein cholesterol value in determining whether patients required dietary or drug therapy and have since been revised.[32] Low density lipoprotein cholesterol levels for initiating treatment and the target levels to be achieved are pitched lower in patients with coronary heart disease than in patients without coronary heart disease, as shown in Table 5.3.

Categorisation of patients according to their risk status is included in the current guidelines of the British Hyperlipidaemia Association.[69] As shown

107

Table 5.3 National Cholesterol Education Program cutpoints for LDL cholesterol[32]

Risk category	Initiation levels for		Minimum therapeutic goal (mmol/L)
	Diet therapy (mmol/L)	Drug therapy (mmol/L)	
Without CHD (and with <2 risk factors)	≥4·1	≥4·9	<4·1
Without CHD (and with >2 risk factors)	≥3·4	≥4·1	<3·4
With CHD	≥2·6	≥3·4	≤2·6

in Table 5.4, the highest priority in therapeutic terms is given to patients with overt coronary heart disease, including those who have undergone coronary artery bypass grafting, angioplasty, and cardiac transplantation. The second category includes patients with multiple risk factors or with genetically determined dyslipidaemia. The third and fourth categories of risk encompass respectively males and postmenopausal females with solitary hypercholesterolaemia, excluding those with hyper-αlipoproteinaemia (high density lipoprotein cholesterol >2 mmol/L) which is usually a benign condition not requiring treatment. The British Hyperlipidaemia Association guidelines proposed that the cut-off levels of total cholesterol for initiating drug therapy in diet resistant patients should be 5·2 mmol/L for category one, 6·5 mmol/L for category two, and 7·8 mmol/L for categories three and four.

The European Atherosclerosis Society has also published guidelines on the prevention of coronary heart disease.[70] Overall ('global') risk of coronary heart disease is defined as high, moderate or low according to the severity of the lipid abnormalities and the presence or absence of non-lipid risk factors. The latter include modifiable traits such as hypertension, cigarette smoking, diabetes, obesity, high fibrinogen, and low density lipoprotein cholesterol, which is defined as <0·8 mmol/L in men and <1 mmol/L in women. Other factors regarded as contributing to risk are the presence of coronary heart disease, a family history of coronary heart disease or peripheral vascular disease and being male or postmenopausal if female.

In the European Atherosclerosis Society guidelines lipid abnormalities are classified into hypercholesterolaemia, hypertriglyceridaemia or mixed

Table 5.4 British Hyperlipidaemia Association categories of risk of development or progression of coronary heart disease ([69])

First	Dyslipidaemic patients with existing coronary heart disease or postcoronary artery bypass graft, angioplasty or cardiac transplant
Second	Patients with multiple risk factors or genetically determined dyslipidaemia
Third	Males with asymptomatic hypercholesterolaemia
Fourth	Postmenopausal females with asymptomatic hypercholesterolaemia

Table 5.5   European Atherosclerosis Society management of hyperlipidaemia ([70])

Risk category	Target levels	
No other risk factors and/or HDL-C ⩾ 1·5	TC 5–6 LDL-C4–4·5	
Moderate overall	TC 5 LDL-C 3·5–4	TG < 2·3 HDL-C > 0·9 TC:HDL-C ⩽ 5
Two non-lipid risk factors or one plus low HDL-C	TC 4·5–5 LDL-C 3–3·5	

TC, TG, LDL-C, HDL-C represent total cholesterol, triglyceride, low density lipoprotein cholesterol and high density lipoprotein cholesterol in mmol/L.

hyperlipidaemia of varying degrees of severity. In general terms milder forms of hyperlipidaemia are treated with diet, weight reduction and exercise unless coronary heart disease is present. In the latter circumstance or if hyperlipidaemia is severe, drug therapy should be used as an adjunct to diet to achieve the recommended target levels, as shown in Table 5.5.

Although there are differences in emphasis between the National Cholesterol Education Program, British Hyperlipidaemia Association and European Atherosclerosis Society guidelines, all agree that dyslipidaemia should be treated more readily and vigorously in patients with coronary heart disease than in those who are at risk but who have not yet manifested it clinically. In addition, all the guidelines emphasise that recourse to lipid-lowering drugs should be reserved for those with coronary heart disease or at high overall risk of its development, taking into account the severity and duration of the lipid abnormalities and the presence of other risk factors. Finally, they all stress the need to achieve lower levels of low density lipoprotein cholesterol when attempting to arrest progression of pre-existing coronary heart disease than when primary prevention is the objective.

The most recent guidelines to be published are those issued jointly by the European Society of Cardiology, European Atherosclerosis Society and European Hypertension Society.[71] These base treatment decisions on the overall absolute risk of coronary heart disease but their recommended levels of serum cholesterol which merit drug treatment, i.e. ⩾7 or occasionally ⩾6 mmol/L, are already outmoded in the light of the results of the WOSCOPS, CARE and 4S trials.

Dietary therapy of dyslipidaemia

Dietary change should always be tried first in the management of dyslipidaemia, accompanied by control of other risk factors such as smoking and physical inactivity. The National Cholesterol Education Program Step One[32] and European Atherosclerosis Society[70] diets both aim to reduce total fat intake to provide <30% calories with no more than 10% being derived from saturated fat, the remainder from mono- and polyunsaturated fats. Cholesterol intake is limited to 300 mg/day. The European Atherosclerosis Society diet also emphasises the importance of consuming around 35 g of fibre/day. This type of diet has been shown to achieve appreciable improvements in lipid profile in patients with mixed hyperlipidaemia attending a lipid clinic,[72] but has been less successful in a general practice setting.[73]

If target levels of serum lipids are not achieved despite at least three months adherence to diet and achievement of ideal body weight, consideration should be given to supplementary lipid lowering drug therapy, assuming this is indicated on the grounds of high risk or presence of coronary heart disease.

Lipid lowering drugs

Of the four main classes of lipid lowering drugs used in Britain, the longest established are the fibrates. Clofibrate, bezafibrate, fenofibrate, gemfibrozil and ciprofibrate are all effective in controlling hypertriglycer-idaemia and in raising high density lipoprotein cholesterol but vary in their ability to reduce low density lipoprotein cholesterol, fenofibrate and ciprofibrate being the most potent in this respect. Both the WHO trial of clofibrate[74] and the Helsinki Heart Study of gemfibrozil[75] provided evidence that this class of drug has the ability to reduce the incidence of coronary heart disease in subjects with moderate hypocholesterolaemia, although this was offset by an increased incidence of gallstones and non-cardiac causes of death.

Anion exchange resins have also been in use for many years, particularly cholestyramine. This drug, together with colestipol, has a greater low density lipoprotein lowering ability than fibrates but raises high density lipoprotein cholesterol less and aggravates hypertriglyceridaemia. The advantage these resins have in being unabsorbed is offset by a high frequency of gastrointestinal side effects, which decreases compliance. Nevertheless the LRC Coronary Primary Prevention Trial demonstrated the ability of cholestyramine to reduce significantly the risk of coronary heart disease in hypercholesterolaemic men, especially those who took the prescribed dose in full throughout the trial.[76]

Nicotinic acid is similar to the fibrates in reducing triglycerides but it raises high density lipoprotein cholesterol to a much greater extent. It reduces low density lipoprotein cholesterol to some extent and, uniquely, Lp(a).[77] Use of the drug is constrained by its frequent side effects but when given alone[78] or in combination with clofibrate,[79] it favourably influenced both total and coronary heart disease mortality in patients with pre-existing coronary heart disease.

The most recently introduced class of lipid lowering drugs are the hydroxy-methylglutaryl coenzyme A reductase inhibitors or statins. Pharmacological inhibition of hydroxy-methylglutaryl coenzyme A reductase blocks endogenous cholesterol synthesis and upregulates low density lipoprotein receptor activity, resulting in a reduction in plasma levels of low density lipoprotein cholesterol. Compounds licensed for use in Britain are simvastatin and pravastatin, which lower low density lipoprotein cholesterol by 25–40%,[80] and more recently fluvastatin. At high doses they also reduce serum triglycerides and induce a small increase in high density lipoprotein cholesterol but are ineffective in reducing Lp(a) levels.[81, 82] Hydroxy-methylglutaryl coenzyme A reductase inhibitors are more effective than anion exchange resins in lowering low density lipoprotein cholesterol but less effective than the fibrates and nicotinic acid in reducing serum triglycerides and raising high density lipoprotein cholesterol. A very recent addition to this class of drug is atorvastatin, which has just been licensed in Britain. This compound has the ability to decrease low density lipoprotein cholesterol by up to 60%[83] and triglycerides by up to 45%.[84] It is also more effective than other statins in patients with familial hypercholesterolaemia, including homozygotes, by virtue of its ability to decrease production as well as stimulate receptor mediated catabolism of low density lipoprotein cholesterol.[85]

Fish oils such as Maxepa, which are rich in very long chain polyunsaturated fatty acids decrease triglyceride synthesis and thereby lower serum triglycerides. They may also have antiarrhythmic properties.

The salient features of all these lipid lowering drugs are shown in Table 5.6. The choice of drug will depend upon the type and severity of the dyslipidaemia, the possible side effects and whether there are any contraindications to use, such as in persons with hepatic dysfunction.

Under certain circumstances a combination of two or more lipid lowering drugs may be necessary. For example, the combined use of an anion exchange resin and a hydroxy-methylglutaryl coenzyme A reductase inhibitor is very effective in heterozygous familial hypercholesterolaemia, decreasing low density lipoprotein cholesterol by more than 50%.[86] Similarly, the combination of simvastatin and bezafibrate is more effective than either drug alone in the treatment of mixed hyperlipidaemia.[87]

Non-pharmacological lipid lowering therapy

Sometimes it is necessary to resort to more radical methods of treatment. Plasma exchange and low density lipoprotein apheresis are of proven value in homozygous familial hypercholesterolaemia,[88] as is liver transplantation,[89] but there is no evidence that low density lipoprotein apheresis is superior to combination drug therapy in heterozygous familial hypercholesterolaemia, despite its ability to lower Lp(a).[90]

Table 5.6 Lipid lowering drugs currently available in Britain

Drug	Dose	Indications	Side effects	Contraindications
Fibrates				
Fenofibrate	100 mg tds	Hypertriglyceridaemia	Myositis (rare)	Renal failure
Bezafibrate (Mono)	400 mg od	Mixed hyperlipidaemia	Increased lithogenicity of bile	Gallstones
Gemfibrozil	600 mg bd			
Ciprofibrate	100 mg od			
Anion exchange resins				
Cholestyramine	8 g bd	Hypercholesterolaemia	Gastrointestinal dysfunction	Hypertriglyceridaemia
Colestipol	10 g bd			Peptic ulcer. Piles
HMG CoA reductase inhibitors				
Simvastatin	10–40 mg od	Hypercholesterolaemia	Hepatic dysfunction	Avoid in liver disease and
Pravastatin	20–40 mg od	Mixed hyperlipidaemia	Myositis	with cyclosporin and in fertile
Fluvastatin	20 mg od–40 mg bd			females
Atorvastatin	10–80 mg od			
Nicotinic acid and analogues				
Acipimox	250 mg tds	Hypertriglyceridaemia	Gastrointestinal dysfunction,	Avoid in liver disease, gout
Nicofuranose	0·5–1 g tds	Mixed hyperlipidaemia	cutaneous flush and rash,	
			hyperuricaemia	
Fish oil				
Maxepa	5–15 g/day	Severe hypertriglyceridaemia	Nausea, odour, raises LDL	Hypercholesterolaemia

Partial ileal bypass is an effective means of reducing low density lipoprotein cholesterol,[47] especially in conjunction with a hydroxy-methyl-glutaryl coenzyme A reductase inhibitor, but has side effects such as diarrhoea which necessitate its reversal in a significant minority of patients.[91]

Conclusions

The evidence that dyslipidaemia plays a major causal role in the pathogenesis of atherosclerosis and coronary heart disease is now incontrovertible. There are also compelling data from angiographic and endpoint trials that treatment of dyslipidaemia reduces the rate of progression and stabilises atherosclerotic lesions in coronary arteries, thereby decreasing the incidence of clinical manifestations of coronary heart disease. The strongest evidence of therapeutic benefit relates to the marked reductions in low density lipoprotein cholesterol achieved by statins, best exemplified by the results of the 4S, CARE and WOSCOPS trials. However, there is also evidence that achieving reductions in triglyceride rich lipoproteins and increasing high density lipoprotein cholesterol may be important.[57]

At the present time the highest priority should be given to secondary prevention of coronary heart disease, which is a cost effective endeavour where the benefits far outweigh the risks.[92] Based on the results of the 4S and CARE studies, all patients with coronary heart disease and with a serum cholesterol $\geqslant 4.5$ mmol/L despite diet should be treated with a lipid lowering drug, preferably a statin. Comparable benefit can be expected in those with a lower low density lipoprotein cholesterol (< 4.4 mmol/L) as in those with a higher low density lipoprotein cholesterol ($\geqslant 5.35$ mmol/L).[93] However, patients with low density lipoprotein cholesterol levels < 3.2 mmol/L did not benefit from treatment in the CARE study.[94] A meta-analysis of trials which used quantitative coronary angiography suggests that progression of disease is arrested completely if low density lipoprotein cholesterol is reduced by 44%.[95]

The case for lipid lowering drug therapy in the primary prevention of coronary heart disease is less strong than for secondary prevention but has received a considerable boost with the publication of WOSCOPS. The latter implies that all men below the age of 65 with moderately severe hypercholesterolaemia (> 6.5 mmol/L) would benefit from treatment with a statin. However, the joint recommendations of the EAS, ESC and EHS suggest that drug treatment should be restricted to those whose absolute risk of CHD is $\geqslant 20\%$ per 10 years, otherwise the cost of primary prevention becomes unacceptably high.

Lp(a) remains an enigmatic risk factor but current evidence suggests that its pathogenicity is markedly reduced if concomitant elevations in low density lipoprotein cholesterol are lowered by appropriate therapy.[90, 96] Thus

113

it should be included along with other risk factors such as diabetes, hypertension, and smoking when estimating the overall risk of coronary heart disease in dyslipidaemic subjects and deciding upon the need to treat.

1 Davies MJ, Woolf N. Atherosclerosis: what is it and why does it occur? *Br Heart J* 1993; **69** (Suppl): S3–S11.

2 Martin MJ, Hulley SB, Browner WS, Kuller LH, Wentworth D. Serum cholesterol, blood pressure, and mortality: implications from a cohort of 361,662 men. *Lancet* 1986; **ii**: 933–6.

3 Hulley SB, Walsh JMB, Newman TB. Health policy on blood cholesterol. Time to change directions. *Circulation* 1992; **86**: 1026–9.

4 Rose G, Reid DD, Hamilton PJS, McCartney P, Keen H, Jarrett RJ. Myocardial ischaemia, risk factors and death from coronary heart disease. *Lancet* 1977; **i**: 105–9.

5 Pekkanen J, Linn S, Heiss G *et al.* Ten-year mortality from cardiovascular disease in relation to cholesterol level among men with and without pre-existing cardiovascular disease. *N Engl J Med* 1990; **322**: 1700–7.

6 Kannel WB, Wilson PWF. Efficacy of lipid profiles in prediction of coronary disease. *Am Heart J* 1992; **124**: 768–74.

7 Stampfer MJ, Sacks FM, Salvini S, Willett WC, Hennekens CH. A prospective study of cholesterol, apolipoproteins, and the risk of myocardial infarction. *N Engl J Med* 1991; **325**: 373–81.

8 Barbir M, Wile D, Trayner I, Aber VR, Thompson GR. High prevalence of hyper-triglyceridaemia and apolipoprotein abnormalities in coronary artery disease. *Br Heart J* 1988; **60**: 397–403.

9 NIH Consensus Development Panel on Triglycerides, High-density Lipoprotein, and Coronary Heart Disease. Triglyceride, high-density lipoprotein, and coronary heart disease. *JAMA* 1993; **269**: 505–10.

10 Ericsson C-G, Hamsten A, Nilsson J, Grip L, Svane B, de Faire U. Angiographic assessment of effects of bezafibrate on progression of coronary artery disease in young male post-infarction patients. *Lancet* 1996; **347**: 849–53.

11 Manninen V, Tenkanen L, Koskinen P *et al.* Joint effects of serum triglyceride and LDL cholesterol and HDL cholesterol concentrations on coronary heart disease risk in the Helsinki Heart Study. *Circulation* 1992; **85**: 37–45.

12 Assmann G, Schulte H. Relation of high-density lipoprotein cholesterol and triglycerides to incidence of atherosclerotic coronary artery disease (the PROCAM experience). *Am J Cardiol* 1992; **70**: 733–7.

13 Berg K, Dahlen G, Frick MH. Lp(a) lipoprotein and pre-β_1-lipoprotein in patients with coronary heart disease. *Clin Genet* 1974; **6**: 230–5.

14 Rosengren A, Wilhelmsen L, Eriksson E, Risberg B, Wedel H. Lipoprotein(a) and coronary heart disease: a prospective case-control study in a general population sample of middle aged men. *Br Med J* 1990; **301**: 1248–51.

15 Kostner GM, Avogaro P, Cazzolato G, Maryn E, Bittolo-Bon G, Quinici GB. Lipoprotein(a) and the risk for myocardial infarction. *Atherosclerosis* 1981; **3**: 51–61.

16 Rhoads GG, Dahlen G, Berg K, Morton NE, Dannenberg AL. Lp(a) lipoprotein as a risk factor for myocardial infarction. *JAMA* 1986; **256**: 2540–4.

17 Seed M, Hoppichler F, Reaveley D *et al.* Relation of serum lipoprotein(a) concentration and apolipoprotein(a) phenotype to coronary heart disease in patients with familial hypercholesterolaemia. *N Engl J Med* 1990; **322**: 1494–9.

18 Wiklund O, Angelin B, Olofsson S-O *et al.* Apolipoprotein(a) and ischaemic heart disease in familial hypercholesterolaemia. *Lancet* 1990; **i**; 1360–3.

19 Sandholzer Ch, Boerwinkle E, Saha N, Tong MC, Utermann G. Apolipoprotein(a) phenotypes, Lp(a) concentration and plasma lipid levels in relation to coronary heart disease in a Chinese population: evidence for the role of the apo(a) gene in coronary heart disease. *J Clin Invest* 1992; **89**: 1040–6.

20 Dahlen GH, Guyton JR, Attar M, Farmer JA, Kautz JA, Gotto AM. Association of levels

of lipoprotein Lp(a), plasma lipids, and other lipoproteins with coronary artery disease documented by angiography. *Circulation* 1986; **74**: 758–65.

21 Armstrong VW, Cremer P, Eberle E *et al.* The association between serum Lp(a) concentrations and angiographically assessed coronary atherosclerosis. Dependence on serum LDL levels. *Atherosclerosis* 1986; **62**: 249–57.

22 Hearn JA, DeMaio SJ Jr, Roubin GS, Hammarstrom M, Sgoutas D. Predictive value of lipoprotein(a) and other serum lipoproteins in the angiographic diagnosis of coronary artery disease. *Am J Cardiol* 1990; **66**: 1176–80.

23 Genest J, Jenner JL, McNamara JR *et al.* Prevalence of lipoprotein(a) [Lp(a)] excess in coronary artery disease. *Am J Cardiol* 1991; **67**: 1039–45.

24 Morgan R, Bishop AJ, Young WT, Ephraim DC, Matthews SB, Rees A. The relationship between apolipoprotein(a), lipid and lipoprotein levels and the risk of coronary artery disease. *Cardiovasc Risk Fact* 1992; **2**: 105–11.

25 Hoff HF, Beck GJ, Skibinski CI *et al.* Serum Lp(a) level as a predictor of vein graft stenosis after coronary artery bypass surgery in patients. *Circulation* 1988; **77**: 1238–44.

26 Hearn JA, Donohue BC, Ba'albaki H *et al.* Usefulness of serum lipoprotein(a) as a predictor of restenosis after percutaneous transluminal coronary angioplasty. *Am J Cardiol* 1992; **69**: 736–9.

27 Barbir M, Kushwaha S, Hunt B *et al.* Lipoprotein(a) and accelerated coronary arterial disease in cardiac transplant recipients. *Lancet* 1992; **340**: 1500–2.

28 Boerwinkle E, Leffert CC, Lin J, Lackner C, Chiesa G, Hobbs HH. Apolipoprotein(a) gene accounts for greater than 90% of the variation in plasma lipoprotein(a) concentrations. *J Clin Invest* 1992; **90**: 52–60.

29 Halvorsen S, Skjonsberg OH, Berg K, Ruyter R, Godal HC. Does Lp(a) lipoprotein inhibit the fibrinolytic system? *Thromb Res* 1992; **68**: 223–32.

30 Rath M, Niendorf A, Reblin T, Dietel M, Krebber J-H, Beisiegel U. Detection and quantification of lipoprotein(a) in the arterial wall of 107 coronary bypass patients. *Arteriosclerosis* 1989; **9**: 579–92.

31 Cushing GL, Gaubatz JW, Nava ML *et al.* Quantitation and localization of apolipoprotein(a) and B in coronary artery bypass vein grafts resected at re-operation. *Arteriosclerosis* 1989; **9**: 593–603.

32 Expert Panel on Detection, Evaluation and Treatment of High Blood Cholesterol in Adults. Summary of the second report of the National Cholesterol Education Program (NCEP) Expert Panel on detection, evaluation, and treatment of high blood cholesterol in adults (Adult Treatment Panel II). *JAMA* 1993; **269**: 3015–23.

33 Thompson GR, Wilson PW. *Coronary risk factors and their assessment.* London: Science Press Ltd, 1992.

34 Rader DJ, Brewer HB Jr. Lipoprotein(a). Clinical approach to a unique atherogenic lipoprotein. *JAMA* 1992; **267**: 1109–12.

35 Holme I. An analysis of randomized trials evaluating the effect of cholesterol reduction on total mortality and coronary heart disease incidence. *Circulation* 1990; **82**: 1916–24.

36 Criqui MH. Cholesterol, primary and secondary prevention, and all-cause mortality. *Ann Intern Med* 1991; **115**: 973–6.

37 Collins R, Keech A, Peto R, Sleight P. Cholesterol and total mortality: need for larger trials. *Br Med J* 1992; **304**: 1689.

38 Oliver M. Might treatment of hypercholesterolaemia increase non-cardiac mortality? *Lancet* 1991; **337**: 1529–31.

39 Rossouw JE, Lewis B, Rifkind BM. The value of lowering cholesterol after myocardial infarction. *N Engl J Med* 1990; **323**: 1112–19.

40 Silberberg JS, Henry DA. The benefits of reducing cholesterol levels: the need to distinguish primary from secondary prevention. 1. A meta-analysis of cholesterol-lowering trials. *Med J Aust* 1991; **155**: 665–70.

41 Law MR, Wald NJ, Thompson SG. By how much and how quickly does reduction in serum cholesterol concentration lower risk of ischaemic heart disease. *Br Med J* 1994; **308**: 367–73.

42 Law MR, Thompson SG, Wald NJ. Assessing possible hazards of reducing serum cholesterol. *Br Med J* 1994; **308**: 373–9.

43 Brensike JF, Levy RI, Kelsey SF *et al.* Effects of therapy with cholestyramine on

progression of coronary arteriosclerosis: results of the NHLBI type II coronary intervention study. *Circulation* 1984; **69**: 313–24.

44 Levy RI, Brensike JF, Epstein SE *et al.* The influence of changes in lipid values induced by cholestyramine and diet on progression of coronary artery disease: results of the NHLBI type II coronary intervention study. *Circulation* 1984; **69**: 325–37.

45 Blankenhorn DH, Nessim SA, Johnson RL, Sanmarco MER, Azen SP, Cashin-Hemphill L. Beneficial effects of combined colestipol-niacin therapy on coronary atherosclerosis and coronary venous bypass grafts. *JAMA* 1987; **257**: 3233–40.

46 Cashin-Hemphill L, Mack WJ, Pogoda JM, Sanmarco ME, Azen SP, Blankenhorn DH. Beneficial effects of colestipol-niacin on coronary atherosclerosis. A 4-year follow up. *JAMA* 1990; **264**: 3013–17.

47 Buchwald H, Varco RL, Matts JP *et al.* Effect of partial ileal bypass surgery on mortality and morbidity from coronary heart disease in patients with hypercholesterolemia. *N Engl J Med* 1990; **323**: 946–55.

48 Brown G, Albers JJ, Fisher LD *et al.* Regression of coronary artery disease as a result of intensive lipid-lowering therapy in men with high levels of apolipoprotein B. *N Engl J Med* 1990; **323**: 1289–98.

49 Kane JP, Malloy MJ, Ports TA, Phillips NR, Diehl JC, Havel RJ. Regression of coronary atherosclerosis during treatment of familial hypercholesterolemia with combined drug regimens. *JAMA* 1990; **264**: 3007–12.

50 Ornish D, Brown SE, Scherwitz LW *et al.* Can lifestyle changes reverse coronary heart disease? *Lancet* 1990; **336**: 129–33.

51 Watts GF, Lewis B, Brunt JNH *et al.* Effects on coronary artery disease of lipid-lowering diet, or diet plus cholestyramine, in the St. Thomas' Atherosclerosis Regression Study (STARS). *Lancet* 1992; **339**: 563–9.

52 Schuler G, Hambrech TR, Schlierf G *et al.* Regular physical exercise and low-fat diet. Effects on progression of coronary artery disease. *Circulation* 1992; **86**: 1–11.

53 Blankenhorn DH, Azen SP, Kramsch DM *et al.* Coronary angiographic changes with lovastatin therapy. The Monitored Atherosclerosis Regression Study (MARS). *Ann Intern Med* 1993; **119**: 969–76.

54 Waters D, Higginson L, Gladstone P *et al.* Effects of monotherapy with an HMG-CoA reductase inhibitor on the progression of coronary atherosclerosis as assessed by serial quantitative arteriography. The Canadian Coronary Atherosclerosis Intervention Trial. *Circulation* 1994; **89**: 959–68.

55 Haskell WL, Alderman EL, Fair JM *et al.* Effects of intensive multiple risk factor reduction on coronary atherosclerosis and clinical cardiac events in men and women with coronary artery disease. The Stanford Coronary Risk Intervention Project (SCRIP). *Circulation* 1994; **89**: 975–90.

56 MAAS Investigators. Effect of simvastatin on coronary atheroma: the Multicentre Anti-Atheroma Study (MAAS). *Lancet* 1994; **344**: 633–8.

57 Thompson GR. Angiographic trials of lipid-lowering therapy: end of an era? *Br Heart J* 1995; **74**: 343–7.

58 Buchwald H, Matts JP, Fitch LL *et al.* Changes in sequential coronary arteriograms and subsequent coronary events. *JAMA* 1992; **268**: 1429–33.

59 Koga N, Iwata Y. Pathological and angiographic regression of coronary atherosclerosis by LDL apheresis in a patient with familial hypercholesterolemia. *Atherosclerosis* 1991; **90**: 9–21.

60 Pitt B, Mancini GBJ, Ellis SG, Rosman HS, Park J-S, McGovern ME, for the PLAC I Investigators. Pravastatin limitation of atherosclerosis in the coronary arteries (PLAC I): reduction in atherosclerosis progression and clinical events. *J Am Coll Cardiol* 1995; **26**: 1133–9.

61 Jukema JW, Bruschke AVG, Van Boven AJ *et al.* Effects of lipid lowering by pravastatin on progression and regression of coronary artery disease in symptomatic men with normal to moderately elevated serum cholesterol levels. The Regression Growth Evaluation Statin Study (REGRESS). *Circulation* 1995; **91**: 2528–40.

62 Furberg CD, Adams HP Jr, Applegate WB *et al*, for the Asymptomatic Carotid Artery Progression Study (ACAPS) Research Group. Effect of lovastatin on early carotid atherosclerosis and cardiovascular events. *Circulation* 1994; **90**: 1679–87.

63 Crouse JR III, Byington RP, Bond MG *et al.* Pravastatin, lipids, and atherosclerosis in the carotid arteries (PLAC II). *Am J Cardiol* 1995; **75**: 455–9.
64 Pravastatin Multinational Study Group for Cardiac Risk Factors. Effects of pravastatin in patients with serum total cholesterol levels from 5·2 to 7·8 mmol/liter (200 to 300 mg/dl) plus two additional atherosclerotic risk factors. *Am J Cardiol* 1993; **72**: 1031–7.
65 Shepherd J, Cobbe SM, Ford I *et al.*, for the West of Scotland Coronary Prevention Study Group. Prevention of coronary heart disease with pravastatin in men with hyper-cholesterolemia. *N Engl J Med* 1995; **333**: 1301–7.
66 West of Scotland Coronary Prevention Group. West of Scotland Coronary Prevention Study: identification of high-risk groups and comparison with other cardiovascular intervention trials. *Lancet* 1996; **348**: 1339–42.
67 Scandinavian Simvastatin Survival Study Group. Randomised trial of cholesterol lowering in 4444 patients with coronary heart disease: the Scandinavian Simvastatin Survival Study (4S). *Lancet* 1994; **344**: 1383–9.
68 Sacks FM, Pfeffer MA, Moye LA *et al.*, for the Cholesterol and Recurrent Events Trial Investigators. The effect of pravastatin on coronary events after myocardial infarction in patients with average cholesterol levels. *N Engl J Med* 1996; **355**: 1001–9.
69 Betteridge DJ, Dodson PM, Durrington PN *et al.* Management of hyperlipidaemia: guidelines of the British Hyperlipidaemia Association. *Postgrad Med J* 1993; **69**: 359–69.
70 European Atherosclerosis Society International Task Force for Prevention of Coronary Heart Disease. Prevention of coronary heart disease: scientific background and new clinical guidelines. *Nutr Metab Cardiovasc Dis* 1992; **2**: 113–56.
71 Pyörälä K, de Backer G, Graham I, Poole-Wilson P, Wood D, on behalf of the Task Force. Prevention of coronary heart disease in clinical practice. Recommendations of the Task Force of the European Society of Cardiology, European Atherosclerosis Society and European Society of Hypertension. *Eur Heart J* 1994; **15**: 1300–31.
72 Jones DB, Lousley S, Slaughter P, Carter RD, Mann JI. Prudent diet: effect on moderately severe hyperlipidaemia. *Br Med J* 1982; **284**: 1233.
73 Neil HAW, Roe L, Godlee RJP *et al.* Randomised trial of lipid lowering dietary advice in general practice: the effects on serum lipids, lipoproteins and antioxidants. *Br Med J* 1995; **310**: 569–73.
74 Committee of Principal Investigators. A cooperative trial in the primary prevention of ischaemic heart disease using clofibrate. *Br Heart J* 1978; **40**: 1069–1118.
75 Frick MH, Elo O, Haapa K *et al.* Helsinki Heart Study: primary-prevention trial with gemfibrozil in middle-aged men with dyslipidemia. Safety of treatment, changes in risk factors, and incidence of coronary heart disease. *N Engl J Med* 1987; **317**: 1237–45.
76 Lipid Research Clinics Program. The Lipid Research Clinics Coronary Primary Prevention Trial results. II. The relationship of reduction in incidence of coronary heart disease to cholesterol lowering. *JAMA* 1984; **251**: 365–74.
77 Carlson LA, Hamsten A, Asplund A. Pronounced lowering of serum levels of lipoprotein Lp(a) in hyperlipidaemic subjects treated with nicotinic acid. *J Int Med* 1989; **226**: 271–6.
78 Canner PL, Berge KG, Wenger NK *et al.* Fifteen year mortality in Coronary Drug Project patients: long-term benefit with niacin. *J Am Coll Cardiol* 1986; **8**: 1245–55.
79 Carlson LS, Rosenhamer G. Reduction of mortality in the Stockholm ischaemic heart disease secondary prevention study by combined treatment with clofibrate and nicotinic acid. *Acta Med Scand* 1988; **223**: 405–518.
80 Maher VMG, Thompson GR. HMG CoA reductase inhibitors as lipid-lowering agents: five years experience with lovastatin and an appraisal of simvastatin and pravastatin. *Q J Med* 1990; **74**: 165–75.
81 Thiery J, Armstrong VW, Schleef J, Creutzfeldt C, Creutzfeldt W, Seidel D. Serum lipoprotein Lp(a) concentrations are not influenced by an HMG CoA reductase inhibitor. *Klin Wochenschr* 1988; **66**: 462–3.
82 Berg K, Leren TP. Unchanged serum lipoprotein(a) concentrations with lovastatin. *Lancet* 1989; **ii**: 812.
83 Nawrocki JW, Weiss SR, Davidson MH *et al.* Reduction of LDL cholesterol by 25% to 60% in patients with primary hypercholesterolemia by atorvastatin, a new HMG-CoA reductase inhibitor. *Arterioscler Thromb Vasc Biol* 1995; **15**: 678–82.
84 Bakker-Arkema RG, Davidson MH, Goldstein RJ *et al.* Efficacy and safety of a new HMG-

CoA reductase inhibitor, atorvastatin, in patients with hypertriglyceridemia. *JAMA* 1996; **275**: 128–33.

85 Naoumova RP, Marais D, Firth JC, Neuwirth CKY, Taylor GW, Thompson GR. Atorvastatin augments therapy of homozygous familial hypercholesterolemia by inhibiting up regulation of cholesterol synthesis after apheresis and bile acid sequestrants. *Circulation* 1996; **94** (Suppl): I–583.

86 Mol MJT, Stuyt PMJ, Demacker PNM, Stalenhoef AFH. The effects of simvastatin on serum lipoproteins in severe hypercholesterolaemia. *Neth J Med* 1990; **36**: 182–90.

87 Kehely A, MacMahon M, Barbir M *et al.* Combined bezafibrate and simvastatin treatment for mixed hyperlipidaemia. *Q J Med* 1995; **88**: 421–7.

88 Thompson GR. *A handbook of hyperlipidaemia*. London: Current Science, 1994.

89 Barbir M, Khaghani A, Kehely A *et al.* Normal levels of lipoproteins including lipoprotein(a) after liver–heart transplantation in a patient with homozygous familial hypercholesterolaemia. *Q J Med* 1992; **85**: 807–12.

90 Thompson GR, Maher VMG, Matthews S *et al.* The Familial Hypercholesterolaemia Regression Study: a randomised trial of LDL apheresis. *Lancet* 1995; **345**: 811–16.

91 Ohri SK, Keane PF, Swift I *et al.* Reappraisal of partial ileal bypass for the treatment of familial hypercholesterolemia. *Am J Gastroenterol* 1989; **84**: 740–3.

92 Goldman L, Gordon DJ, Rifkind BM *et al.* Cost and health implications of cholesterol lowering. *Circulation* 1992; **85**: 1960–8.

93 Scandinavian Simvastatin Survival Study Group. Baseline serum cholesterol and treatment effect in the Scandinavian Simvastatin Survival Study (4S). *Lancet* 1995; **345**: 1274–5.

94 Sacks FM, Rouleau J-L, Moye LA *et al.*, for the CARE Investigators. Baseline characteristics in the Cholesterol and Recurrent Events (CARE) trial of secondary prevention in patients with average serum cholesterol levels. *Am J Cardiol* 1995; **75**: 621–3.

95 Thompson GR, Hollyer J, Waters DD. Percentage change rather than plasma level of LDL-cholesterol determines therapeutic response in coronary heart disease. *Curr Opin Lipidol* 1995; **6**: 386–8.

96 Maher VMG, Brown BG, Marcovina SM, Hillger LA, Zhao X-G, Albers JJ. Effects of lowering elevated LDL cholesterol on the cardiovascular risk of lipoprotein(a). *JAMA* 1995; **274**: 1771–4.

6: Hypertension: the influence of age and pressure on treatment options

CJ BULPITT AND AE FLETCHER

Introduction

Hypertension has been defined as the blood pressure above which treatment does more good than harm. This is the definition that we shall adopt in this chapter. Trials have varied in the method of taking diastolic blood pressure but have usually taken the point of disappearance of phase 5 Korotkoff sound and this is the measure taken here.

There are three main options for the treatment of hypertension. The first is no treatment or at least delayed treatment, the second is treatment but without using drugs and the third is the drug option. The decision to adopt any one of these options depends, as with the whole of medicine, on the balance between the benefits and risks. With hypertension, the balance between benefit and risk varies with age, blood pressure, and, probably to a lesser extent, on the actual drug treatment employed.

There are some areas of agreement between practising clinicians as to when drug treatment must be employed. The first is the treatment of malignant or accelerated hypertension. Untreated, this leads to a life expectancy of only six months.[1] The benefits of treatment in terms of survival were proved many years ago and active treatment is never withheld from these patients. Similarly, patients with either severe heart failure or subarachnoid haemorrhage and hypertension are treated with anti-hypertensive drugs.

Treatment may also be considered for patients who have less to gain. To take an extreme example, a young woman who does not smoke with a diastolic blood pressure of 90 mmHg is not at a high risk of a stroke. Even if active drug treatment reduced this risk by 40% (and this is probable) then a reduction of a very rare event by 40% is still not an attractive proposition.

119

Added to this, the adverse effects of drug treatment will still be present and the benefit to risk evaluation does not favour immediate treatment.

The need to decide whether or not to treat patients at intermediate risk has led to the publication of many guidelines over the years.[2-4] They have many features in common as they have to consider the same but accumulating body of evidence in making their recommendations. This evidence provides information on the benefits of treating mainly diastolic hypertension in patients of middle age or up to 79 years. Less evidence is available for the treatment of levels of systolic blood pressure, for younger patients or for the very elderly. We shall consider the treatment of hypertension (diastolic and systolic) in patients aged 40–59, the treatment of diastolic hypertension between ages 60 and 79, the treatment of systolic hypertension in this age group, and finally the treatment of diastolic or systolic hypertension over the age of 80.

In the following discussion we will be considering "sustained" levels of blood pressure, levels recorded at repeated visits. A minimum of three visits is required and it could be argued that the time lapse between the first and last visit should be at least three months. The objective is to exclude, from possibly lifetime treatment, patients with only transient levels of high blood pressure. Similarly, the patient should be well rested in the sitting position before the blood pressure is recorded and most recommendations include a resting period of at least five minutes. In the very elderly there are reasons to suggest that the blood pressure should also be taken in the standing position as at this age blood pressure may fall markedly on rising and treatment may not then be indicated.

Hypertension at age 40–59

Table 6.1 considers the results in terms of stroke and myocardial infarction incidence and all-cause mortality for three large trials. The trials included some young patients and some aged 60–69 but predominantly the results are applicable to the age group under discussion. The Australian[6] and Medical Research Council (MRC)[7] trials compared active treatment with placebo. In the MRC Trial randomisation was to two different active treatments and the results are combined in Table 6.1. The Hypertension Detection and Follow-up Programme (HDFP)[8] compared usual care with more efficient care that reduced blood pressure to a greater extent.

For every 1000 patients followed for a year in these trials, one or two had a stroke event avoided by active or intensive treatment. The benefits applied to both men and women. For a combination of fatal and non-fatal myocardial infarction the reductions were less marked but probably one event per 1000 patient-years was avoided in men although this was not proven in women. It has to be remembered that women have fewer episodes of myocardial infarction than men and the possibility of benefit, recorded by the HDFP, may have accrued from activities associated with special care and not simply from a reduction in blood pressure. In the HDFP non-cardiovascular mortality was also reduced by intensive treatment which suggests additional activity in the specialised care clinics. The trials also showed some evidence for a reduction in total mortality for men but no evidence for middle aged women.

In order to put these benefits in context, Table 6.2 gives the adverse effects which were observed in one of these trials, the MRC Trial, and again expressed as events per 1000 patient-years. In this table the excess of events over the events observed in the placebo group is given and it can be seen

Table 6.1   Effects of treatment compared with placebo in the Australian[6] and MRC (middle aged)[7] trials and with controls in the HDFP[8]

| | Rate per 1000 patient years | | Reduction in risk per 1000 patient years |
	Treatment	Control	
All strokes			
Both sexes			
Australian	1·9	3·2	1·3
MRC	1·4	2·6	1·2
Men			
MRC	1·7	2·9	1·2
HDFP*	2·9	5·1	2·2
Women			
MRC	1·1	2·1	1·0
HDFP*	3·2	4·5	1·3
Fatal and non-fatal MI			
Both sexes			
Australian	4·7	4·8	0·1
MRC	5·2	5·5	0·3
Men			
MRC	8·3	9·0	0·7
HDFP +	4·8	5·7	0·9
Women			
MRC	1·8	1·7	–
HDFP +	3·9	4·6	0·7
All-cause mortality			
Both sexes			
Australian	3·6	5·1	1·5
MRC	5·8	5·9	0·1
Men			
MRC	7·1	8·2	1·1
HDFP*	2·9	3·4	0·5
Women			
MRC	4·4	3·5	–
HDFP*	2·4	2·4	–

Reduction in risk gives the events prevented by active treatment.
HDFP = Hypertension Detection and Follow-up Program, intensive treatment compared, not with placebo, but with usual care. Table based on Isles *et al.*[9]
* White only; + includes whites and blacks and additional diagnoses from questionnaire data alone.

121

Table 6.2 Adverse effects observed in the MRC trial in middle aged persons[7] in events/1000 patient-years (reproduced with permission from *Postgrad Med J* 1993; **69**: 764–74)

	Men		Women	
	Bendrofluazide	Propranolol	Bendrofluazide	Propranolol
Impaired glucose tolerance	4·4	0	3·9	0
Gout or SUA >500 (men) or 450 μmol/L (women)	12·1	0	1·5	0
Impotence	11·3	5·0	–	–
Raynaud's	0	5·1	0	4·5
Skin disorder	0	1·2	0	1·1
Dyspnoea	0	6·7	0	6·9
Lethargy	3·1	4·8	1·4	8·0

All entries are significant at the 1% level and represent the difference between the rate on active treatment and the rate on placebo. A zero entry means no statistically significant excess or deficit.

that the adverse events due to treatment can occur with a high frequency. For example, impaired glucose tolerance affects four per 1000 per year in the patients given bendrofluazide in the trial. This adverse effect was not observed with propranolol. Similarly, 11 per 1000 men per year reported impotence due to bendrofluazide and this was considered to be twice the incidence on propranolol. The well known adverse effects of β-blockers are also demonstrated in the table with a high incidence of Raynaud's phenomenon, dyspnoea, and lethargy.

It is not easy to compare Tables 6.1 (benefits) and 6.2 (risks) for several reasons. The first is that a stroke or myocardial infarction may be a devastating event and the benefit can be expected to accumulate year by year. In contrast, certain events in Table 6.2, such as the development of a high uric acid or impaired glucose tolerance, may or may not be accompanied by clinical problems and therefore may not concern the patient. In addition, although 11 men per 1000 per year may report impotence it is unlikely that this proportion will accumulate year by year. However, the benefits may accumulate through time.

A patient may be unwilling to tolerate adverse effects if their risk of stroke or myocardial infarction is very low. Collins *et al.*, in an overview,[10] estimated that coronary events may be reduced by 14% by treatment and strokes by 40%. Table 6.3 gives the coronary and stroke events at different ages in the MRC Trial. It is probable that a man over the age of 45 would consider that his risk of stroke was high enough (2·4 per 1000 person-years)

Table 6.3 Coronary and stroke events/1000 patient-years on placebo in the Medical Research Council Trial in middle aged patients.[7,11] Figures in parentheses are for patients presenting with a diastolic pressure > 100 mmHg

Sex	Age	Rate on placebo/1000 person years Coronary events	All strokes	Strokes DBP > 100 mmHg
Men	35-44	3·3	0·4	(1·0)
	45-54	7·5	2·4	(3·8)
	55-64	12·2	5·3	(6·4)
Women	35-44	0·3	1·6	(2·4)
	45-54	1·1	1·3	(1·7)
	55-64	2·6	3·1	(4·9)

to justify taking active treatment. This view will be shared by a woman aged 55–64 (3·1 per 1000 person-years). A man aged 45–54 would also realise that a 14% reduction in the more frequent coronary events (7·5 per 1000 person-years) would be an additional incentive to take active treatment.

Miall and Greenberg[11] have also published the MRC results for stroke according to whether the diastolic pressure was above or below 100 mmHg. These rates are also given in Table 6.3. When considering only those with a diastolic over 100, stroke rates were increased at 1·0 per 1000 person-years for men aged 35–44 and 1·7–2·4 per 1000 person-years for women aged 35–54. As the rate of 2·4 occurred in young women with a negligible chance of a coronary event, it is possible that the benefits do not exceed risks for women aged less than 54 and men aged less than 44, even for diastolic pressures of 100–105 mmHg. Guidelines recommend treatment irrespective of age for diastolic blood pressures in excess of 100 mmHg.[2]

If treatment is not to be immediately offered to men under the age of 45 or women under the age of 55 with mild hypertension, what should be the treatment plan for these people? We discuss later the role of non-pharmacologic treatment and these patients must still be followed as their blood pressure may rise further. Eventually they will probably enter the older and higher risk age groups.

Diastolic hypertension at age 60–79

A meta-analysis by Amery et al.[12] suggested that stroke events in the trials in the elderly were reduced by 40%. Table 6.4 gives the percentage reduction in events in five trials of antihypertensive treatment in the elderly. The consistency of the results is striking with percentage reductions ranging from 25% to 47%. The treatment regimes employed were based on a diuretic regime in the Australian (a subset aged 60–69),[13] and the European Working Party on High Blood Pressure in the Elderly (EWPHE)[14] trials. The Hypertension in the Elderly Persons (HEP) Trial[15] was based on atenolol and the STOP Hypertension Trial[16] was based on either a diuretic

Table 6.4   Percentage reduction in stroke and cardiac events and reduction in total mortality in trials of antihypertensive treatment in the elderly with diastolic hypertension

	Stroke			Cardiac			
	Non-fatal	Fatal	All	Non-fatal	Fatal	All	Total mortality
Australian (13)	− 37	− 1	− 34	− 10	− 75	− 19	− 23
EWPHE (14)	− 35	− 32	− 36*	− 9	− 38*	− 20	− 23
Coope and Warrender (15)	− 27	− 70*	− 42*	− 26	+ 1	− 15	− 3
STOP (16)	− 38*	− 73*	− 47*	–	− 25	− 13	− 43*
MRC (17)	− 30	− 12	− 25*	− 13	− 22	− 19	− 3

* $p < 0.05$

or one of several β-blockers. In the event the vast majority of patients in this trial ended up on a diuretic plus β-blocker. The MRC Trial in the elderly[17] randomised active treatment to be based either on the β-blocker atenolol or a hydrochlorothiazide/amiloride diuretic combination. The trials were concerned predominantly with diastolic hypertension but the HEP and MRC trials included a proportion of patients with isolated systolic hypertension (see below).

In the MRC Elderly Trial, total coronary events were reduced by 44% with a hydrochlorothiazide/amiloride combination but not by atenolol.[17] In other studies employing a β-blocker the reductions in total cardiac events were 15% (the HEP Trial)[15] and 13% (the STOP Trial).[16] The corresponding reductions when a diuretic was employed were 19% (Australian Trial age 60–69)[13] and 20% (EWPHE Trial).[14] In the MRC Elderly Trial[17] the investigators have reported benefits with a diuretic over and above the effects of lowering blood pressure. Any benefits from treatment with a β-blocker were confined to non-smokers. In view of these findings, Beard et al.[18a] recommended diuretics rather than β-blockers for elderly patients with uncomplicated hypertension. This may be good advice as the earlier MRC Trial indicated doubt concerning the ability of propranolol to reduce stroke events or coronary events in smokers.

The cardiovascular event rate is much higher in the elderly and these persons have more to gain from treatment. Table 6.5 gives the number of patients that need to be treated for five years to prevent one event. The returns from treating the elderly are much greater than for younger persons. In the more hypertensive patients in the EWPHE Trial (average untreated pressure 182/101 mmHg) only 10–25 have to be treated for five years to prevent either a stroke event or a cardiac event.

The Prospective Studies Collaboration reviewed 42 prospective observational cohorts during which 13,397 strokes were observed.[18b] Six blood pressure categories were compared in three age at screening groups, < 45, 45–64, and 65 +. The relative risks of stroke between the highest and lowest

Table 6.5   Number of patients needed to be treated for five years to save one event, stroke or cardiac, in the MRC Trials[7, 17] and the EWPHE Trial[13]

	MRC Trials		
Basic treatment	Younger patients (mean age 52)	Older patients (mean age 70)	EWPHE Trial (mean age 72)
	Stroke event		
Diuretic	110	60	10–20+
β-blocker	280	110	–
	Cardiac event		
Diuretic	No benefit	40	10–25#
β-blocker	No benefit	No benefit	–

+Lower estimate includes transient ischaemic attack
Lower estimate includes arrhythmias and heart block.

pressure groups were 10, 5 and 2 respectively. However, the absolute increases in stroke rates on going from the lowest to the highest blood pressure group were two per 1000 per year at age <45, five per 1000 per year at age 45–64 and eight per 1000 per year at age 65+, supporting greater returns from treating the elderly.

However high the benefits, the risks must be appraised. In the trials the risks of treatment depend on the exact nature of the antihypertensive treatment and include potentially life threatening events, biochemical changes not known to be associated with symptoms, and adverse effects on quality of life. The risks in the EWPHE and MRC Elderly Trials are given in Table 6.6. In the EWPHE Trial important consequences of diuretic treatment included gout, four per 1000 per year, and diabetes mellitus, nine per 1000 per year.[14] The latter was associated with starting oral hypoglycaemic drugs in seven per 1000 per year. Active treatment was also associated with a need for peripheral vasodilators in seven per 1000 per year.[19] Table 6.6 also indicates that a certain degree of mild hypokalaemia and an elevated serum creatinine will be expected in actively treated patients. As deaths from cardiac causes and renal failure were not increased on active treatment these biochemical changes were presumably, on balance, of little clinical importance. An excess of 12% of patients reported dry mouth and 7% diarrhoea. These symptoms appeared to be mainly due to the methyldopa treatment received by a third of patients on active treatment.

These risks must be contrasted with the benefits. For example, in the EWPHE Trial four per 1000 will get gout in one year, nine diabetes and over 120 per 1000 will get side effects of drugs. Set against this is the saving of six per 1000 for fatal strokes, 11 per 1000 for non-fatal strokes, 11 per 1000 for fatal cardiac events and eight per 1000 for episodes of severe congestive heart failure.

In the MRC Trial the adverse events leading to withdrawal have been

Table 6.6   Risk estimates: differences between active and placebo treatment in the EWPHE[14] and MRC Elderly[17] Trials (expressed as number/1000/year) (reproduced with permission from *Postgrad Med J* 1993; **69**: 764–74)

	EWPHE	MRC Diuretic	MRC Atenolol
Gout	+4*	+4*	0
Mild hypokalaemia (K$^+$ <3·5 mmol/L)	+71*	–	–
Elevated serum creatinine (>180 μmol/L)	+23*	–	–
Diabetes	+9	+4*†	+3*†
Dry mouth	+124*	–	–
Diarrhoea	+71*	–	–
Need for hypoglycaemic drugs	+7	–	–
Need for peripheral vasodilators	+7	–	–
Skin disorders	–	+3*	–
Muscle cramp	–	+5*	+1
Nausea	–	+6*	+3*
Dizziness	–	+6*	+9*
Raynaud's	–	+1	+11*
Dyspnoea	–	+1	+22*
Lethargy	–	+4	+17*
Headache	–	+3	+6*

* $p > 0.05$, for difference between active and placebo rates: † impaired glucose tolerance. The MRC data are reasons for withdrawal. – = data not published.

published and are also given in Table 6.6. The burden of adverse events appears similar to that in the EWPHE Trial. The side effects appear to be less frequent as these adverse events had to be severe enough to cause withdrawal of the patient from the treatment. These risks have to be compared with the gains in all treated patients of three per 1000 patient-years for all strokes and two per 1000 for all coronary events. For diuretic treatment the gains were four per 1000 and five per 1000 patient-years, respectively.

The risk–benefit analysis in the EWPHE Trial is clearly in favour of treatment. In the MRC Elderly Trial, the results are less convincing but do support a policy of treating the patients entered in the EWPHE Trial – those with sustained DBP $\geqslant 90$ mmHg plus SBP $\geqslant 160$ mmHg.

Diastolic hypertension over age 80

Although epidemiological data support a positive relationship between both systolic and diastolic blood pressure and mortality up to the age of 74 years in both men and women, over the age of 80, epidemiological data suggest that the higher the blood pressure, the longer the subject will live.[20]

It is probable that the negative relationship between blood pressure and total mortality implies that the sick elderly with a poor myocardium, cancer, weight loss due to chronic disease or early dementia will have a fall in blood pressure. The epidemiological data may not imply that such a negative

126

relationship exists between blood pressure and stroke. It is possible that the very elderly with high levels of blood pressure do still experience an excess of stroke events. Even if the very elderly hypertensive do live longer than average they may live even longer if their blood pressure is lowered.

In order to investigate this possibility the Hypertension in the Very Elderly Trial (HYVET) is being started, as we need to see the results of an experimental reduction in blood pressure over the age of 80 in order to determine treatment options. In the meantime the problem arises of the hypertensive patient who has been treated for many years and who reaches the age of 80. If the blood pressure is normal on treatment it is reasonable to suggest that antihypertensive treatment be withheld for a period. If the original hypertension returns then treatment may be indicated. Experimental evidence is lacking on the need to continue treatment but trials have found that when a benefit has been observed, this advantage has been true for both previously treated and previously untreated patients. The results of HYVET are expected to throw further light on the need to continue treatment in the 80s and the need to start treatment at this age.[21]

Isolated systolic hypertension

Isolated systolic hypertension is currently defined as a sustained systolic pressure ≥ 160 mmHg in the presence of a diastolic pressure < 95 mmHg or < 90 mmHg. Only one large trial has investigated the effects of treating isolated systolic hypertension, the Systolic Hypertension in the Elderly Program (SHEP) Trial.[22] This trial included persons over the age of 60, with an average age of 72 years.

Fatal cerebrovascular events were little influenced by treatment but non-fatal strokes were reduced by five per 1000 patient-years. Fatal coronary events were reduced by two per 1000 patient-years, non-fatal myocardial infarction also by two per 1000 per year, left ventricular failure by five per 1000 per year and coronary artery bypass grafting by two per 1000 per year. Forty-three percent of the MRC Elderly Trial also had isolated systolic hypertension and the trial reports 'There is no reason to doubt the applicability of the overall trial results to those with isolated systolic hypertension'.[17]

The biochemical adverse effects were qualitatively and quantitatively similar to those observed in other trials. In view of the fact that cardiac morbidity and mortality were reduced by active treatment, the increases in serum glucose and cholesterol and reductions in serum potassium did not produce a net increase in adverse cardiac events. However, from the patient's point of view the increase in serum uric acid and glucose are likely to have had clinical consequences in some patients, namely those who developed gout or symptoms due to diabetes mellitus.

The SHEP research group reported on 29 symptoms, 27 of which were more frequent in the actively treated group. The exceptions were 'heart beating fast or skipping beats' and 'severe headaches'. The nine symptoms with the greatest excess in the actively treated group were passing out, chest pain, memory problems, sexual problems, change in bowel habits, pain in the joints, ankle swelling, heart beating slowly and cold hands. The last three symptoms may have been due to the fact that 20% of actively treated patients were given a β-adrenergic blocking drug. In a separate publication the trial has reported that active treatment increased the time to complete the Reitan Trial Making Test B by three seconds.[23] This test of psychomotor speed and attention is compatible with the report of an excess of memory problems in the main trial.

The risks from treating isolated systolic hypertension appear to be as great as for treating combined systolic and diastolic hypertension, yet the absolute benefits are less, at least for mortal events. In proportional terms the evidence so far suggests a worthwhile benefit from treating isolated hypertension, but in view of the lower absolute gains, more evidence is being accrued in further trials.[24]

The SHEP Trial concerned patients over the age of 60 and no evidence is available for treating isolated systolic hypertension at younger ages.

Control of blood pressure by non-pharmacological approaches

Non-pharmacological approaches may be targeted both at the whole population or at those at high risk of CVD, either by virtue of blood pressure alone or because of multiple risk factors. The population approach, most clearly promulgated by Rose,[25] is based on the view that, since the majority of cardiovascular events occur at slightly elevated levels of blood pressure below the range normally considered "hypertensive", small reductions across the entire blood pressure distribution would result in a greater benefit to the population than approaches targeted only at "hypertensives". The high risk strategy acknowledges that for individuals at the upper end of the blood pressure distribution, the increase in absolute risk necessitates more intensive intervention. The population and high risk strategies should not be seen as alternatives but complementary approaches. The management of hypertensive patients must include an assessment of other CVD risk factors and implementing control of these where appropriate, in addition to control of blood pressure. In particular, attention is drawn to the importance of trying to stop hypertensive patients from smoking.

Non-pharmacological approaches to the control of hypertension are based on evidence from epidemiological studies and clinical trials. These studies have identified weight loss, reduction in sodium intake, increased physical activity and reduction of excessive alcohol intake as the principal non-pharmacological approaches for the control of blood pressure, both in the population and for the management of individuals with high blood pressure. Weight loss and reduction in alcohol intake have been identified as Health of the Nation Targets,[26] but in the absence of legislation on the labelling or restriction of sodium content of prepared foods, it seems unlikely that a population approach to the control of sodium intake will be effective. Moreover, at present there have been disappointing results from one community programme, the North Karelia Salt Project, the aim of which is to reduce salt intake among the whole population.[27] There is some weak evidence for the benefits from community interventions aimed at reducing sodium intake in studies carried out in Belgium[28] and Portugal.[29]

There is at present inadequate positive evidence to support other non-pharmacological approaches to the management of hypertension, such as potassium, calcium or magnesium supplements, fish oil or high fibre consumption and stress management.

In this chapter we will consider the use of non-pharmacological approaches to manage patients with high blood pressure levels, either in the range usually recommended for treatment by international societies[5] or to prevent a further rise in blood pressure in those with borderline hypertension.

Physical exercise

Many observational studies have described an inverse relationship between blood pressure and physical activity or objective measures of physical fitness.[30] The strength and magnitude of the association are difficult to determine from such studies because of possible confounding factors, in particular the self selection of "fitter" individuals into the high physical activity groups, and because of considerable variation between studies in the definitions of physical activity. In a follow-up study of college alumni, vigorous exercise was protective against the development of hypertension in later life.[31] Controlled studies of exercise training programmes have generally used regimens with a high energy expenditure. Fagard,[30] in a review of 36 studies in both hypertensive and normotensive individuals, reported that the average intensity of training varied between 50% and 85% of maximal exercise capacity (median 65%). The training consisted mainly of walking, running, jogging or bicycling.

The pooled analysis of the results of these studies is shown in Table 6.7 and is the blood pressure response to the programme after adjustment for control observations and grouped by the pretraining blood pressures as normotensive, borderline hypertensive, and hypertensive. Significant reductions in both systolic and diastolic blood pressure were observed in all three groups. The blood pressure lowering effect of exercise was more pronounced at higher baseline pressures with reductions of an average of 10/8 mmHg in hypertensives, 6/7 mmHg in borderline hypertensives, and 3/3 mmHg in normotensives. The results were independent of age and

Table 6.7   The training induced changes in blood pressure and 95% confidence limits in various groups of subjects, classified according to World Health Organisation (WHO) criteria

WHO classification	Trained groups (n)	Systolic mean	Weighted net change in blood pressure (mmHg) (95% CI)	Diastolic mean	(95% CI)
Normotension	27	−3·2	(−5·4 to −0·9)	−3·1	(−4·5 to −1·7)
Borderline hypertension	7	−6·2	(−9·3 to −3·2)	−6·8	(−10·8 to −2·8)
Hypertension	14	−9·9	(−14·0 to −5·7)	−7·6	(−10·9 to −4·3)

weight loss. Attempts to identify optimal training programmes from the results of these and other studies have not been successful and it remains unclear whether prolonged low intensity exercise or short bursts of high or moderate intensity confer the greatest benefits. As a general guideline, the level and type of exercise prescribed should be appropriate for the individual's condition and circumstances but should be at a level to exceed 50% of maximal exercise capacity, for example brisk walking five times a week for 30 minutes or jogging for 30 minutes three times a week. β-blockers may be contraindicated in the exercising patient because of their unfavourable effects on sustained submaximal exercise. The long term effects of physical exercise on blood pressure are not well established although there is some limited evidence for a favourable influence on left ventricular hypertrophy.[32]

Physical exercise also confers benefits on other CVD risk factors which are often present in hypertensive patients. Weight reduction and an increase in HDL cholesterol are well established effects.[33] The biological benefits of physical exercise support the well documented inverse association between physical activity and CHD.[34] Recent studies in UK populations have also shown the protective effects of exercise on stroke risk.[35, 36] The level of physical activity required to halve the stroke risk in one study was engaging in sporting activities at least once a week.[35] In the United Kingdom, with generally low levels of exercise and high levels of sedentary occupations, the population attributable risk of physical inactivity for CHD and stroke may be high and hence the potential benefit of increased exercise considerable. The adverse effects of exercise have not been determined in the long term but may include osteoarthritis and repetitive strain injuries. Conversely, osteoporosis may be prevented.

Alcohol Consumption

Many studies have consistently described a relationship between alcohol consumption and blood pressure.[37] In some studies the relationship was linear across the entire range of alcohol consumption, while other studies have suggested a threshold effect of around three units a day. J curves have also been described, perhaps as a result of the inclusion of previously heavy drinkers in the non-drinking group. In the large Kaiser Permanente Study of 80,000 men and women aged 15–79 years, systolic pressure increased by 1 mmHg for each daily unit of alcohol.[38] The pressor effect of alcohol appears to be due to ethanol as it has been found irrespective of whether the alcohol consumed is wine, beer or spirits. Randomised controlled studies varying the intake of alcohol consumption have confirmed the effects of alcohol on increasing blood pressure both in normotensive and hypertensive men.[39, 40]

Recommendations on optimal intakes for the control of blood pressure also need to take account of the considerable evidence on alcohol intake and mortality. Studies have shown J or U shaped relationships suggesting that intakes of 1–2 units daily are associated with the lowest CHD risks[41] while in some studies inverse associations have been reported for increasing alcohol consumption and decreased CHD risk, at least in men.[42, 43] The relationship between alcohol consumption and stroke is less well established. Modest alcohol consumption has been reported to increase the risk of haemorrhagic stroke,[44-46] while for ischaemic strokes J shape, inverse associations and negative associations have been reported.[45-47] Recommendations on alcohol consumption must also take account of any increased risk in non-cardiovascular mortality and social and psychological problems which may be associated with high intakes. In a US population, the overall mortality risk associated with different amounts of alcohol consumption was optimal at 1–2 drinks per day for men and at intakes less than this but more than once a month for women. Men consuming more than six drinks a day had a relative risk of 1·3 compared with those who never drank while women drinking this amount had an excess risk of 2·2 compared with non-drinkers, in part reflecting the added risk of breast cancer for women drinkers, a finding confirmed in other studies.[46]

In summary, it is likely that excess alcohol consumption, more than six drinks daily, does more harm than good since the beneficial effects on CHD may be outweighed by adverse effects on other causes of death, especially in women. For any individual, the risks and benefits of high alcohol intake depend on the absolute risks of different causes of mortality. At present the evidence continues to support recommendations of 1–2 drinks daily as the optimum intake, at least in the young. Hypertensive patients, however, are older and at a greater risk of CHD. In treated hypertensives there is evidence that the reduction in CHD and stroke compensates for the increase in non-circulatory deaths, at least for 3–4 drinks a day in men.[48]

Sodium reduction

Evidence for a relationship between sodium and blood pressure has been provided by studies between populations, within populations and from randomised trials of sodium reduction. There is general agreement that sodium influences blood pressure, but less agreement on the magnitude of the relationship from individual studies. Problems in the accurate estimation of sodium from a single 24 hour measurement means that estimates of effect are likely to be underestimated (regression dilution bias). Several studies and pooled overviews of data have estimated an increase of 4–5 mmHg systolic and 2 mmHg diastolic for every 100 mmol increase of sodium in both between population and within population studies.[49-51] The effect of sodium on blood pressure increases with age and with level of blood pressure; for example, at 60–69 years an increase of 100 mmol of sodium is associated with a 10 mmHg rise in systolic blood pressure and for persons of this age on the 95th centile of the blood pressure distribution, there is an associated 15 mmHg increase in systolic blood pressure.[49]

Overviews of randomised controlled trials of reducing dietary salt have supported these predictions.[52, 53] A median reduction of 74 mmol sodium was associated with an average 4·9 mmHg systolic fall in studies in hypertensive subjects and an average 1·7 mmHg fall in normotensive subjects. These data confirm that hypertensives and in particular older hypertensives should be encouraged to restrict their salt intake. Sodium restriction may also be useful in the management of patients with borderline hypertension. In the Trials of Hypertension Prevention (TOPH) in middle aged people with a high normal blood pressure (DBP 80–89 mmHg), a reduction of 56 mmol of sodium was observed in patients randomised to the sodium reduction group and associated with a small fall of 1·7 mmHg systolic compared with the control group whose sodium intakes did not alter.[54]

Weight control

Cross-sectional studies have shown a strong relationship between body weight and blood pressure.[55-57] The INTERSALT Study found that for a given average height, a 10 kg difference in body weight was associated with a 3 mmHg difference in systolic blood pressure and a 2·2 mmHg difference in diastolic pressure.[57] Body weight in adolescence is a strong predictor of blood pressure in later life and may explain blood pressure tracking.[58] Intervention trials have shown that with reduction of calorie intake, the blood pressure decreases within a few weeks and this is maintained over several months.[59] This reduction is independent of reduced sodium intake and increased physical activity. The blood pressure reduction per kilogram of weight loss is greater for hypertensive subjects (4 mmHg systolic) compared with normotensives (1·2 mmHg systolic).[60] Weight loss in addition to drug treatment has also been shown to be more effective than drug treatment alone in obese hypertensives.[61]

In the TOPH Trial of the prevention of primary hypertension, weight reduction was the most effective of the three strategies tested for reducing blood pressure in subjects with high normal pressures (DBP 80–89 mmHg). A fall in weight of 6 kg over a six month period was associated with a 3 mmHg systolic difference in blood pressure adjusted for the fall in the control blood pressure.[54] Weight loss in combination with a sodium restriction diet and reduced alcohol consumption has also been shown to slow the rate of rise in blood pressure in patients with well controlled blood pressures taken off drug treatment.[62] Although body weight can be reduced short term, it is difficult to maintain the weight loss over time and considerable encouragement may be required in the maintenance of weight loss. Psychological factors may play a role in obesity and counselling of the obese patient may be required to assist weight loss programmes. As with physical activity, weight loss also favourably influences other CVD risk factors including lipids, glucose intolerance and diabetes.

Cost effectiveness and drug comparisons

The key economic issue is the level of blood pressure at which antihypertensive treatment becomes "affordable". This relates to the absolute size of the risk associated with a particular level of pressure (measured for any population by the stroke, coronary heart disease rate, and congestive heart failure rate), the magnitude of the benefit derived from antihypertensive treatment, the costs of antihypertensive treatment including detection, evaluation and management, and the consequences (economic and quality of life) of not treating. Cost effectiveness analyses of the treatment of hypertension have shown that the gains in cost effectiveness are greatest where absolute risk is increased, for example at higher levels of blood pressure (DBP of 100+), at older ages, and when other risk factors are present.[63a]

Cost effectiveness ratios for age groups over 60 are not available for most studies but are likely to be even more favourable due to the increase in absolute risk. Assuming that all treatments produce an equal benefit on stroke reduction (an assumption which, as discussed above, has not yet been substantiated in randomised controlled trials), then the most cost effective drugs are the cheapest, currently the diuretics. Costs of antihypertensive treatment impact on individuals as well as policy and treatment cost has been shown to contribute to poor compliance and poor hypertension control. Other opportunities for cost containment in hypertension management include a rational use of costly investigations such as ambulatory blood pressure monitoring and echocardiograms, until the benefit of the routine use of such techniques has been established.

The impact of different antihypertensive treatments on quality of life should also be considered in treatment recommendations. Although quality of life considerations are important there are methodological concerns about the adjustment of life expectancy by quality of life (Quality Adjusted

133

Life Year, QALY). Arbitrary values have been used to describe the quality of life resulting from side effects of treatment, after a stroke or myocardial infarction. Cost effectiveness ratios are extremely sensitive to these values and even minor variations cancel the life expectancy gains from treatment. The lack of robustness of the methodology suggests that the results of costs per QALY analyses for hypertension should be treated with caution.

The actual magnitude of cost effectiveness ratios for hypertension treatment varies considerably between studies since widely different estimates of benefit have been used and have not included all trial results. Cost effectiveness analyses have underestimated the potential benefit from the treatment of the elderly by exclusion of elderly people and their ability to benefit in the models. Moreover, antihypertensive treatment may also improve other common conditions in the elderly, such as heart failure and vascular dementia.

Certain categories of antihypertensive drugs are only now being fully evaluated in randomised control trials with morbidity and mortality as outcomes. Short acting dihydropyridines do not appear to be appropriate postmyocardial infarction and it has been suggested that they may be associated with an excess of myocardial infarction in hypertensive subjects.[63b] Additional concern arose from a suggestion that there was an excess of cancer deaths in patients treated with all classes of calcium channel blocker for hypertension.[63c] However, the STONE Trial,[63d] the Boston Collaborative Drug Surveillance Program,[63e] and a large pharmacoepidemiological investigation[63f] have failed to confirm any cancer association or increased infarction risk in patients treated with these drugs.

Optimal levels of treated blood pressure

Epidemiological data in predominantly middle aged populations show a continuous positive relationship between blood pressure level and cardiovascular risk.[64] As a consequence it would appear that the goal of antihypertensive treatment should be to lower blood pressure as far as possible, but two factors appear to refute this. First, there is a popular misconception that blood pressure levels below the cutpoints used to define hypertension are "normal" and therefore safe. Second, and more seriously, is the data showing that when CHD mortality is plotted against treated diastolic blood pressure, an increase at lower pressure levels is observed: the so-called J curve phenomenon.[65] Similar relationships do not appear to occur for stroke or for treated systolic pressure and CHD.[66, 67] As both CHD and stroke are important outcomes in hypertensive patients, the physician is faced with the dilemma of whether to aim for maximal blood pressure lowering or to treat with caution.

The main concern is whether the J shape relationships observed for treated diastolic pressure and CHD represent an adverse effect of blood pressure lowering by drug treatment or some other association reflected by a low blood pressure, for example a poor myocardial function associated with a poor survival.[68]

The strongest evidence against a causal relationship between treatment, low pressure, and CHD mortality is the existence of similar relationships in patients whose "treatment" was placebo or who were randomised to the control group in a clinical trial. The Hypertension in Elderly Patients in Primary Care Trial found an increased CHD rate for the lowest diastolic pressures during the trial (less than 80 mmHg) in both actively treated patients and the untreated controls.[69] The trial of the European Working Party on High Blood Pressure in the Elderly (EWPHE) showed an increased mortality in the lowest strata of the treated diastolic blood pressure distribution.[70] The same phenomenon was observed for patients on placebo and for non-cardiovascular mortality. It is likely that in the elderly hypertensives, such as in the EWPHE Trial, the association between low blood pressure levels and mortality reflected deteriorating health.

It has been suggested that the adverse effect of a treated low diastolic pressure is observed only in patients with ischaemia, although the studies are not consistent in this finding. The SHEP Trial provided reassurance that low diastolic pressures can be safely reduced in patients with existing CHD.[22] In actively treated patients the reductions in systolic pressures from an average of 171 mmHg to 142 mmHg, accompanied by a lowering of diastolic pressure from 77 mmHg to 68 mmHg, were associated with a significant 27% reduction in myocardial infarction. Sixty percent of patients had baseline ECG abnormalities and in these the reduction in CHD events was 31%. It must be remembered, however, that the mean blood pressure of subjects with isolated systolic hypertension was high.

In conclusion, it would appear reasonable to lower diastolic pressures to below 85 mmHg. This gives maximum benefit for stroke reduction, while for myocardial infarction the rate is reduced compared to pressures over 100 mmHg. On balance, we consider that the J shaped curve is likely to be a consequence and not a cause of CHD. Systolic pressure in middle aged fit hypertensive patients should be lowered to below 125 mmHg since there is no indication of any adverse effects of so doing, although this may prove difficult or take a long time in patients with very high levels of untreated pressure. There may, however, be subsets of patients in whom the effects of blood pressure lowering are uncertain, such as the very frail elderly or those with markedly reduced LV function. Rapid reductions in blood pressure should probably be avoided. In particular, a large and sudden fall in pressure unrelated to treatment may predict a poor prognosis.

How far the diastolic blood pressure should be lowered below 85 mmHg is unclear. In most studies the target diastolic blood pressure has been below 90 mmHg and little is known about outcome with treated pressures below 80 mmHg. Although the SHEP Trial provides evidence that in the elderly diastolic pressures may be safely lowered to below 70 mmHg, these low diastolic pressures were in the presence of raised systolic pressures and all were below 90 mmHg at the start of the trial. When systolic pressure is not high we do not know the optimal levels to which we can reduce diastolic blood pressure.

Management strategies

All patients with hypertension should be given advice on the importance of weight loss if obese, dietary salt restriction, regular exercise, and moderation of alcohol intake. In patients with mildly elevated BP (systolic 140–159, diastolic 90–100 mmHg), this non-pharmacological treatment may suffice, though careful follow-up (twice yearly BP measurement) will be required.

The presence of mild hypertension, diastolic BP 100–105 mmg, should be confirmed by repeated measurements of a period of three months. With higher BP measurements and/or evidence of organ damage (e.g. left ventricular hypertrophy) this time interval may be shortened. There is evidence of benefits such as a reduced stroke incidence from treating hypertension when diastolic BP is greater than 95 mmHg and systolic BP greater than 160 mmHg. The benefits are seen particularly in older patients, patients with higher BP and those with other cardiovascular risk factors (e.g. diabetes or hypercholesterolaemia). Most trials with morbidity and mortality as outcomes have used diuretics and β-blockers, which are inexpensive but have recognised side effect profiles which sometimes limit their application. The risks and benefits from treatment with alternative drugs need to be determined. Even very elderly patients may benefit from BP reduction and a clinical trial to examine this is underway. The treatment of isolated systolic hypertension is also likely to be advantageous but further trials are under way to confirm that benefits of treatment exceed risks.

In patients treated for hypertension, the therapeutic aim is to lower diastolic BP to below 85 mmHg. Where possible systolic BP is best lowered to 125 mmHg. Even partial achievement of therapeutic targets appears to be important.

1 Pickering GW, Cranston WI, Peers MA. *The treatment of hypertension.* Springfield: Charles C. Thomas, 1961.
2 Swales JD. Guidelines on guidelines. *J Hypertens* 1993; **11**: 899–903.
3 Sever P, Beevers G, Bulpitt CJ *et al.* Management guidelines in essential hypertension: report of the second working party of the British Hypertension Society. *Br Med J* 1993; **306**: 983–7.
4 The Fifth Report of the Joint National Committee on Detection, Evaluation, and Treatment of High Blood Pressure. *Arch Intern Med* 1993; **153**: 154–83.
5 WHO/ISH. Guidelines for the management of mild hypertension: memorandum from a World Health Organization/International Society of Hypertension Meeting. *J Hypertens* 1993; **11**: 905–18.
6 Report by the Management Committee. The Australian Therapeutic Trial in Mild Hypertension. *Lancet* 1982; **i**: 1261–7.

7 Medical Research Council Working Party. MRC trial of treatment of mild hypertension: principle results. *Br Med J* 1985; **2**: 97–104.

8 Hypertension Detection and Follow-up Program Cooperative Group. Five-year findings of the Hypertension Detection and Follow-up Program I. Reduction in mortality in persons with high blood pressure, including mild hypertension. *JAMA* 1979; **242**: 2562–71.

9 Isles CG, Brown JJ, Lever AF, Murray GD. What clinical trials have taught us. In: Bühler FR and Laragh JH. eds. *Handbook of hypertension. The management of hypertension.* Amsterdam: Elsevier, 1990, Ch 13.

10 Collins R, Peto R, MacMahon S *et al.* Blood pressure, stroke and coronary heart disease. *Lancet* 1990; **335**: 827–38.

11 Miall WE, Greenberg G. *Mild hypertension: is there pressure to treat?* Cambridge: Cambridge University Press, 1987.

12 Amery A, Staessen J, Fagard R, van Hoof R. Hypertension in the elderly. In: Bühler FR and Laragh JH. eds. *Handbook of hypertension. The management of hypertension.* Amsterdam: Elsevier, 1990, Ch. 13.

13 Management Committee. Treatment of mild hypertension in the elderly. *Med J Aust* 1981; **ii**: 398–402.

14 Amery A, Birkenhäger WH, Brixko P *et al.* Mortality and morbidity results from the European Working Party on High Blood Pressure in the Elderly Trial. *Lancet* 1985; **i**: 1349–54.

15 Coope J, Warrender TS. Randomised trial of treatment of hypertension in elderly patients in primary care. *Br Med J* 1986; **293**: 1145–51.

16 Dahlof B, Lindholm LH, Hanson L, Schersten B, Ekbom T, Wester P-O. Morbidity and mortality in the Swedish Trial in Old Patients with Hypertension (STOP Hypertension). *Lancet* 1991; **338**: 1281–5.

17 Medical Research Council Working Party. MRC trial of treatment of hypertension in older adults: principle results. *Br Med J* 1992; **304**: 405–12

18a Beard K, Bulpitt C, Mascie-Taylor H, O'Malley K, Sever P, Webb S. Management of elderly patients with sustained hypertension. *Br Med J* 1992; **304**: 412–16.

18b Prospective Studies Collaboration. Cholesterol, diastolic blood pressure and stroke: 13,000 strokes in 450,000 people in 45 prospective cohorts. *Lancet* 1995; **346**: 1647–53.

19 Fletcher AE, on behalf of EWPHE. Adverse treatment effects in the trial of the European Working Party on High Blood Pressure in the Elderly. *Am J Med* 1991; **90**: 42–4.

20 Bulpitt CJ, Fletcher AE. Aging, blood pressure and mortality. *J Hypertens* 1992; **10**: S45–S49.

21 Bulpitt CJ, Fletcher AE, Amery A *et al.* The Hypertension in the Very Elderly Trial (HYVET): Rationale, methodology and comparison with previous trials. *Drugs Ageing* 1994; **5**: 171–83.

22 SHEP Cooperative Research Group. Prevention of stroke by antihypertensive drug treatment in older persons with isolated systolic hypertension. *JAMA* 1991; **265**: 3255–64.

23 Gurland BJ, Teresi J, McFate Smith W, Black D, Hughes G, Edlavitch S. Effects of treatment for isolated systolic hypertension on cognitive status and depression in the elderly. *J Am Geriatr Soc* 1988; **36**: 1015–22.

24 Staessen J, Bert P, Bulpitt CJ *et al.* Nitrendpine in older patients with isolated systolic hypertension: second progress report on the SYST-EUR trial. *J Hum Hypertens* 1993; **7**: 265–71.

25 Rose GA. Strategy of prevention: lessons from cardiovascular disease. *Br Med J* 1981; **282**: 1847–51.

26 Department of Health. *Health of the nation.* London: HMSO, 1992.

27 Nissinen A, Tuomilheto J, Enlund H, Kottke TE. Costs and benefits of community programmes for the control of hypertension. *J Hum Hypertens* 1992; **6**: 473–9.

28 Staessen J, Bulpitt CJ, Fagard R, Joosens KV, Lijnen P, Amery A. Salt intake and blood pressure in the general population: a controlled intervention trial in two towns. *J Hypertens* 1988; **6**: 965–73.

29 Forte JG, Miguel JMP, Miguel MJP, de Padua F, Rose G. Salt and blood pressure: a community trial. *J Hum Hypertens* 1989; **3**: 179–84.

30 Fagard RH. Physical fitness and blood pressure. *J Hypertens* 1993; **11** (Suppl 5): S47–

S52.

31 Paffenbarger RS, Wing AL, Hyde RT, Jung DL. Physical activity and incidence of hypertension in college alumni. *Am J Epidemiol* 1983; **117**: 245–57.

32 Jennings GL, Deakin G, Dewar E, Laufer E, Nelson L. Exercise, cardiovascular disease and blood pressure. *Clin Exp Hypertens* 1989; **11**: 1035–52.

33 Wood PD, Stefanick MI, Williams PT, Haskell WI. The effects on plasma lipoproteins of a prudent weight reducing diet with or without exercise in overweight men and women. *N Engl J Med* 1991; **325**: 461–6.

34 Powell KE, Thompson PD, Caspersen CJ, Kendrick JS. Physical activity and the incidence of coronary disease. *Annu Rev Public Health* 1987; **8**: 253–87.

35 Wannamethee G, Shaper AG. Physical activity and stroke in middle aged men. *Br Med J* 1992; **304**: 587–601.

36 Shinton R, Sagar G. Lifelong exercise and stroke. *Br Med J* 1993; **307**: 231–4.

37 World Hypertension League. Alcohol and hypertension: implications for management. *WHO Bulletin* 1991; **69**(4): 377–82.

38 Klatsky AL, Friedman GD, Spiegelaub AB, Gerard MJ. Alcohol consumption and blood pressure: Kaiser-Permanente Multiphasic Health Examination data. *N Engl J Med* 1977; **296**: 1194–200.

39 Puddey IB, Beilin LJ, Vandongen R, Rouse IL, Rogers P. Evidence for a direct effect of alcohol consumption on blood pressure in normotensive man – a randomised controlled trial. *Hypertension* 1985; **7**: 707–13.

40 Puddey IB, Beilin LJ, Vandongen R. Regular alcohol use raises blood pressure in treated hypertensive subjects – a randomized controlled trial. *Lancet* 1987; **i**: 647–51.

41 Marmot B, Brunner E. Alcohol and cardiovascular disease: the status of the U shaped curve. *Br Med J* 1991; **303**: 565–8.

42 Klatsky AL, Armstrong MA, Friedman GD. Alcohol and mortality. *Ann Intern Med* 1992; **117**: 646–54.

43 Rim EB, Giovannucci EL, Willett WC *et al.* Prospective study of alcohol consumption and risk of coronary disease in men. *Lancet* 1991; **338**: 464–8.

44 Klatsky AL, Armstrong MA, Friedman GD. Risk of cardiovascular mortality in alcohol drinkers, ex drinkers and non drinkers. *Am J Cardiol* 1990; **66**: 1237–42.

45 Donahue RP, Abbott RD, Reed DM, Yano K. Alcohol and haemorrhagic stroke. The Honolulu Heart Program. *JAMA* 1986; **255**: 2311–14.

46 Stampfer MJ, Colditz GA, Willett WC, Speizer FE, Hennekens CH. A prospective study of moderate alcohol consumption and the risk of coronary disease and stroke in women. *N Engl J Med* 1988; **319**: 267–73.

47 Gorelick PB, Rodin MB, Lamgenberg P, Hier DB, Costigan J. Weekly alcohol consumption, cigarette smoking and the risk of ischaemic stroke: results of a case control study at three urban medical centers in Chicago, Illinois. *Neurology* 1989; **39**: 339–43.

48 Palmer AJ, Fletcher AE, Bulpitt CJ *et al.* Alcohol intake and cardiovascular mortality in hypertensive patients: a report from the Department of Health Hypertension Care Computing Project (DHCCP). *J Hypertens* 1995; **12**: 957–64.

49 Law MR, Frost CD, Wald NJ. By how much does dietary salt reduction lower blood pressure? I Analysis of observational data among populations. *Br Med J* 1991; **312**: 811–15.

50 Law MR, Frost CD, Wald NJ. By how much does dietary salt reduction lower blood pressure? II Analysis of observational data within populations. *Br Med J* 1991; **312**: 815–18.

51 Elliott P. Observational studies on salt and blood pressure. *Hypertension* 1991; **17**: 13–18.

52 Law MR, Frost CD, Wald NJ. By how much does dietary salt reduction lower blood pressure? III Analysis of trials of sodium reduction. *Br Med J* 1991; **312**: 819–24.

53 Cutler J, Follman D, Elliott P, Suh I. An overview of randomised trials of sodium reduction and blood pressure. *Hypertension* 1991; **17**: 127–33.

54 The Trials of Hypertension Prevention Collaborative Research Group. The effects of non pharmacologic interventions on blood pressure of persons with high normal levels. Results of the trials of hypertension prevention, Phase 1. *JAMA* 1992; **267**: 1213–20.

55 Stamler R, Stamler J, Riedlinger WF *et al.* Weight and blood pressure: findings in hypertension screening of 1 million Americans. *JAMA* 1978; **240**: 1607–10.

56 Chiang B, Perlman L, Epstein F. Overweight and hypertension: a review. *Circulation* 1969; **89**: 413–21.
57 Dyer AR, Elliott P. The INTERSALT study: relations of body mass index to blood pressure. *J Hum Hypertens* 1989; **3**: 299–308.
58 Worynarowska B, Mukherjee D, Roche AF, Siervogel RM. Blood pressure changes during adolescence and subsequent adult blood pressure level. *Hypertension* 1985; 7: 695–701.
59 Sims EAH, Berchtold P. Obesity and hypertension. Mechanisms and implications for management. *JAMA* 1982; 247: 49–52.
60 Schotte DE, Stunkard AJ. The effects of weight reduction on blood pressure in 301 obese patients. *Arch Intern Med* 1990; **150**: 1701–4.
61 Reisin E, Abel R, Modan M, Silverberg DS, Eliahou HE, Modan B. Effect of weight loss without salt restriction on the reduction of blood pressure in overweight hypertensive patients. *N Engl J Med* 1978; **298**: 1–6.
62 Blaufox MD, Langford HG, Oberman A, Hawkins CM, Wassertheil Smoller W, Cutler GR. Effect of dietary change on the return of hypertension after withdrawal of prolonged antihypertensive therapy. *J Hypertens* 1984; 2: 179–81.
63a Fletcher AE. *Economics of hypertension control.* Geneva: World Hypertension League, 1994.
63b Psaty BM, Heckbert BR, Keepsell TD *et al.* The risk of myocardial infarction associated with antihypertensive drug therapies. *JAMA* 1995; **274**: 620–5.
63c Pahor M, Guralnik JM, Ferruci L *et al.* Calcium channel blockade and incidence of cancer in aged populations. *Lancet* 1996; **348**: 493–7.
63d Gong L, Zhang W, Zhu Y *et al.* Shanghai Trial of Nifedipine in the Elderly (STONE). *J Hypertens* 1996; **14**: 1237–45.
63e Jick H, Jick S, Derby LE, Vasilakis C, Wald Myers M, Maier CR. Calcium channel blockers and risk of cancer. *Lancet* 1997; **349**: 525–8.
63f Bulpitt CJ, Palmer AJ, Beevers DG *et al.* Calcium channel blockers and cardiac mortality in the treatment of hypertension. A report from the DOH Hypertension Care Computing Project (DHCCP). *J Hum Hypertens* 1997; **11**: 205–11.
64 MacMahon S, Peto R, Cutler J *et al.* Blood pressure, stroke and coronary heart disease. Part 1 Prolonged differences in blood pressure: prospective observational studies corrected for the regression dilution bias. *Lancet* 1990; **335**: 765–74.
65 Cruickshank JM. Coronary flow reserve and the J curve relation between diastolic blood pressure and myocardial infarction. *Br Med J* 1988; **297**: 1227–30.
66 Waller PC, Isles CG, Lever AF *et al.* Does therapeutic reduction of blood pressure cause death from coronary heart disease? *J Hum Hypertens* 1988; 2: 7–10.
67 Fletcher A, Beevers DG, Bulpitt CJ *et al.* The relationship between a low treated blood pressure and IHD mortality. A report from the DHSS Hypertension Care Computing Project (DHCCP). *J Hum Hypertens* 1988; 2: 11–15.
68 Fletcher AE, Bulpitt CJ. How far should blood pressure be lowered? *N Engl J Med* 1992; **326**: 251–4.
69 Coope J, Warrender TS. Lowering blood pressure. *Lancet* 1987; **ii**: 518.
70 Staessen J, Bulpitt C, Clement D *et al.* The relationship between mortality and treated blood pressure in elderly patients with hypertension: report of the European Working Party on High Blood Pressure in the Elderly. *Br Med J* 1989; **298**: 1552–6.

7: Heart failure

NC DAVIDSON AND AD STRUTHERS

Introduction

Chronic heart failure is an extremely common clinical syndrome which is characterised by left ventricular dysfunction, fluid retention, limited exercise tolerance, and reduced life expectancy. The development of clinical symptoms and signs may be preceded by a prolonged period of asymptomatic cardiac dysfunction, during which the progression to heart failure may be delayed by drug treatment. Although major advances in our understanding of the pathophysiology of this disorder have resulted in a variety of new treatment options, the prognosis for a patient with heart failure remains poor. This chapter will assess the therapeutic implications of recent developments in the field and the prospects for further improvements in the immediate future.

In this context we will deal mainly with heart failure which is due to left ventricular systolic dysfunction although it should be recognised that abnormalities of diastolic filling frequently accompany systolic impairment and may contribute to the symptoms of breathlessness in patients with heart failure. Isolated diastolic dysfunction may rarely occur, especially in the presence of hypertensive left ventricular hypertrophy. At present, there are no established specific therapies for diastolic dysfunction.

Pathophysiology

The initial event in the development of heart failure is myocardial injury, caused by ischaemia, infection, toxins or mechanical stress, leading to a significant reduction in the mass of functional myocytes. This results in the activation of a range of homoeostatic mechanisms in the heart, the peripheral vasculature and the kidneys (Figure 7.1).

Damage to the myocardium causes a reduction in the volume of blood ejected from the left ventricle during systole and an increase in the end diastolic volume which, according to the Frank–Starling principle, would result in an increased stroke volume in a normal heart. This fall in cardiac output is accompanied by an increase in sympathetic tone[1] and stimulation of β-adrenergic receptors in the non-injured myocardium, resulting in

140

positive inotropic and chronotropic effects. A rise in ventricular wall stress during diastole causes induction of specific proto-oncogenes (c-fos and c-myc), which stimulate the synthesis of myofibrillar proteins, causing the viable areas of myocardium to increase in thickness;[2] the new tissue adopts the biochemical characteristics and superior energy efficiency of foetal myocardium. The net result of these changes is to limit the extent of ventricular dilation and reduce the energy expenditure of the failing heart.

Increased sympathetic activity and a fall in the renal perfusion pressure both stimulate the production of renin by juxtaglomerular cells in the kidney,[3] although it is uncertain whether this precedes the initiation of diuretic therapy. Renin catalyses the conversion of angiotensinogen to angiotensin I, which is then converted in vascular beds by angiotensin converting enzyme (ACE) to the potent vasoconstrictor angiotensin II. This stimulates adrenal production of aldosterone which causes retention of salt and water, increasing intravascular volume. Further increases in vascular tone are caused by vasopressin[4] and by the endothelins,[5] locally active potent vasoconstrictor peptides which are secreted from the vascular endothelium.

Recent evidence suggests that apoptosis, or programmed cell death, occurs in the cardiac myocytes of failing human hearts, particularly in idiopathic dilated cardiomyopathy[6] and this may be an important factor in the progression to heart failure. In contrast to cell necrosis, apoptosis is a closely regulated sequence of molecular and biochemical events which are energy dependent and genetically programmed. Characteristically apoptosis occurs in isolated cells with no associated inflammatory response. There are several potential stimuli for apoptosis in the failing heart, including nitric oxide, reactive oxygen species, cytokines, hypoxia, and mechanical stretch[7] but the relative importance of these stimuli is not known. This area of research is at an early stage but as our knowledge of the mechanisms of apoptosis in the failing human myocardium improves this may lead to important novel therapeutic strategies.

The degree of vasoconstriction and fluid retention in early heart failure is limited to some extent by counter-regulatory mechanisms. Decreased renal blood flow results in the release of prostaglandins which promote natriuresis and diuresis,[8] increased atrial pressures reduce sympathetic activity and stimulate secretion of atrial natriuretic peptide (ANP) which antagonises the renin–angiotensin–aldosterone system at three separate sites[9, 10] and inhibits the secretion of endothelins.[11] However, although the production of ANP increases with the progression of heart failure, there is evidence that its natriuretic properties are attenuated,[12] possibly due to receptor downregulation and reduced renal blood flow.[13]

In the early stages of heart failure the mechanical and neurohormonal compensatory mechanisms described above maintain the resting cardiac output at normal levels, although this may be at the expense of increased

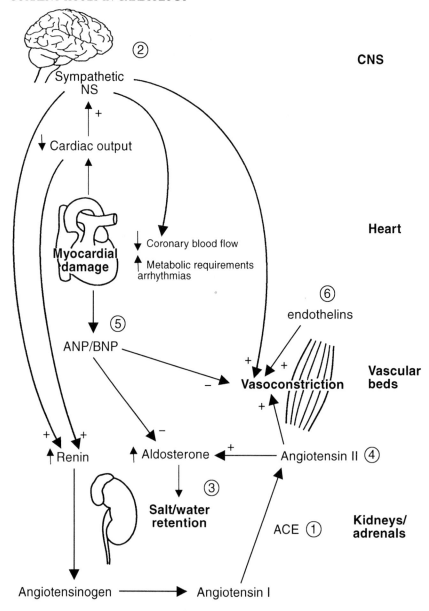

Fig 7.1 Neurohormonal mechanisms in heart failure. Numbers indicate the sites of action of drugs currently in clinical or experimental use in the treatment of heart failure: 1. ACE inhibitors; 2. β-blockers; 3. aldosterone antagonists; 4. angiotensin II receptor antagonists; 5. neutral endopeptidase inhibitors; 6. endothelin receptor antagonists.

pulmonary and systemic venous pressures. Peripheral vasoconstriction causes a rise in the afterload and therefore increases the stress on the ventricular wall, until ultimately the heart loses its ability to augment the stroke volume in response to increased end diastolic pressures. This causes myocardial thinning and necrosis with dilation of the ventricular cavity and may result in functional mitral regurgitation due to loss of support for the mitral valve annulus. Chronic stimulation of the sympathetic nervous system results in downregulation of cardiac β1-adrenoreceptors and a functional "uncoupling" of the remaining receptors such that their inotropic responses are reduced.[14]

The adverse effects of excessive neurohormonal activation are well documented. Increased activity of the cardiac sympathetic nerves results in higher metabolic requirements of the myocardium, reduced coronary blood flow and a lower threshold for arrhythmias; stimulation of α-adreno-receptors in the peripheral vasculature contributes to the profound vasoconstriction and decreased tissue perfusion observed in patients with heart failure[15] while high levels of circulating catecholamines may also be directly toxic to the myocardium.[16] Prolonged activation of the renin–angiotensin–aldosterone system has several potential adverse effects in addition to vasoconstriction. High levels of angiotensin II may cause myocardial necrosis[17] and acceleration of atheroma[18] while excessive aldosterone promotes urinary potassium and magnesium excretion with a resultant decrease in arrhythmia threshold.[19] In animal studies, aldosterone has also been shown to stimulate myocardial collagen deposition.[20]

Patients with heart failure have an extremely high mortality rate despite recent therapeutic advances. This is illustrated by the results of recent large trials shown in Table 7.1. Deaths occur either due to a progressive deterioration or, in many cases, suddenly and unexpectedly at an early stage of the disease process. The mechanism of the latter form of death is controversial but is likely to be distinct from that of deaths due to gradual deterioration.

Diagnosis

In the later stages of the disease the diagnosis of heart failure is relatively simple. The patient will usually have symptoms of exertional breathlessness and orthopnoea and on examination will have an elevated jugular venous pressure, gallop rhythm, pulmonary crepitations, hepatomegaly, and ankle oedema. The identification of patients with mild left ventricular dysfunction provides a greater challenge and several studies have demonstrated that clinical methods are insensitive in this situation.[21, 22] Many patients with significant impairment of systolic function will be asymptomatic or will have non-specific symptoms such as generalised weakness and lethargy and will have no signs of heart failure. Ideally, all patients with suspected left

Table 7.1 Major trials of angiotensin converting enzyme inhibitors in heart failure

Acronym	No. patients	Treatment period (mean)	Entry criteria	Drug	1° endpoint	No. deaths/no. randomised patients		p value
						Active treatment	Control	
CONSENSUS	253	6 months	NYHA IV	Enalapril	Survival	50/127 (39%)	68/126 (54%)	0·003
SOLVD Treatment	2569	3·5 years	Symptomatic LVEF ≤35%	Enalapril	Survival	452/1285 (35·2%)	510/1284 (39·7%)	0·0036
Prevention	4228	3 years	Asymptomatic LVEF ≤35%	Enalapril	Survival/ onset CHF	313/2111 (14·8%)	334/2111 (15·8%)	0·30
VHeFT II	804	2·5 years	NYHA II-III	Enalapril v ISDN/ hydralazine	Survival/ ex. tolerance	132/403 (32·7%) (enalapril)	153/401 (38·2%)	0·08

CHF = congestive heart failure; NYHA = New York Heart Association grading; LVEF = left ventricular ejection fraction; ISDN = isosorbide dinitrate ventricular dysfunction should be assessed by two-dimensional and Doppler echocardiography which will provide definitive information on ventricular contractility, in addition to important information on valvular function, allowing the detection of unsuspected aortic or mitral stenosis. Obviously such a policy would not be possible with the current level of provision of echocardiography services in the UK and it is possible that, as has recently been suggested, measurement of plasma levels of natriuretic peptides may in the future provide a useful screening test to decide which patients require further investigation.[23]

When left ventricular dysfunction has been confirmed, treatable underlying causes should be excluded. In the developed world the vast majority of cases will be due to ischaemic heart disease and this will nearly always be associated with electrocardiographic abnormalities. Other possible aetiologies to consider include haemochromatosis, alcohol, hyperthyroidism, phaeochromocytoma, and viral infections. Cardiac biopsy was previously performed in patients with suspected idiopathic dilated cardiomyopathy but this is no longer indicated since it has been demonstrated that these patients do not benefit from corticosteroid treatment.

Therapeutic goals

The basic therapeutic goals in heart failure are to postpone death and to improve the quality of life. One of the most important lessons of the past decade of heart failure research is that many current treatments have divergent effects on these two objectives and therefore it is sometimes necessary to decide for an individual patient whether prolongation of life or reduction of symptoms is more important. This decision should ideally be taken jointly by the doctor and the patient and depends upon the functional capacity of the patient, the presence of concurrent disease, and the possibility of future "curative" treatment, i.e. cardiac transplant. For a younger patient with ventricular dysfunction and normal exercise capacity, the slowing of the progression to heart failure and the prevention of lethal arrhythmias are extremely important, but for an older patient with severe dyspnoea a relatively minor symptomatic improvement may be very significant while an increase in longevity, with no associated functional improvement, would not necessarily be desirable.

Until recently the standard method for assessing a new treatment for heart failure was to study the acute haemodynamic changes produced by the drug. This is no longer appropriate in view of well documented examples of drugs which produce acute haemodynamic improvements but which increase mortality or make patients feel worse (Table 7.2). Chronic changes in haemodynamic parameters such as left ventricular ejection fraction (LVEF) appear to correlate with subsequent mortality[24] and have been used as a surrogate measurement for this. The only totally objective

Table 7.2 Effects of drug treatment on mortality, symptoms, and haemodynamic indices in patients with heart failure

Drug class	Mortality	Symptoms	Haemodynamic indices	
			Acute	Chronic
Diuretics	?	+ +	+ +	+ / −
ACE inhibitors	+ +	+	+ +	+ +
Digoxin	0	+	+	+
β-blockers	+	+	−	+ +
Nitrates	?	+	+ +	+
Calcium antagonists				
Old	?	−	−	−
New	0	+	+	+
Flosequinan	−	+	+	+
Prazosin	0	+ / −	+	+ / −
Phosphodiesterase inhibitors	−	+	+ +	+ / −

+ + large benefit; + small benefit; + / − equivocal effect; 0 neutral effect; ? unknown

endpoint is survival and this has been used extensively in recent large clinical trials but there remains a need for methods which assess possible changes in the functional status of the patient. Many exercise testing protocols have been developed and it is now accepted that those protocols which involve submaximal rather than maximal exercise are more representative of the daily activities of the patient. The use of questionnaires to measure quality of life is increasing but the validation of such methods remains problematic.

Treatment

General principles

Prior to the initiation of drug treatment for heart failure the current therapy of the patient should be assessed to determine whether it includes any drugs which may exacerbate the problem. These include non-steroidal anti-inflammatory drugs and corticosteroids which can aggravate fluid retention and class I antiarrhythmic agents which can cause reversible myocardial depression. If possible, any such medication should be reduced or stopped before starting further treatment. Patient education is an extremely important part of treatment and time spent explaining the nature of the problem, preferably with diagrams and printed instructions, is likely to be rewarded later by improved compliance. All patients with heart failure should be advised to reduce their dietary sodium intake and certainly to add no salt to their food; in a few cases this alone will be sufficient to alleviate fluid retention. The short life expectancy of patients with established heart failure has meant that little attention has been given to the modification of risk factors such as smoking and hyperlipidaemia but as patients are treated at an earlier stage of the disease and mortality is decreased by therapeutic interventions, secondary prevention of athero-matous disease will assume greater importance.

Exercise training

In the past, patients with heart failure were advised to limit their activities but this situation is now reversed as the evidence for beneficial effects of regular exercise is accumulating. The size, structure and function of skeletal muscle are all abnormal in these patients and several small studies have suggested that the muscle changes can be reversed with exercise training.[25] Two recent studies using supervised training programmes in patients with symptomatic heart failure have demonstrated significant improvements in exercise time and peak oxygen consumption.[26, 27] Whether this translates into a worthwhile symptomatic or survival benefit for the patient and whether unsupervised exercise is beneficial remains uncertain but further studies will clarify the issue. In the meantime patients with heart failure should be encouraged to remain active and to exercise on a regular basis.

Diuretics

Diuretics remain a first line treatment for patients with established heart failure. Their ability to improve symptoms is undisputed but it is unlikely that their effect, when prescribed alone, on disease progression and survival will ever be formally assessed in a large trial. These agents inhibit the reabsorption of sodium and chloride at specific sites in the renal tubule and alleviate sodium retention, thereby reducing left ventricular wall stress.

Diuretics can be broadly divided according to their site of action: thiazides and potassium sparing diuretics act on the distal convoluted tubule; frusemide and bumetanide act on the loop of Henle. The former group increase the fractional excretion of sodium by only 5–10% and are ineffective at low glomerular filtration rates (<30 ml/min). Loop diuretics are more potent, increasing fractional excretion of sodium by up to 25% and retaining their activity until the GFR drops below 5 ml/min. Treatment with loop and especially thiazide diuretics occasionally results in significant hypokalaemia and serum potassium should routinely be checked after starting or increasing the dose of a diuretic. There has been a debate over the need for the addition of a potassium sparing diuretic, such as amiloride or triamterene. Some claimed that this was only necessary if hypokalaemia developed, if the patient had a history of arrhythmias or was taking digoxin (which is more likely to produce toxicity in the presence of hypokalaemia). This debate has been defused by the use of ACE inhibitors in most patients with heart failure on diuretic therapy.

In mild heart failure, when renal function is preserved, a thiazide diuretic is often sufficient to alleviate fluid retention although as the disease progresses a loop diuretic will provide greater symptomatic benefit at the

147

cost of hyponatraemia and increased activation of the renin–angiotensin system. If appropriate, patients should be encouraged to manipulate their own diuretic dosage according to their daily weight, the presence of oedema and symptoms of breathlessness. Patients with normal glomerular filtration rates usually respond adequately to a daily dose of 40 mg of frusemide per day or its equivalent but with advanced heart failure diuretic resistance is common. It has been suggested that this is partly due to diminished absorption of the oral preparation from the oedematous intestinal mucosa but pharmacokinetic data indicate that adequate doses of loop diuretics are delivered to the kidneys in patients with heart failure who are resistant to diuretics.[28] It seems more likely that pharmacodynamic factors such as increased reabsorption of solute from the distal nephron are responsible for the impaired drug effect. This is the rationale for the cautious use of segmental nephron blockade with the combination of a loop diuretic and a thiazide diuretic in patients with persistent oedema.

ACE inhibitors

Angiotensin converting enzyme (ACE) inhibitors are now well established as a treatment for patients with left ventricular dysfunction regardless of symptoms. This is based on the results of several large multicentre trials which have used mortality as the primary endpoint. CONSENSUS[29] and the SOLVD Treatment Trial[30] have demonstrated improved survival in patients with symptomatic heart failure and impaired left ventricular function treated with ACE inhibitors as compared to placebo. VHeFT II[31] used a similar patient group and demonstrated that ACE inhibitors produced mortality benefits over and above another vasodilator regime of isosorbide dinitrate and hydralazine. In the SOLVD Prevention Trial the study group consisted of patients with left ventricular dysfunction but no symptoms of heart failure.[32] The results showed a non-significant reduction in mortality but a significant reduction in hospitalisations or pharmacological treatment for heart failure in those patients who received an ACE inhibitor. It is likely that the degree of benefit attributed to ACE inhibitors in these trials has been underestimated as they were all analysed on an "intention to treat" basis and in the SOLVD Treatment Trial, for example, 30% of the patients in the placebo group were treated with open label ACE inhibitors at the end of the study.

The mechanisms of action of ACE inhibitors remain controversial. Angiotensin converting enzyme is a non-specific enzyme which facilitates the degradation of several peptides, including bradykinin and encephalins, in addition to the conversion of angiotensin I to angiotensin II. The findings of the VHeFT II Study, which demonstrated that enalapril produced a greater reduction in mortality than an isosorbide dinitrate/hydralazine combination, suggest that ACE inhibitors do not simply act as vasodilators. It is possible that part of the benefit attributable to these agents is due to potentiation of the activity of endogenous bradykinin, which is a potent vasodilator and modulator of vascular growth.

The most common side effects associated with ACE inhibitors are cough, which is caused by increased concentrations of kinins in the pulmonary vasculature, and symptomatic hypotension. Both are related to the mechanism of action of the drug and are likely to occur with all drugs in the class, while rarer idiosyncratic reactions such as rash and neutropenia may be alleviated by changing to a different ACE inhibitor. First dose and subsequent hypotension are most common in patients who are on high doses of diuretics and those with hyponatraemia, both of which are associated with activation of the renin–angiotensin system. This can usually be avoided by the reduction or omission of diuretics for 48 hours prior to the first dose of an ACE inhibitor.

There are several important practical issues regarding treatment of heart failure with an ACE inhibitor which are as yet unresolved. Firstly, it should be noted that the patient groups used in the above studies are not necessarily representative of patients with heart failure in the general population, especially with regard to age and sex. In SOLVD the average age was 59 years and 88% of the patients were men. VHeFT II studied only male patients, with an average age of 60·5 years. Conversely, a general practice based study of diuretic treated patients in the UK found that the median age of diagnosis of heart failure was 71 years in men and 76 years in women.[21] Further studies are required to assess whether the beneficial effects of ACE inhibitors are evident in elderly and female patients with heart failure.

Secondly, it is uncertain whether a diuretic is a necessary adjunct to treatment with an ACE inhibitor in all patients with heart failure. The SOLVD Prevention Trial, in which all patients were asymptomatic and therefore were not taking a diuretic, demonstrated a reduction in progression to heart failure in patients treated with enalapril. However, in several small studies comparisons of the effects of diuretic therapy alone and an ACE inhibitor alone in patients with symptomatic heart failure have demonstrated symptomatic and haemodynamic benefits in the diuretic group.[33,34] Therefore current evidence suggests that although ACE inhibitors may be beneficial when prescribed alone in patients with asymptomatic left ventricular dysfunction, they should be given in conjunction with a diuretic in patients with symptomatic heart failure.

Thirdly, are the beneficial effects of ACE inhibitors drug specific or due to a class effect? Although the large mortality trials in heart failure described above have all used enalapril, there is evidence from the post-MI studies SAVE,[35] AIRE[36] and GISSI-3[37] that treatment with captopril, ramipril and lisinopril is associated with a reduced mortality. This suggests that pharmacokinetic differences between ACE inhibitors are not of major importance and that the benefits observed are due to a class effect. Further trials involving direct comparisons of the drugs would be required to answer this question fully.

Lastly, which is the correct dose of ACE inhibitor for patients with ventricular dysfunction and/or heart failure? There is a discrepancy between the high dosages that have been used in clinical trials and the low doses which are generally used in clinical practice. Current evidence suggests that the efficacy of ACE inhibitors increases with dose[38, 39] and it is notable that in both the SOLVD and VHeFT II studies a dose of 10 mg twice daily of enalapril was used. A community based study, NETWORK, compared the effects of three doses of enalapril on mortality, hospitalisation rate and the need for medical intervention over a six month period.[40] The relative risk of a primary event in the group treated with enalapril 10 mg bd compared to those treated with 2·5 mg bd was 1·14 but the confidence intervals were wide (0·83–1·57) and so little can be deduced from the results of this study. The ongoing ATLAS Trial is a large scale international comparison of low dose (5 mg daily) versus high dose (35 mg daily) of lisinopril with the primary endpoint of mortality. This trial will have greater statistical power than NETWORK and follow-up will be completed by the end of 1997. Therefore, until the results of ATLAS are available, based on the results of the mortality studies to date, patients with heart failure should be treated with the maximum tolerated dose of ACE inhibitor up to the equivalent of 20 mg daily of enalapril. In order to achieve these higher doses and to avoid symptomatic hypotension or a deterioration in renal function, it may be necessary to reduce the dose of diuretic.

Calcium channel antagonists

The use of calcium channel antagonists in chronic heart failure was prompted initially by their potent systemic vasodilatory properties and the theoretical benefit of a reduction of the myocardial intracellular calcium overload which has been observed in failing hearts. Despite this, haemodynamic and clinical deteriorations have been reported in patients with heart failure during long term and short term treatment with verapamil, diltiazem and nifedipine.[41] This effect was attributed to a negative inotropic effect caused by an excessive reduction of the influx of calcium into myocardial cells. However, the symptomatic hypotension produced by these agents causes significant neurohormonal activation and it is likely that this is a major factor in their detrimental effects. The effect of the newer sustained release preparations of these calcium antagonists in patients with ventricular dysfunction remains uncertain.

Recognition of the key role of neuroendocrine activity in the progression of heart failure has led to optimism regarding the therapeutic potential of newer calcium channel antagonists such as felodipine and amlodipine, which might suppress rather than stimulate neurohormonal activity. These agents have greater vascular selectivity than their predecessors and in small,

150

long term, placebo controlled trials in patients with heart failure have been associated with improved exercise capacity and a significant reduction in plasma noradrenaline levels.[42, 43] However, the larger VHeFT III Trial demonstrated no significant effect of felodipine on exercise tolerance, mortality or on noradrenaline levels in patients with heart failure who were already treated with an ACE inhibitor.[44] The PRAISE Trial has demonstrated an overall neutral effect of amlodipine on survival in patients with heart failure[45] but in the subgroup of patients with non-ischaemic cardiomyopathy, amlodipine significantly reduced both sudden deaths and deaths due to pump failure. Thus, on the basis of current evidence, patients with heart failure due to ischaemic heart disease should not routinely be given a calcium antagonist but if there is coexistent angina then either amlodipine or felodipine should be used.

Other vasodilators

The first trial to show objective evidence of a reduction in mortality with vasodilators in heart failure was VHeFT I[46] which used a combination regime of isosorbide dinitrate and hydralazine, designed to produce balanced reductions in preload and afterload. A subsequent comparison of this regime with enalapril in VHeFT II demonstrated a significant advantage in terms of exercise tolerance for nitrates/hydralazine, but the ACE inhibitor produced a greater mortality benefit. Since the death rates were different between the groups it is difficult to directly compare the effects of the treatments on exercise tolerance of the survivors. Thus, although ACE inhibitors are the current first choice vasodilator, the combination of a nitrate and hydralazine should be considered in patients unable to tolerate them. It is not certain whether nitrates produce any additional benefit in patients already treated with an ACE inhibitor.

Other vasodilators which have been assessed for their therapeutic efficacy in heart failure include prazosin, an α-adrenergic blocker, and flosequinan, which is thought to act by attenuating the effects of the second messenger compound inositol triphosphate. Both of these agents have now been largely abandoned as therapeutic options in heart failure. Prazosin did not show any benefit over placebo in terms of patient survival in VHeFT I and the initial haemodynamic improvements produced by the drug did not persist with chronic treatment. Flosequinan was marketed as an agent which could produce symptomatic improvements in patients who were already on or who were unable to tolerate an ACE inhibitor. Although the results of initial haemodynamic and symptom based studies appeared favourable,[47] a large scale survival trial, PROFILE, was terminated early because of excess mortality in the high dose flosequinan group. Whether such a drug, which can improve symptoms but may reduce life expectancy, should have a role in the treatment of selected patients remains controversial. One possible option for such drugs is to use them in lower doses which may produce the symptomatic benefits without the adverse effects on mortality.

Digoxin

Cardiac glycosides have been used in the treatment of heart failure for centuries but the role of digoxin for patients in sinus rhythm remains controversial. Digitalis glycosides inhibit the enzyme sodium potassium adenosine triphosphatase, resulting in an accumulation of intracellular sodium and an increase in calcium influx via the sodium–calcium exchanger in sarcolemmal membranes. This results in increased myocardial contractility and traditionally this has been accepted as the mechanism by which digoxin produces beneficial haemodynamic effects. Recently it has become evident that cardiac glycosides are also neurohormonal modulators; digoxin appears to restore the sympathetic/parasympathetic autonomic balance towards normal and to improve baroreflex function in patients with heart failure. Moreover, cardiac glycosides inhibit renin secretion and stimulate secretion of ANP experimentally,[48] both of which would have beneficial effects in heart failure.

The ability of digitalis glycosides to produce short term and sustained improvements in haemodynamic indices has been well established and there is now good evidence that they also produce symptomatic benefits. Support for the use of digoxin has come from the recent RADIANCE Study which demonstrated that the withdrawal of digoxin from patients with moderate heart failure, on ACE inhibitors, resulted in significant adverse haemodynamic and symptomatic effects.[49] The results of such a withdrawal study should be interpreted with caution as the patients were a selected group who were, at least, tolerant of treatment with digoxin prior to entry into the study.

Despite the strong evidence that digoxin can reduce symptoms in patients with heart failure who are in sinus rhythm, there is no convincing evidence that it improves the survival of these patients. This issue was addressed in the Digitalis Investigators Group (DIG) Trial[50] which demonstrated no significant effect of digoxin on the mortality of patients with heart failure who were already treated with an ACE inhibitor. Therefore, digoxin should be considered in patients with heart failure who are in sinus rhythm if they remain symptomatic on treatment with a diuretic and an ACE inhibitor, but it should not be used routinely.

β-blockers

The level of activation of the sympathetic nervous system as measured by plasma levels of catecholamines is a good predictor of mortality in patients with heart failure.[51] Knowledge of the detrimental effects of prolonged sympathetic activation and the success of neurohormonal suppression that has been demonstrated by ACE inhibitors provides the theoretical basis for the use of β-adrenoreceptor antagonists in heart failure. This has been tempered by studies which have consistently demonstrated adverse short term haemodynamic effects of β-blockade[52] and for this reason these drugs have generally been avoided in patients with ventricular dysfunction. Interest in the potential beneficial effects of β-blockers in heart failure was stimulated by the results of the β-Blockers Heart Attack Trial[53] which suggested that the observed overall mortality benefits associated with propanolol postmyocardial infarction were even more prominent in patients with a history of heart failure. This has been further supported by the findings of other postinfarction trials, but obviously these study groups do not represent all patients with chronic heart failure.

Long term studies of β-blockers in heart failure have generally shown beneficial effects on haemodynamic indices and variable effects on exercise tolerance. The largest randomised placebo controlled trial to date, the MDC Trial,[54] has demonstrated a significant increase in LVEF and a reduction in hospitalisations with metoprolol, but no effect on mortality, over a period of 12–18 months. This trial, in common with several previous studies, included only patients with idiopathic dilated cardiomyopathy. The relevance of these findings to the majority of heart failure patients with ischaemic heart disease is uncertain, especially as the aetiology appears to influence the pattern of β-adrenoreceptor downregulation in the heart.[55] It is notable that in the MDC Trial approximately 96% of patients with heart failure were able to tolerate the introduction of metoprolol. In the CIBIS Trial, patients with chronic heart failure of varying aetiologies were treated with bisoprolol in a randomised, placebo controlled design.[56] There was a significant reduction in hospitalisation rate and an improvement in functional status in the bisoprolol treatment group, but no significant effect on overall mortality or on the incidence of sudden death.

Recently, attention has focused on carvedilol, a third generation β-blocker with ancillary properties as an $\alpha1$-adrenoreceptor blocker (resulting in vasodilation) and as an antioxidant. This agent has been tested in five placebo controlled trials, four of which were prospectively linked studies in the USA[57] and the other based in Australia and New Zealand (the ANZ trial).[58] In the US trials, carvedilol reduced hospital admissions and worsening of heart failure in patients with mild heart failure and improved the symptomatic status of patients with moderate and severe heart failure. The LVEF rose significantly by about 7% in the carvedilol treated group but there was no change in exercise capacity. The ANZ Trial recruited mainly patients with mild heart failure and demonstrated a reduction in hospital admissions in the treatment group but there was no effect on the development of worsening heart failure or on symptomatic status. Combined analysis of the US trials demonstrated a reduction in mortality of 67% for the carvedilol treated group compared to placebo during a mean

153

follow-up period of 8·7 months (2·9% versus 8·2%). This effect was not obviously influenced by the aetiology or the severity of heart failure, but the mortality benefit for carvedilol was dose related (patients on 25 mg bd fared better than those on 6·25 mg bd). The follow-up period in the ANZ Trial was 18 months with few deaths and no significant difference between mortality rates for carvedilol and placebo, but a significant fall of 41% in the primary endpoint of death or hospital admission in the carvedilol treated patients. The results of the carvedilol trials are consistent with the MDC Trial in that 95% of heart failure patients were able to tolerate the gradual initiation of β-blocker treatment.

The results of the above trials with carvedilol are very encouraging, but they must be interpreted with some caution for several reasons. Firstly, although the mortality benefits associated with carvedilol treatment in the US trials appear impressive, they are based on a total of only 53 deaths during the median follow-up period of less than seven months. Secondly, the trial design excluded from the final mortality analysis those patients who died or who developed worsening heart failure during the run-in period; if these events were included in the overall analysis then the mortality benefit for carvedilol would be considerably diluted[59] (but still significant). Thirdly, the US studies do not demonstrate a reduction in mortality in the subgroup of 105 patients with severe heart failure (in whom there were only four deaths during follow-up) and it is this group of patients who would be most at risk from an early haemodynamic deterioration following the initiation of β-blocker therapy. Lastly, in common with the large ACE inhibitor trials, relatively young patients were recruited in to the carvedilol studies. The mean age in the US studies was 58 years and therefore the results are not necessarily applicable to the majority of heart failure patients, who are elderly.

More research into the effects and the mechanisms of action of carvedilol and other similar agents is clearly needed. This should clarify the contribution of carvedilol's ancillary vasodilator and antioxidant properties to its therapeutic effect. As with ACE inhibitors and thrombolytic agents, clinical practice is unlikely to change until the beneficial effects of the new treatment have been confirmed by further studies. The ongoing Beta-Blocker Evaluation Survival Trial will test the effects of bucindolol (a non-selective β-blocker with vasodilatory properties) on survival in 2800 patients with heart failure over a minimum of 18 months with no run-in period.

On the basis of the available evidence, treatment with carvedilol might be considered in patients with mild to moderate symptomatic heart failure who do not have contraindications to β-blocker therapy (asthma, brady-cardia, severe hypotension). At present this is problematic as carvedilol does not yet have a licence for the treatment of heart failure and the smallest tablet of carvedilol available is 12·5 mg which precludes the administration of the 3·125 mg bd initiation dose used in the trials described above. Presumably these matters will be addressed in the near future. It should be recognised that, contrary to conventional teaching, β-blockers can be safely initiated in the majority of patients with left ventricular dysfunction and that patients may derive long term benefit despite an initial deterioration.[60] The initiation of β-blocker therapy in patients with heart failure should be performed in hospital.

Antiarrhythmic agents

The high incidence of sudden death in patients with heart failure suggests that they may benefit from specific antiarrhythmic therapy. These patients have many arrhythmogenic factors including myocardial fibrosis, which may provide a substrate for re-entrant arrhythmias, activation of the sympathetic nervous system and electrolyte disturbances caused by diuretic treatment and increased activity of the renin–angiotensin–aldosterone system. Holter ECG monitoring has demonstrated a high frequency of ventricular ectopic beats in patients with heart failure although the correlation between such abnormalities and survival is poor.[61] Following the CAST Study,[62] which demonstrated an increased mortality from treatment of asymptomatic abnormalities on Holter monitoring, there is no justification for the routine treatment of ventricular extrasystoles and it is imperative that all clinical studies of antiarrhythmic drugs use all-cause mortality rather than electrophysiological criteria as the primary endpoint.

Class I antiarrhythmic drugs all have negative inotropic effects and have therefore been avoided in patients with left ventricular dysfunction. The use of β-blockers as antiarrhythmic agents in heart failure is theoretically attractive but in the MDC Trial discussed previously there was a slightly higher (non-significant) incidence of sudden death in the treatment group than in the placebo group. There are also good theoretical reasons for considering magnesium as an antiarrhythmic agent in heart failure: depletion of magnesium is common in patients on diuretics and hypo-magnesaemia is associated with an adverse prognosis in patients with heart failure.[63] A small trial has demonstrated a reduction in the frequency of ventricular ectopic beats with oral magnesium in patients with heart failure;[64] magnesium has additional vasodilatory properties which may be due to calcium channel antagonism. Further evidence of the tolerability and efficacy of oral magnesium is required to determine whether this treatment is likely to be useful.

The antiarrhythmic agent which looks most promising in heart failure is amiodarone which has recently been studied in the large multicentre placebo-controlled GESICA Trial conducted in Argentina.[65] This study used mortality as the primary endpoint and demonstrated a risk reduction of 28% in patients with advanced heart failure treated with amiodarone over an average of 13 months. The findings of this trial were surprising for two reasons: firstly, there was a low incidence of side effects requiring withdrawal from treatment (although there was no monitoring for asymptomatic side effects) and secondly, the beneficial effects of amiodarone were not restricted to the prevention of arrhythmias as there was a significant improvement in functional capacity and a reduction in deaths due to progressive heart failure in the treatment group. The latter findings may be due to the diverse pharmacological actions of amiodarone which has additional properties of β blockade and calcium channel antagonism. Unfortunately these results were not replicated in the CHF-STAT Study which was based in the United States.[66] This demonstrated that, in patients with symptomatic heart failure, amiodarone treatment resulted in a significant improvement in left ventricular ejection fraction but there was no associated improvement in symptomatic status or survival.

Thus although amiodarone is well tolerated in patients with heart failure, at present there is no justification for empirical amiodarone treatment in all patients. Further study of the tolerability of the drug in these patients is required to determine the incidence of major side effects (such as pulmonary fibrosis) and more minor but troublesome problems such as photosensitivity. Increased understanding of the mechanisms by which amiodarone may produce the benefits described above may facilitate the development of similar agents which have lower toxicity. It was this concept that led to the SWORD Trial which tested d-sotalol, a potassium channel blocker with the class III antiarrhythmic actions of amiodarone but with no β-blocking activity, in patients with previous myocardial infarction and LVEF below 40%. However, the trial was terminated early due to excess mortality in the patients treated with d-sotalol, presumably due to arrhythmic deaths.[67] This result reinforces the lesson of the previous CAST Study[62] that all antiarrhythmic agents are potentially lethal, especially when given to unselected patients. Moreover, it suggests that the diverse effects of amiodarone, which acts as both a β-blocker and a calcium antagonist as well as a class III agent, may play an important role in its beneficial therapeutic effect.

The role of implantable cardioverter defibrillators in patients with heart failure remains controversial. There is now good evidence from the MADIT Trial that if high risk patients are selected, prophylactic treatment with an implanted defibrillator results in improved patient survival as compared to conventional medical therapy with amiodarone.[68] In MADIT all patients underwent invasive electrophysiological testing to demonstrate inducible, non-suppressible ventricular tachycardia prior to enrolment. Further trials are needed to determine whether antiarrhythmic treatment can be successfully targeted to patients at risk by using simpler methods of risk assessment. Two measurements which are promising in this role are QT dispersion (the interlead variability of the QT interval on a standard ECG), which is a powerful predictor of the risk of sudden death in patients with heart failure,[69] and heart rate variability, which is an indicator of autonomic tone.[70]

Positive inotropic agents

As the primary abnormality in heart failure is a reduction in cardiac performance, a logical therapeutic strategy is to attempt to improve this performance directly. Many positive inotropic agents have been tested in heart failure and virtually all have been abandoned due to excessive mortality.[71] Sympathomimetic agents such as dobutamine have a beneficial haemodynamic effect in acute heart failure but attempts to translate this into treatment for chronic heart failure have been unsuccessful due to an increased incidence of ventricular arrhythmias. Similar problems have occurred with agents such as enoximone and milrinone which are inhibitors of cyclic adenosine monophosphate (cAMP) phosphodiesterase. These agents increase the myocardial concentrations of cAMP, which is an important second messenger in mediating the inotropic response. Despite significant short term haemodynamic benefits, long term studies have consistently demonstrated reduced survival with these drugs which appears to be related to a proarrhythmic effect.

Two newer inotropic agents, vesnarinone and pimobendan, have been investigated but results so far are not encouraging. The precise mechanism of action of these drugs is uncertain; vesnarinone has complex and diverse effects on ion channels and phosphodiesterase and increases the intracellular flux of calcium while pimobendan inhibits phosphodiesterase but also appears to sensitise the myocardial contractile apparatus to the effects of calcium. Preliminary mortality data with vesnarinone indicate that it has a narrow therapeutic window[72] but a subsequent study (as yet unpublished) has found that low dose vesnarinone was also associated with increased mortality. Pimobendan may merit further investigation but at present its potential role in the treatment of patients with heart failure is unclear.

Anticoagulants

In patients with ventricular dysfunction and atrial fibrillation warfarin should routinely be prescribed, if there are no contraindications, to reduce the high incidence of stroke. Several recent studies have demonstrated that in such patients the benefits of anticoagulation greatly outweigh the risks and treatment with warfarin is clearly more effective in stroke prevention than treatment with aspirin. The situation with regard to anticoagulation in patients with heart failure who are in sinus rhythm is less clear; this issue will be addressed by the ongoing Warfarin Aspirin Study of Heart Failure (WASH).

Surgery

The role of surgery in the management of heart failure has generally been restricted to those patients with advanced disease resistant to medical therapy. It should be realised that in the presence of active myocardial ischaemia patients with abnormal ventricular function have a high perioperative mortality from coronary bypass surgery but that the potential survival benefits from revascularisation are also high. This has been clearly demonstrated by a recent meta-analysis of the large trials comparing medical and surgical management of stable angina pectoris.[73]

Cardiac transplantation is the only potentially curative procedure for the vast majority of patients with heart failure. The prognosis of patients following a heart transplant has been dramatically improved since the introduction of cyclosporin but the main limiting factor on this form of treatment has been, and is likely to remain, the limited availability of donor organs. Currently the main criteria for acceptance onto a transplant programme are chronic stable heart failure which is not controlled by optimal medical treatment, age less than 60 years, and the absence of irreversible pulmonary hypertension (other criteria will apply but may vary between centres). The problem of organ availability may be solved in the future by the use of xenografts (i.e. hearts from other species) or by the development of artificial ventricular-assist devices, whose main role at present is to provide short term support until an organ becomes available for transplantation.

Another surgical option currently undergoing clinical trial is cardiomyoplasty, a technique which involves manipulation and electrical stimulation of the latissimus dorsi muscle to provide support for the failing left ventricle. The role of this technique is not yet determined but one precondition is that the patient retains reasonable function of the right ventricle.

Future prospects

Attempts to improve the treatment of patients with heart failure have consistently demonstrated the importance of the neuroendocrine response to medication. The therapeutic value of a drug appears to depend mainly on the effect which it has on both adverse and beneficial aspects of the neurohormonal response to left ventricular dysfunction. Accordingly there has been a resurgence of interest in agents, in addition to ACE inhibitors, which reduce the activity of the renin–angiotensin–aldosterone system. During chronic ACE inhibition the suppression of angiotensin II and aldosterone activity is often incomplete and it is possible that specific antagonists of these hormones may have additional beneficial effects. Antagonists of the angiotensin II receptor are now available for clinical use and the recent ELITE Study suggests that they may even be superior to

ACE inhibitors in terms of reducing mortality. These drugs, in contrast with ACE inhibitors, will not result in an increase in kinin activity, which avoids the side effect of cough. Increasing bradykinin activity was thought of as a potentially beneficial effect of ACE inhibitors but the ELITE Study casts doubt on this idea; it may be significant that bradykinin can stimulate noradrenaline release in some situations. There is increasing recognition of the detrimental effects of excessive aldosterone activity in heart failure, which can persist despite ACE inhibitor treatment. This has prompted a multicentre trial, entitled RALES, which is ongoing and which will assess the effects of the aldosterone antagonist spironolactone in patients already treated with an ACE inhibitor.

A new type of diuretic agent which potentially suppresses rather than activates the renin–angiotensin system is currently under investigation. Neutral endopeptidase (NEP) inhibitors block the metabolism of atrial natriuretic peptide and other related natriuretic peptides and should therefore potentiate their unique diuretic and vasodilatory properties. Drugs which are combined inhibitors of NEP and ACE have also been developed and are now undergoing long term clinical trials in patients with heart failure. Endothelin receptor antagonists are at an early stage of development, but as the precise role of endothelin in cardiovascular and renal homoeostasis is not yet defined the effect of such antagonists cannot be accurately predicted.

Another promising therapeutic area in heart failure is the correction of metabolic abnormalities in the failing myocardium. A recent small study assessed the short term effects of sodium dichloroacetate on haemodynamic function in patients with heart failure.[74] Dichloroacetate stimulates pyruvate dehydrogenase, causing inhibition of free fatty acid metabolism and stimulation of glucose and lactate consumption by the heart. The results suggested an increase in left ventricular mechanical efficiency which was not observed when the same patients were treated with dobutamine. It is unclear whether this will be of any practical benefit in the treatment of patients with acute or chronic heart failure, but this area clearly merits further investigation.

Current management strategies

Any patient who, on clinical grounds, is suspected of having ventricular dysfunction should ideally be investigated by echocardiography (Figure 7.2). This will not only provide assessment of ventricular function but may identify an underlying cause such as aortic stenosis. If the echocardiogram shows evidence of regional wall motion abnormalities and there is electrocardiographic evidence of previous MI then the cause of heart failure is likely to be coronary artery disease. However, if there is global ventricular dysfunction and the ECG shows non-specific changes then alcoholic

159

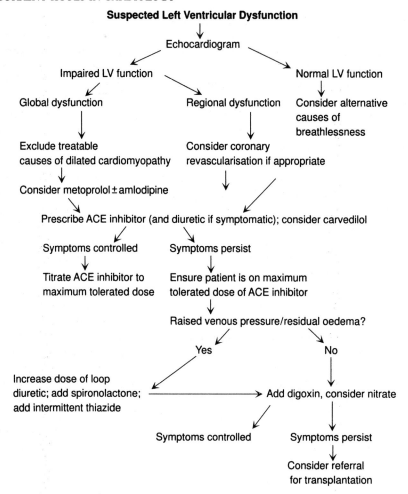

Suspected Left Ventricular Dysfunction

Fig 7.2 Algorithm for the management of patients with suspected left ventricular dysfunction.

cardiomyopathy, thyrotoxicosis and haemochromatosis should be considered.

Advice should be given about restriction of dietary sodium intake, avoidance of excessive alcohol consumption and the importance of regular exercise. All patients with proven ventricular dysfunction should be started on an ACE inhibitor unless there is a clear contraindication such as aortic stenosis. The dose should be titrated up to the equivalent of enalapril 10 mg bd or the maximum tolerated dose. This alone will be sufficient for patients with no symptoms and may alleviate minimal symptoms but patients with fluid retention and/or pulmonary oedema will require the addition of a loop diuretic (e.g. frusemide 40 mg od). The combination of a diuretic and an ACE inhibitor will control the symptoms of many patients with heart failure but if there is little or no improvement then compliance with medication and dietary salt intake should be reassessed. In patients who are unable to tolerate an ACE inhibitor the combination of isosorbide dinitrate and hydralazine may be useful. The results of the CHF-STAT Trial suggest that amiodarone should not be used routinely, but it is at least clear that amiodarone is the drug of choice in patients with heart failure who have documented ventricular arrhythmias.

If a patient remains breathless on a diuretic and an ACE inhibitor then digoxin may be of symptomatic benefit. The addition of an oral nitrate may also provide symptomatic relief provided that the patient does not develop significant hypotension. Resistant oedema should be treated initially with increased doses of loop diuretics followed by the introduction of a low dose of thiazide diuretic on a short term or intermittent basis. Further treatment will depend on the situation and the wishes of the patient; a younger patient may be considered for cardiac transplantation at this stage.

The precise role of β-blockers in the treatment of patients with ischaemic cardiomyopathy has yet to be clearly defined but if there are no contraindications and the patient has symptomatic heart failure, then the cautious introduction of carvedilol should be considered. At present there is no compelling evidence for the use of other β-blockers, except in patients with idiopathic dilated cardiomyopathy, in whom treatment with metoprolol (as described in the MDC Trial)[54] and also amlodipine (as described in the PRAISE Study)[45] should be considered. The coexistence of angina and ventricular dysfunction in patients with ischaemic heart disease is common and can cause therapeutic problems. All such patients should receive standard treatment for their heart failure as detailed above and a logical initial treatment for the angina is an oral nitrate. If this is not effective then a β-blocker may be introduced with the knowledge that most patients with heart failure will be tolerant of it. Older calcium channel antagonists should be avoided in favour of agents such as amlodipine and felodipine. In general there should be a low threshold for coronary angiography and revascularisation in patients with angina and ventricular dysfunction. An unresolved issue is the importance of hibernating myocardium, i.e. viable ischaemic myocardium, the function of which can be significantly improved by revascularisation. We do not yet know how common this is, what is the best method for its detection or how effective revascularisation would be.

The treatment of acute heart failure has not been scrutinised by large clinical trials in the same way as the therapy of chronic heart failure. The standard treatment remains intravenous diuretics and vasodilators, guided when necessary by invasive haemodynamic monitoring. In severe cases, short term treatment with inotropic agents such as dobutamine or enoximone may be useful. Left ventricular-assist devices may be used to provide short term support prior to cardiac transplantation.

Summary

The treatment of patients with heart failure continues to develop at a rapid rate. Further improvements are essential in view of the increasing incidence of the condition and the high mortality which is still associated with it. Effective identification and treatment of the early stages of ventricular dysfunction are paramount in the attempt to reduce the impact of heart failure in the population. Previous experience suggests that drugs which modify the neurohormonal and metabolic abnormalities associated with heart failure are more likely to produce therapeutic benefit than those which stimulate the heart directly.

1 Leimbach WN, Wallin BG, Victor RG, Aylward PE, Sundlof G, Mark AL. Direct evidence from intraneural recordings for increased central sympathetic outflow in patients with heart failure. *Circulation* 1986; **73**: 913–19.

2 Nadal-Ginard B, Mahdavi V. Molecular basis of cardiac performance: plasticity of the myocardium generated through protein isoform switches. *J Clin Invest* 1989; **84**: 1693–700.

3 Eiskjaer H, Bagger JP, Danielsen H *et al*. Mechanisms of sodium retention in heart failure: relation to the renin–angiotensin–aldosterone system. *Am J Physiol* 1991; **260**: F883–9.

4 Creager MA, Faxon DP, Cutler SS, Kohlman O, Ryan TG, Gavras H. Contribution of vasopressin to vasoconstriction in patients with congestive heart failure: comparison with the renin–angiotensin system and the sympathetic nervous system. *J Am Coll Cardiol* 1986; **7**: 758–65.

5 Kiowski W, Sutsch G, Hunziker P *et al*. Evidence of endothelin-1-mediated vasoconstriction in severe chronic heart failure. *Lancet* 1995; **346**: 732–6.

6 Narula J, Haider N, Renu V *et al*. Apoptosis in myocytes in end-stage heart failure. *N Engl J Med* 1996; **335**: 1182–9.

7 Colucci WS, Braunwald E. Pathophysiology of heart failure. In: Braunwald E, ed. *Heart disease*, 5th edn. Philadelphia: W.B. Saunders, 1997.

8 Packer M. Interaction of prostaglandins and angiotensin II in the modulation of renal function in congestive heart failure. *Circulation* 1988; 77(Suppl I): 64–73.

9 Delkers W, Kleiner S, Bähr V. Effects of incremental infusions of atrial natriuretic factor on aldosterone, renin and blood pressure in patients with essential hypertension. *Hypertension* 1988; **12**: 205–13.

10 Kawaguchi H, Ito K, Takamura I. ANF inhibits ACE activity stimulated by endothelin. *J Hypertens* 1992; **10**(Suppl 4): S98.

11 Kohno M, Yasunari K, Yokokawa K *et al*. Inhibition by atrial and brain natriuretic peptides of endothelin-1 secretion after stimulation with angiotensin II and thrombin of cultured human endothelial cells. *J Clin Invest* 1991; **87**: 1999–2004.

12 Molina CR, Fowler MB, McCrory S *et al*. Haemodynamic, renal and endocrine effects of atrial natriuretic peptide infusion in severe heart failure. *J Am Coll Cardiol* 1988; **12**: 175–86.

13 Schiffrin EL. Regulation of receptors for atrial natriuretic peptide in the rat and human. *Cardiovasc Drugs Ther* 1988; **2**: 493–500.

14 Homcy CJ, Vatner SF, Vatner DE. β-adrenergic receptor regulation in the heart in pathophysiological states: abnormal adrenergic responsiveness in cardiac disease. *Annu Rev Physiol* 1991; **53**: 137–59.

15 Mancia G. Sympathetic activation in congestive heart failure. *Eur Heart J* 1990; **11** (Suppl A): 3–11.

16 Szakacs JE, Cannon A. Norepinephrine myocarditis. *Am J Clin Pathol* 1958; **30**: 425–35.

17 Tan LB, Jalil JE, Pick R, Janicki JS, Weber KT. Cardiac myocyte necrosis induced by angiotensin II. *Circ Res* 1991; **69**: 1185–95.

18 Daeman MJ, Lombardi DM, Bosman FT, Schwartz SM. Angiotensin II induces smooth muscle cell proliferation in the normal and injured rat arterial wall. *Circ Res* 1991; **68**: 450–6.

19 Leier CV, Dei Cas L, Metra M. Clinical relevance and management of the major electrolyte abnormalities in congestive heart failure: hyponatraemia, hypokalaemia, and hypomagnesaemia. *Am Heart J* 1994; **128**: 564–74.

20 Weber KT, Brilla CG. Pathological hypertrophy and the cardiac interstitium: fibrosis and the renin–angiotensin–aldosterone system. *Circulation* 1990; **83**: 1840–65.

21 Wheeldon NM, MacDonald TM, Flucker CJ et al. Echocardiography in chronic heart failure in the community. *Q J Med* 1993; **86**: 17–23.

22 Remes J, Miettinen H, Reunanen A, Pyorala K. Validity of clinical diagnosis of heart failure in primary health care. *Eur Heart J* 1991; **12**: 315–21.

23 Lerman A, Gibbons RJ, Rodeheffer RJ et al. Circulating N-terminal atrial natriuretic peptide as a marker for symptomless left-ventricular dysfunction. *Lancet* 1993; **341**: 1105–9.

24 Cintron G, Johnson G, Francis G et al. Prognostic significance of serial changes in left ventricular ejection fraction in patients with congestive heart failure. *Circulation* 1993; **87**(Suppl VI): VI-17–VI-23.

25 Clark A. Is exercise training a practical therapeutic option in heart failure? *Br J Cardiol* 1994; **1**: 189–90.

26 Sullivan MJ, Higginbotham MB, Cobb FR. Exercise training in patients with severe left ventricular dysfunction: haemodynamic and metabolic effects. *Circulation* 1988; **78**: 506–16.

27 Coats AJS, Adamopolous S, Radaelli A et al. Controlled trial of physical training in chronic heart failure: exercise performance, haemodynamics ventilation and autonomic function. *Circulation* 1992; **85**: 2119–31.

28 Brater DC. Pharmacokinetics of loop diuretics in congestive heart failure. *Br Heart J* 1994; **72**(Suppl 2): S40–S43.

29 CONSENSUS Trial Study Group. Effects of enalapril on mortality in severe congestive heart failure: results of the Cooperative New Scandinavian Enalapril Survival Study. *N Engl J Med* 1987; **316**: 1429–35.

30 The SOLVD Investigators. Effect of enalapril on survival in patients with reduced left ventricular ejection fractions and congestive heart failure. *N Engl J Med* 1991; **325**: 293–302.

31 Cohn JN, Johnson G, Ziesche S et al. A comparison of enalapril with hydralazine-isosorbide dinitrate in the treatment of chronic congestive heart failure. *N Engl J Med* 1991; **325**: 303–10.

32 The SOLVD Investigators. Effect of enalapril on mortality and the development of heart failure in asymptomatic patients with reduced left ventricular ejection fractions. *N Engl J Med* 1992; **327**: 685–91.

33 Richardson A, Bayliss J, Scriven AJ et al. Double-blind comparison of captopril alone against frusemide plus amiloride in mild heart failure. *Lancet* 1987; **ii**: 709–11.

34 Anand IS, Kalra GS, Ferrari R et al. Enalapril as initial and sole treatment in severe chronic heart failure with sodium retention. *Int J Cardiol* 1990; **28**: 341–6.

35 Pfeffer MA, Braunwald E, Moyé LA et al. Effect of captopril on mortality and morbidity in patients with left ventricular dysfunction after myocardial infarction. Results of the Survival and Ventricular Enlargement Trial. *N Engl J Med* 1992; **327**: 669–77.

36 The AIRE Study Investigators. Effect of ramipril on mortality and morbidity of survivors of acute myocardial infarction with clinical evidence of heart failure. *Lancet* 1993; **342**: 821–8.

37 GISSI Investigators. GISSI-3: effects of lisinopril and transdermal glyceryl trinitrate singly and together on six week mortality and ventricular function after acute myocardial infarction. *Lancet* 1994; **343**: 1115–22.

38 Pouleur H. High or low dose of angiotensin-converting enzyme inhibitor in patients with left ventricular dysfunction. *Cardiovasc Drugs Ther* 1993; 7: 891–2.

39 Nussberger J, Fleck E, Bahrmann H, Delius W, Schultheiss HP, Brunner HR. Dose-related effects of ACE inhibitor in man: quinapril in patients with moderate congestive heart failure. *Eur Heart J* 1994; **15**(Suppl D): 113–22.

40 Poole-Wilson PA, on behalf of the NETWORK Investigators. The NETWORK study. The effect of dose of an ACE inhibitor on outcome in patients with heart failure (abstract). *J Am Coll Cardiol* 1996; **27** (Suppl I): 141A.

41 Packer M, Kessler PD, Lee WH. Calcium channel blockade in the management of severe chronic congestive heart failure: a bridge too far. *Circulation* 1987; **75** (Suppl V): V56–V64.

42 Kassis E, Amtorp O. Long-term clinical, haemodynamic, angiographic and neuro-hormonal responses to vasodilatation with felodipine in patients with chronic congestive heart failure. *J Cardiovasc Pharmacol* 1990; **15**: 347–52.

43 Packer M, Nicod P, Bijoy N *et al.* Randomized, multicentre double-blind placebo-controlled evaluation of amlodipine in patients with mild to moderate heart failure. *J Am Coll Cardiol* 1991; **17**: 274A.

44 The VHeFT III Study Group. Effect of felodipine on short term exercise and neurohormone response and long term mortality in heart failure: results of VHeFT III. *Circulation* 1995; **92**(Suppl I): I–143.

45 The PRAISE Study Group. Effect of amlodipine on morbidity and mortality in severe chronic heart failure. *N Engl J Med* 1996; **335**: 1107–14.

46 Cohn JN, Archibald DG, Ziesche S *et al.* Effect of vasodilator therapy on mortality in chronic congestive heart failure: results of a veterans administration cooperation study. *N Engl J Med* 1986; **314**: 1547–52.

47 Packer M, Narahara KA, Elkayam U *et al.* Double-blind, placebo-controlled study of the efficacy of flosequinan in patients with chronic heart failure. *J Am Coll Cardiol* 1993; **22**: 65–72.

48 Gheorghiade M, Ferguson D. Digoxin. A neurohormonal modulator in heart failure? *Circulation* 1991; **84**: 2181–6.

49 Packer M, Gheorghiade M, Young JB *et al.* Withdrawal of digoxin from patients with chronic heart failure treated with angiotensin-converting enzyme inhibitors: RADIANCE study group. *N Engl J Med* 1993; **329**: 1–7.

50 The Digitalis Investigators Group. The effect of digoxin on mortality and morbidity in patients with heart failure. *N Engl J Med* 1997; **336**: 525–33.

51 Cohn JN, Levine TB, Olivari MT *et al.* Plasma norepinephrine as a guide to prognosis in patients with chronic congestive heart failure. *N Engl J Med* 1984; **311**: 819–23.

52 Haber HL, Simek CL, Gimple LW *et al.* Why do patients with congestive heart failure tolerate the initiation of β blocker therapy? *Circulation* 1993; **88**: 1610–19.

53 Chadda K, Goldstein S, Byington R, Curb JD. Effect of propanolol after acute myocardial infarction in patients with congestive heart failure. *Circulation* 1986; **73**: 503–10.

54 Waagstein F, Bristow MR, Swedberg K *et al.* Beneficial effects of metoprolol in idiopathic dilated cardiomyopathy. *Lancet* 1993; **342**: 1441–6.

55 Bristow MR, Anderson FL, Port D *et al.* Differences in β-adrenergic neuroeffector mechanisms in ischaemic versus dilated cardiomyopathy. *Circulation* 1991; **84**: 1024–39.

56 CIBIS Investigators. A randomized trial of β-blockade in heart failure. *Circulation* 1994; **90**: 1765–73.

57 Packer M, Bristow MR, Cohn JN *et al.* The effect of carvedilol on morbidity and mortality in patients with chronic heart failure. *N Engl J Med* 1996; **334**: 1349–55.

58 Australia New Zealand Heart Failure Research Collaborative Group. Effects of carvedilol, a vasodilator β-blocker, in patients with heart failure due to ischaemic heart disease. *Circulation* 1995; **92**: 212–18.

59 Packer M, Cohn JN, Colucci WS. Carvedilol in patients with heart failure (letter). *N Engl J Med* 1996; **335**: 1319.

60 Sackner-Bernstein JD, Krum H, Goldsmith RL *et al.* Should worsening heart failure early after initiation of beta-blocker therapy for chronic heart failure preclude long-term treatment? *Circulation* 1995; **92** (Suppl I): I–395.

61 Packer M. Lack of relation between ventricular arrhythmias and sudden death in patients with chronic heart failure. *Circulation* 1992; **85** (Suppl I): I50–I56.

62 The CAST Investigators. Preliminary report: effect of encainide and flecainide on

mortality in a randomized trial of arrhythmia suppression after myocardial infarction. *N Engl J Med* 1989; **321**: 406–12.

63 Gottlieb SS, Baruch L, Kukin ML *et al.* Prognostic importance of the serum magnesium concentration in patients with congestive heart failure. *J Am Coll Cardiol* 1990; **16**: 827–31.

64 Bashir Y, Sneddon JF, Staunton HA *et al.* Effects of long-term oral magnesium chloride replacement in congestive heart failure secondary to coronary artery disease. *Am J Cardiol* 1993; **72**: 1156–62.

65 Doval HC, Nul DR, Grancelli HO *et al.* Randomised trial of low-dose amiodarone in severe congestive heart failure. *Lancet* 1994; **344**: 493–8.

66 Massie BM, Singh SN, Fletcher RD, Fisher SG, for the CHF-STAT Investigators. Effect of amiodarone on ejection fraction and CHF status in the VA cooperative study of amiodarone for congestive heart failure. *Circulation* 1995; **92** (Suppl I): I–143.

67 Waldo AL, Camm AJ, deRuyter H *et al.*, for the SWORD Investigators. Effect of d-sotalol on mortality in patients with left ventricular dysfunction after recent and remote myocardial infarction. *Lancet* 1996; **348**: 7–12.

68 Moss AJ, Hall J, Cannom DS *et al.* Improved survival with an implanted defibrillator in patients with coronary disease at high risk for ventricular arrhythmia. *N Engl J Med* 1996; **335**: 1933–40.

69 Barr CS, Naas A, Freeman M *et al.* QT dispersion and sudden unexpected death in chronic heart failure. *Lancet* 1994; **343**: 327–9.

70 Karemaker JM. Heart rate variability: why do spectral analysis? *Heart* 1997; **77**: 99–101.

71 Curfman GD. Inotropic therapy for heart failure: an unfulfilled promise. *N Engl J Med* 1991; **325**: 1509–10.

72 Feldman AM, Bristow MR, Parmley WW *et al.* Effects of vesnarinone on morbidity and mortality in patients with heart failure. *N Engl J Med* 1993; **329**: 149–55.

73 Yusuf S, Zucker D, Peduzzi P *et al.* Effect of coronary artery bypass graft surgery on survival: overview of 10-year results from randomised trials by the Coronary Bypass Surgery Trialists Collaboration. *Lancet* 1994; **344**: 563–70.

74 Bersin RM, Wolfe C, Kwasmas M *et al.* Improved haemodynamic function and mechanical efficiency in congestive heart failure with sodium dichloroacetate. *J Am Coll Cardiol* 1994; **23**: 1617–24.

8: Management of the postprocedure patient

P YIU AND JR McEWAN

Introduction

Ischaemic heart disease is the leading cause of death in the Western world. Percutaneous transluminal coronary angioplasty (PTCA) with or without stenting and coronary artery bypass surgery (CABG) are now popular treatments with a safe and predictable outcome. Consequently, the number of procedures carried out each year is escalating. In 1982, 6008 isolated coronary artery bypass operations were carried out in the UK.[1] A decade later, the figure has tripled to 19,241 (Figure 8.1). This represents a CABG rate of 306 per million.[2] In 1990, 8500 PTCA were carried out in the UK.[3] By 1994 this had increased to 202 per million. The demand for cardiac interventions still far exceeds supply and the British Cardiac Society has recommended a target for 1996/7 of 600 CABGs and 400 PTCAs per million.[3] Provision of effective health care in this specialised field depends not only on the number of interventions that can be completed per year but

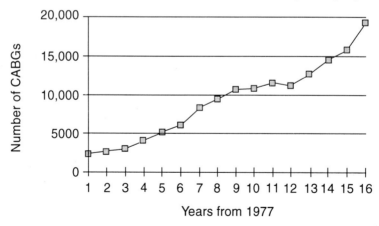

Fig 8.1   The number of isolated coronary artery bypass operations performed each year from 1977 (reproduced from UK Cardiac Register 1992 with permission).

also the ability to provide adequate aftercare of the postprocedure patient.

Recent technical advances are leading to earlier discharge of patients and most general physicians and general practitioners are coming into contact with patients soon after such procedures. Efficient use of the surgeon's or interventional cardiologist's skills may not necessarily involve long term follow-up of these patients. A knowledge of the procedure, the subsequent adjuvant drug therapy and the predictable short and long term outcomes should allow devolution of almost all follow-up to the referring doctor. Indeed, it can be left to some patients to re-refer themselves for specific problems or events. In addition, the long term success of PTCA and CABG depends upon halting progression of native coronary artery disease which relies on active risk factor management.

In this chapter, we will discuss the follow-up and management of the postprocedure patient. Based on outcome results of established trials, simple guidelines on patient care can be drawn up, making long term routine visits to hospital outpatients unnecessary. Unpredictable appointment dates and long waiting times are frustrating for patients and interrupt the smooth continuity of care present in the general practice setting.

Post-PTCA and related procedures

PTCA is popular with patients because of the rapid relief of symptoms afforded and the early return to normal activities. In the UK in 1992 12,701 PTCA were carried out and this was supplemented by "bail out" stent placement in a further 731 and relative stents in 813 (Grey, Chairman, British Cardiac Intervention Society, personal communication). Worldwide, in excess of one million endovascular coronary procedures are carried out annually. The care of patients following such interventions requires an understanding of the nature of the procedures and the anticipated course.

The procedures

Prior to a standard angioplasty the patient will have been prescribed aspirin. PTCA is usually carried out from an access point in the femoral artery, though the brachial approach is also feasible. After vascular access is achieved the patient is anticoagulated with heparin for the procedure. A soft tipped guide catheter is used to selectively intubate the coronary ostium and a fine guidewire (0·3 mm) passed through it into the coronary artery and beyond the target lesion. An appropriately sized (2–4 mm) balloon catheter is passed over the guidewire (either "over the wire" or suspended in "monorail" fashion from the wire) to the lesion (Figure 8.2). Brief inflations of the balloon for periods of about two minutes, at maximum pressures of around eight atmospheres, squash the atheroma into the vessel wall which is probably torn in the process.

167

PTCA can be supplemented in vessels of 3 mm or greater diameter with a stent (Figure 8.3). These are either self expanding or balloon expanded meshes or tubes of fine metal which support the wall, holding back dissection flaps (a process for which they are sometimes employed following a complicated standard PTCA – "bail out stenting"[4]).

Elective stenting of suitable vessels is gaining popularity because of the low rate of restenosis[5] (see below) but a perceived requirement for systemic anticoagulation after employment of stents has led to more access site haemorrhage than is seen with standard PTCA. However, technical and pharmacological modifications of the technique are resolving some of these limitations.

Following a brief period of observation in the catheter laboratory the patient is returned to the ward with access lines still in place. For standard angioplasties, without extensive dissection, the lines are removed four hours later after the APTT is measured at <150 sec. In current (early 1997) practice in the UK, following stent placement, the lines are similarly removed but heparin restarted six hours later at a dose to keep the APTT twice normal. Ticlopidine (see Chapter 3) 250 mg bd is begun immediately after the procedure but because therapeutic effects take 48 hours to develop, heparin is usually continued during that period. There is therefore a rationale for beginning ticlopidine 48 hours before an elective stenting

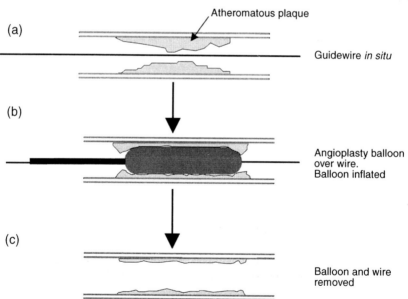

Fig 8.2   PTCA. (a) The stenotic lesion is crossed by a guidewire. (b) The balloon is inflated at the site of the stenosis, compressing the atheroma. (c) The lumen diameter is increased.

procedure, as this obviates the requirement for heparin other than during the procedure.

In the immediate period after the procedure the patient is observed for acute complications such as sudden coronary occlusion or access site problems. When the lines are removed femoral bleeding is prevented by compression. In a small percentage of patients local haemorrhage at the access site causes a pseudoaneurysm which forms a tender expansile lump. This complication is more common when the patient has been anti-coagulated prior to the procedure or when access lines are of a larger diameter. If the neck of pseudoaneurysm can be occluded for 30–40 minutes under ultrasound guidance, the sac will thrombose and the alternative treatment of surgical repair can be avoided[6] (Figure 8.4).

Sudden onset of chest pain and ECG changes suggest coronary occlusion which merits immediate return to the catheter laboratory for re-evaluation. If access lines have already been removed a new access site may be required.

There is remarkable parity between the rates of immediate complications with PTCA and elective stent placement. In all, current figures suggest that

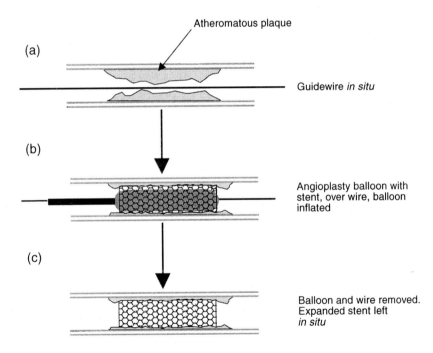

Fig 8.3   Stent placement. (a) The stenotic lesion is crossed by a guidewire. (b) The deflated balloon, inside the stent, is inflated at the stenosis, compressing the atheroma. (c) The stent remains after the balloon is deflated and withdrawn. The lumen diameter is increased.

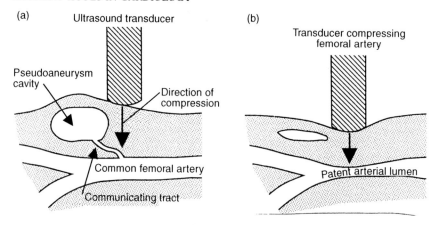

Fig 8.4 Technique for non-surgical closure of pseudoaneurysm of the femoral artery. (a) The transducer is positioned directly over the defect in the femoral artery (which may be displaced from the aneurysm cavity). (b) The artery is compressed so that flow into the cavity ceases while flow within the arterial lumen is maintained. Reproduced from Currie[6] with permission.

immediate technical success is achieved in >90% of standard PTCA and elective stenting procedures. Emergency or urgent bypass grafting or a further endovascular procedure is necessary in about 7% of patients while procedural mortality is less than 1% for either procedure.

Discharge and driving

The standard PTCA patient in whom the procedure is uncomplicated will be discharged the day following the procedure. Patients with a stent will remain in hospital for a variable time after the procedure depending on the antithrombotic regime prescribed, but with preprocedural prescription of ticlopidine, discharge next day is possible.

In the UK, driving by those with a Group I licence is not allowed for seven days after an angioplasty (stents and related procedures are not particularly singled out within the guidelines). Patients with a Group II licence must complete three stages of a Bruce protocol exercise test without chest pain or ECG changes whilst untreated with any antianginal medication before they can drive again.[7]

Outcome

No studies of PTCA or related procedures have been sufficiently powerful to allow assessment of mortality. PTCA is therefore offered for symptomatic relief of patients with technically feasible lesions whose anginal symptoms are not controlled medically and who do not have a pattern of disease which would indicate prognostic benefit from surgery

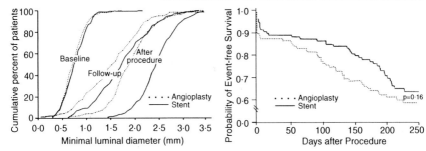

Fig 8.5 (a) Minimal diameter of the lumen at baseline, immediately after stent placement or angioplasty, and at follow-up. There was no difference in baseline values between the stent and angioplasty groups. Immediately after the procedure, the patients in the stent group had a larger minimal luminal diameter than those in the angioplasty group. Six months later, both groups had reduced values and a significant difference in diameter persisted between the two groups. (b) Kaplan–Meier survival curves for major cardiac events (death, myocardial infarction, coronary artery bypass surgery, and repeated angioplasty). Reproduced from Greunzig[8] with permission.

(e.g. main stem disease or severe three vessel disease with an impaired ventricle or multivessel disease in a diabetic).

The major limitation of basic angioplasty has been the rate of restenosis. Careful angiographic analysis confirms its presence in greater than 30% of patients (Figure 8.5) and its clinical importance is confirmed by the requirement for further intervention in at least as high a percentage of patients during the first year following the procedure.[8]

Coronary artery stenting is currently applicable only to relatively large arteries (>3 mm diameter). Recent comparative trials suggest significant benefits over basic PTCA with lower restenosis 22%[5,9] (Figure 8.5). These benefits of stenting are maintained over longer periods of observation of up to three years.[10] Size constraints means stents are not applicable to all clinically significant lesions and some of the long term advantages have in the past been offset by increased bleeding and access site problems, largely related to the use of systemic anticoagulation following stent placement. There is evidence that more effective stent expansion and confirmation of a good result by intravascular ultrasound (IVUS) can identify patients who need not be anticoagulated.[11] IVUS facilities remain limited, so most UK interventional cardiologists, while attempting to optimise stent expansion, will still opt for a postprocedural anticoagulant or antithrombotic regime.

Several recent innovations are likely to help resolve bleeding and access site problems. Like a primary coronary thrombus in MI, stent thrombus is platelet rich and more aggressive antiplatelet therapy using ticlopidine with aspirin has been demonstrated to be more effective than heparin and warfarin with aspirin in preventing acute or subacute stent thrombosis, with fewer systemic or access site bleeding problems.[12] In addition, heparin

171

bonded stents are now available and appear less thrombogenic (and possibly may inhibit the intimal hyperplasia that contributes to restenosis). Initial safety studies suggest they are safe to use in conjunction with aspirin and ticlopidine.[13] New devices are available to plug arterial puncture sites, e.g. Angioseal, which despite their additional costs may save money by allowing early discharge.

Established and new adjuvant drug therapy for PTCA and stent patients

Aspirin

All patients will have been started on aspirin before an endovascular procedure and will be maintained on it indefinitely. When required, it can be given in conjunction with warfarin though usually at a lower but constantly maintained dose of 75 mg daily so that protein binding is kept constant.

Warfarin

Systemic anticoagulation with warfarin is now used infrequently after stent placement as prevention against subacute stent thrombosis. An INR of 3·45–4·5 is currently recommended but this level may confer few benefits over lower levels of anticoagulation (e.g. 2·5–3·5) and almost certainly contributes to the high rate of vascular and bleeding complications which has been reported. If warfarin use remains relevant for stent deployment in the future, optimization of the level of anticoagulation will require examination in further clinical trials.

Hirudin

Hirudin is a 65 amino acid anticoagulant peptide which was originally isolated from leech salivary gland. It is now available from recombinant DNA technology. Hirulog is another synthetic version. Hirudin specifically inhibits thrombin activity (irreversibly), acting within the circulation and also on thrombin already within clot, thus limiting both thrombosis and thrombus extension. Platelets have thrombin receptors and their function is also reduced by hirudin. It seems likely to be a useful adjunct to other antithrombosis therapy during angioplasty and indeed, in comparison with heparin in controlled trials it reduced early cardiac events by more than 50%, though without effect on late restenosis rates.[14] Further studies to optimise its use or define specific indications are awaited.

Abciximab

A chimeric monoclonal antibody of low antigenicity targeting the platelet glycoprotein GpIIb/IIIa has also been examined in high risk angioplasties (unstable angina and recent thrombosis). This expensive monoclonal antibody is given as a single dose at the time of the procedure followed by a 12 hour infusion in conjunction with heparin. The EPIC Study demonstrated a reduction in immediate occlusion rate following angioplasty and the advantages still persisted some weeks later but the benefit was again offset by a high access site complication rate.[15] A reduction in the level of heparin anticoagulation used with abciximab is reported to reduce the number of vascular and bleeding complications to that seen with standard heparin anticoagulation alone (Eli Lilly and Company, circulated communication).

Ticlopidine

In mainland Europe ticlopidine has been used instead of warfarin after stent placement for several years with anecdotal reports of success and a recent controlled trial supports its use in conjunction with aspirin.[12] Ticlopidine inhibits ADP induced platelet aggregation, inhibits fibrinogen binding with platelets and increases bleeding time. It is usually given at a dose of 250 mg bd for one month and effects on platelet function are demonstrated within 48 hours of it being started so it has to be started three days before elective stent placement. The major side effects are haematological, with 2·4% of patients developing neutropenia which is severe in a quarter. The peak incidence is at 2–3 months after starting and it does reverse when the drug is stopped. Careful outpatient monitoring of blood count at two week intervals is advised. In a recent trial of 500 patients neutropenia was not identified, perhaps because of the short duration of the treatment.[12] Other complications include bleeding problems, as would be predicted, but diarrhoea, nausea and skin rashes have also been reported infrequently. Ticlopidine is not yet licensed for use in the UK but if approved, it will eventually be prescribed and monitored in the community.

Outpatient review

In current practice patients are often reviewed in outpatients at six weeks, 12 weeks and 26 weeks. Only the first of these is worthwhile in PTCA patients and could in fact be carried out by a conscientious general practitioner. Anticoagulation regimens for stent patients are still under review so it is likely that for the next few years these patients will continue to be reviewed at six and 12 weeks as part of audit processes. The situation will change as experience is gained. At each visit the current symptoms and current medications are reviewed. Effective revascularisation should obviate any requirement for antianginal medication though some patients may require antihypertensive agents. Aspirin treatment is maintained effectively for life and in stented patients, warfarin anticoagulation for three months or additional antiplatelet therapy with ticlopidine for one month will be required. Ticlopidine is not available except on a named patient basis in the UK and its use requires careful haematological monitoring so such patients will continue to be reviewed at the hospital at least until the drug is discontinued. In the absence of any additional indication for its use, warfarin is discontinued three months after stenting.

In the absence of any new acute event it is unusual for new ECG changes to be identified but it is usual to re-establish the baseline ECG after a procedure. The value of an exercise ECG (or indeed, a thallium perfusion scan) to confirm or refute revascularisation and coronary reserve is debatable. As stated earlier, PTCA and related procedures are carried out to relieve symptoms. Restenosis becomes relevant only if symptoms recur, so ischaemia need not be sought by any other means. An exception might be seen in a patient who has had an endovascular treatment of a proximal LAD lesion, a lesion of prognostic significance and for which alternative therapy (e.g. LIMA CABG) might need to be offered at an early stage.[16, 17] Clinically significant restenosis usually manifests itself within six months of the procedure. New symptoms after this time may be due to the disease progression rather than a late complication of the angioplasty. A most important aspect of the postprocedural consultation is education, particularly with respect to secondary prevention. Risk factors for disease progression and further events should be addressed and treated, e.g. hypertension and hyperlipidaemia.

Indications for re-referral

Recurrent symptoms should merit further assessment for invasive investigation and intervention if, as before, the symptoms are unacceptable on medical therapy. Our impression is that having been previously offered the prospect of complete relief of symptoms, patients are keen for recurrent symptoms to be investigated early and further attempts to revascularise made, if feasible.

Coronary artery bypass surgery

Survival

The VA, European and CASS studies have shown that surgery improves survival in patients with three vessel disease, especially where the ventricle is impaired. Patients with left main stem stenosis[18, 19] and those with two vessel disease involving a >75% stenosis in the LAD[20] fare better with bypass surgery. The Coronary Artery Bypass Graft Surgery Trialists Collaboration analysed data from seven randomised trials comparing a strategy of initial CABG with one of initial medical therapy for stable angina.[20] The CABG group (n=1324) had significantly lower mortality than the medical treatment group (n=1325) at five years (10·2 versus 15·8%, p=0·001), seven years (15·8 versus 21·7%, p<0·001) and 10 years (26·4 versus 30·5%, p=0·03) (Figure 8.6). The risk reduction was greater in patients with left main artery disease than in those with disease in three

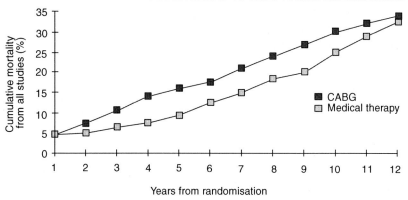

Fig 8.6 Survival curve for overall population from all studies. n = 1325 (CABG group); n = 1324 (medical treatment group) (adapted from *Lancet* 1994; **344**: 566 with permission).

vessels or one and two vessels (odds ratios at five years 0·32, 0·58 and 0·77 respectively). The absolute benefits of CABG surgery were most pronounced in patients in the higher risk categories.

Graft patency

The long term success of surgery in any particular patient depends on graft patency and the progression of native coronary artery disease. Saphenous veins have been used since the inception of CABG in the 1960s and the use of the internal mammary artery took off from the mid-1980s. Currently, a combination of the internal mammary artery (IMA) and saphenous vein grafts is used in typical patients needing two or more bypasses. The internal mammary artery is resistant to atherosclerosis and >90% of grafts remain patent on 10 year follow-up.[21] Recent results of long term studies have confirmed the superiority of IMA grafts in bypassing severe proximal lesions. In patients with diffuse coronary atheroma LAD grafting with an IMA improved survival, reduced the frequency of new coronary events and requirement for further revascularisation.[22] Twenty-six percent of vein grafts stenose or occlude within one year and up to 50% in 10 years. For this reason the internal mammary artery is used whenever possible and depending on local expertise other arterial conduits such as the inferior epigastric artery or gastroepiploic artery are often advocated instead of saphenous vein grafts. The long term results of the latter arterial conduits are awaited.

Prolonging graft patency

Early graft occlusion (within one year) is often due to thrombosis. Several placebo controlled clinical trials have established the efficacy of aspirin therapy in preventing vein graft occlusion. Various doses of aspirin ranging from 100 mg[25] to 975 mg daily[18] have been shown to be beneficial. For practical purposes, aspirin 150 mg should be commenced as soon as the patient has been extubated following CABG and continued for life. There is no convincing evidence that the addition of dipyridamole is superior to aspirin therapy alone. Oral anticoagulants have been shown to reduce the incidence of graft occlusion but are no better than aspirin and have the added hazard of increased bleeding complications.

Van der Meer et al.[26] assessed one-year angiographic vein graft patency after aortocoronary bypass surgery in 948 patients assigned to receive ultra low dose aspirin 50 mg, aspirin 50 mg plus dipyridamole 200 mg twice a day or oral anticoagulants (aiming at INR 2·8–4·8). Clinical outcome was assessed by the incidence of myocardial infarction, thrombosis, major bleeding or death. All three treatments provided protection against graft occlusion of a degree similar to other trials on aspirin therapy alone against placebo. The occlusion rate of distal anastomoses was comparable between the three treatments with 11% in the aspirin plus dipyridamole group, 15% in the aspirin only group and 13% in the oral anticoagulant group. However, clinical events were lowest in the aspirin group with 13·9% compared to 20·3% of patients receiving aspirin plus dipyridamole and 16·9% of the oral anticoagulant group. A recent study has shown conclusively that warfarin treatment is of no value in maintaining graft patency and emphasised the importance of lowering the cholesterol (see below).[30b]

NSAID associated peptic ulceration is related to dosage.[27] Thus, the risk with low dose aspirin 150 mg is small. A patient with a history of duodenal ulceration will benefit from H_2 antagonist prophylaxis[28] whereas miso-prostol is useful for prophylaxis against gastric ulceration.[29] If an ulcer is diagnosed during aspirin therapy, the ulcer can be healed with omeprazole even with continuation of the NSAID.[30a] Dipyridamole is not a proven alternative to aspirin therapy in preventing vein graft occlusion. It is anticipated that some of the novel drugs recently in use for the post-PTCA/stenting patient (e.g. ticlopidine) may also be introduced to cardiac surgery for preventing graft thrombosis in the near future.

At present, there is no specific therapy that can prevent late vein graft occlusion (>1 year). Nevertheless, aspirin therapy should be continued beyond the first year postoperatively. This is because grafting bypasses critical lesions that are responsible for a patient's angina but does not prevent native coronary artery disease progression and aspirin is of proven value in reducing the incidence of myocardial infarction in patients with coronary artery disease.

Symptoms

From the CASS Registry of 24,958 patients, 9557 who underwent CABG were followed up annually for a mean of six years by Cameron et *al.*[23] for recurrence of angina. Angina recurred in 24% of patients in the first year and in 40% by the sixth year. The presence of angina in the first postoperative year was associated with more frequent myocardial infarction ($p = 0.04$) and greater need for reoperation ($p = 0.003$) but did not affect survival during the six year follow-up period. The cumulative survival rate at the sixth postoperative year was 88% for patients both with and without angina during the first postoperative year. Angina was reported as present even if just *one episode* occurred per year, which may explain why the incidence of angina recurrence here is higher than in other studies; the one, five and 10 year rates of survival free from angina amongst a group of 1025 CABG patients at the Cardiovascular Unit of the Rikshospitalet in Oslo[24] were 97·8%, 91·8% and 80·6%. Another important reason contributing to the discrepancy of angina is the period of CABG. In the CASS Study, patients were operated between 1975 and 1979 whereas in the Oslo Study, CABG was performed much later, between 1982 to 1986, when operative skills and perioperative management would have improved.

Modifying risk factors

Risk factors for recurrence of angina and prognosis were studied for the 9557 patients who underwent isolated CABG in the CASS Study.[23] It was found that the significant predictors for recurrence of angina in the first year in a multivariate analysis were minimal coronary artery disease, preoperative angina, use of vein grafts only, previous myocardial infarction, incomplete revascularisation, female gender, smoking, and younger age. In subsequent years, important predictors were angina in the first post-operative year, female gender, younger age, and incomplete revascularisation. The presence of angina in the first postoperative year was associated with more frequent myocardial infarction ($p = 0.04$) and greater need for reoperation ($p = 0.003$) but did not affect survival during the six year follow-up period. When predictors of mortality in multivariate analysis were studied, the significant predictors in order of relative risk estimate were current *smoker* (defined as smoking >half pack per week), non-elective bypass surgery, *diabetes*, vein grafts only, *hypertension*, incomplete revascularisation and multivessel disease. Thus, the CASS Study would suggest that control of smoking, diabetes and hypertension is important for long term survival post-CABG and that control of smoking may reduce the risk of early angina recurrence.

The role of hyperlipidaemia and prognosis in the CASS surgical group was not mentioned in Cameron's study. Nevertheless, the Cholesterol Lowering Atherosclerosis Study has shown that active lowering of LDL with medical therapy can decrease atherosclerosis in native coronaries as well as retard progression of vein graft disease.[31] A large study by Sergeant *et al.*[32] involving 5880 patients who underwent CABG between 1971 and 1987 demonstrated hyperlipidaemia to be a positive risk factor in late angina recurrence and myocardial infarction. Even in the extreme subgroup, patients with familial hypercholesterolaemia, long term survival after CABG can be good and comparable to results in heterogeneous groups of patients within the European and CASS study groups, as shown by Kawasuji et al.[33] They assessed the long term results of CABG performed during 13 years in 62 patients with heterozygous familiar hypercholester-olaemia. After operation, all patients consumed a cholesterol lowering diet and received drug therapy with pravastatin, probucol or cholestyramine. The cholesterol lowering therapy reduced plasma cholesterol level by 37%, LDL by 42% and LDL/HDL cholesterol ratio by 37%. During a mean follow-up (mean = 52 months, range = 10–157 months), actuarial freedom from recurrent angina was 90% at five years and 53% at 11 years after operation. The actuarial survival rate was 95% at five years and 89% at 12 years.

The Post Coronary Artery Bypass Graft Trial investigators have recently reported on their comparison of low dose anticoagulation with warfarin and lipid lowering for prevention of graft atherosclerosis.[30b] All 1351 patients in the trial took 81 mg aspirin a day. Aggressive lowering of LDL cholesterol with lovastatin (and cholestyramine if necessary) aimed at achieving an LDL level of less than 2·56 mmol/L, while moderate treatment aimed for LDL levels between 3·4 and 3·6 mmol/L. The more aggressive regime resulted in angiographically demonstrated atherosclerosis in 27% of grafts, compared with 39% of grafts in those allocated to the moderate regime. In keeping with this highly significant effect, the revascularisation rate at four years was 29% lower in those allocated to the aggressive regime. The potential for additional effects from low dose anticoagulation with warfarin was also examined. A mean normalised international ratio of 1·4 was achieved with daily warfarin doses of between 1 and 4 mg, but no further effect on angiographically defined atherosclerosis was demonstrated. This important study emphasises the importance of lipid lowering therapy in preventing graft failure. The aim of cholesterol lowering should be an LDL level of less than 3·4 mmol/L and a total cholesterol level below 5·2 mmol/L.[34]

Outpatient follow-up

In current practice CABG patients are routinely seen in outpatients at six weeks postoperation and most are seen by junior doctors in training. However, a review by a general practitioner briefed about the expected findings would not be an inappropriate alternative.

At the initial visit, the skin wounds are examined for satisfactory healing and the sternum checked for union. A chest X-ray is performed to ensure adequate re-expansion of the lungs since all patients develop a variable degree of basal collapse during the early postoperative period. A small pleural effusion is common, occurring in 40% of cases in a study by Peng *et al.*[35] In a minority of cases, the effusion is significant and fails to resolve despite repeated needle aspirations. The aetiology of chronic post-CABG effusions is not understood but appears to be more common in patients with an impaired left ventricle.[36] Patients with a compromising effusion, an effusion which increases in size or recurs after aspiration should be followed up in outpatients. Small to moderate effusions which are stable in a non-dyspnoeic patient are left alone and the chest X-ray reviewed again at 12 weeks postoperation.

Drug therapy is reviewed. The importance of continuing aspirin for life is stressed. Coronary endarterectomy is infrequently performed. However, if an extensive endarterectomy was carried out during CABG, some surgeons advocate adding a three month course of warfarin aiming at an INR level of between 2 and 3·8.

An ECG is carried out; 30% or more of CABG patients develop new atrial fibrillation (AF) postoperation.[37] The arrhythmia is almost always transient. Various antiarrhythmic agents are often started during hospitalisation for rate control (e.g. digoxin, metoprolol, verapamil) or attempted cardioversion (e.g. amiodarone, sotalol). These drugs are stopped at the postoperative check-up if the patient is back in sinus rhythm. If the patient is still in AF formal anticoagulation prior to referral for elective cardioversion is appropriate. Antianginal therapy should have ceased immediately after successful CABG. Antihypertensives, medications for cardiac failure and other non-cardiac medications are continued.

Driving

Driving should be avoided for eight weeks to allow a stable union of the sternum. For drivers of heavy goods vehicles and passenger carrying vehicles, the DVLC needs to be notified as such driving is allowed to continue only after successfully completing stage 3 of the Bruce exercise test without chest pain or ST changes, in the absence of antianginal medication. Patients whose functional status has improved at the six week review are discharged to their general practitioner for ongoing care. Well patients can resume work from eight weeks postoperation.

Ongoing care

Successful CABG will have cured a patient of critical ischaemia. Improvement of functional status is well documented and extends to patients of all age groups. There are no restrictions on activities. On the contrary, a gradual stepping up of exercise should be encouraged since exercise is associated with an improvement in lipid profile by raising the HDL/LDL ratio. Moderate exercise sustained for periods of about 20 minutes and repeated regularly, rather than high intensity exercise, is advised.[38] A meta-analysis of trials suggests a potential overall mortality reduction of about 20% in individuals with ischaemic heart disease who exercise regularly.[39] Modifying risk factors for ischaemic heart disease is the primary aim in the ongoing care as this influences the late outcomes of surgery. During the course of ongoing care, a patient may present to their general practitioner with various postprocedure problems. Some of the more common problems and their management are outlined below.

Wound healing

Irritating stitch granulomas associated with the absorbable skin suture and sterile discharges are common around the ends of the sternal wounds, vein harvesting site and also around the knee. Discharges at these sites are often intermittent but usually settle within weeks and occasionally within a few months. Any excess suture material protruding from the wound should be cut off, discharges should be swabbed and infections treated. Antibiotic therapy before microbiology results are available should cover for staphylococcus and enterobacteria. Sternal wound infections, other than a superficial skin infection responding to therapy, and chronic symptomatic granulomas (>3 months) should be referred back to the surgeon. Sternal wires that protrude can occasionally cause localised pain and discomfort. If this becomes troublesome, elective removal can be arranged as a day case.

Peripheral nerve injuries

Injury to the saphenous nerve below the knee is common as the nerve is in apposition to the long saphenous vein at this level. Harvesting the internal mammary will also inevitably damage fine peripheral sensory nerves innervating the anterior chest wall. The numbness and paraesthesia from both nerve injuries are usually well tolerated and may improve over a period of months. Rarely, a constant burning pain from the denervated internal mammary site requires continued analgesia. A small percentage of unfortunate patients develop a brachial plexus injury affecting the lower roots from excessive sternal retraction or pressure induced common peroneal nerve palsy causing foot drop. The resulting motor dysfunctions are debilitating and will need prolonged physiotherapy and sympathy. Recovery is to be expected within 3–5 months.[40]

Tailoring drug therapy post-CABG

Tailoring drug therapy postprocedure needs care and attention to detail and familiarity with the patient's preoperative clinical background. This is best achieved by the patient's general practitioner. Medications for hypertension, hyperlipidaemia, diabetes, heart failure, and non-cardiac drugs are continued. For a variable period from days to weeks postoperatively, drug requirement and dosage will fluctuate whilst bodily systems readjust to the effects of major surgery. Thus, a patient previously on oral hypoglycaemics for diabetes may initially require insulin until the stress response of hyperglycaemia tails off or a known hypertensive patient on calcium antagonists preoperatively may initially require a smaller dosage until the blood pressure re-establishes its preoperative levels. In some patients, the left ventricular function is found at operation to be worse than had been reported at angiography. On symptomatic or prognostic grounds, ACE inhibitors are sometimes begun before discharge, starting with a test dose. The dosage should be increased to therapeutic levels according to patient response and tolerance and continued. A survey of ACE inhibitor treatment by Fox[41] has highlighted that dosages prescribed are suboptimal in a high percentage of cases (68% in the study) despite excluding patients for whom the target dose was limited by hypotension or renal impairment.

Peripheral oedema

Mild peripheral oedema without evidence of cardiac failure commonly occurs post-bypass surgery. Mobilisation, leg elevation, and a short course of diuretics are usually sufficient in resolving this benign condition.

Recurrence of angina

Ten years after CABG, limiting angina will have returned in 20–40%[23, 24] of cases (Figure 8.7). The functional status of the patient rather than the presence of angina influences management.

Antianginal therapy should be started. Referral to a cardiologist for an opinion is indicated when angina is poorly controlled by medication, where exercise tolerance is low or symptoms significantly disrupt lifestyle. Although exercise ECG is poor at providing information regarding graft patency,[42, 43] it is still commonly used as an initial outpatient investigation as it can help identify a subgroup of patients with poor angina status where further investigations are indicated. Thus, a patient whose Bruce protocol exercise test is terminated in under five minutes due to angina or ST changes will probably require either an exercise thallium scan or angiography to assess graft patency and native coronary artery disease. On the other hand, a patient who can perform more than 10 minutes of the Bruce protocol has a good prognosis and can usually be managed with medical therapy.[44] Patients considered for repeat revascularisation are carefully selected since mortality of redo coronary artery bypass surgery is four times that of first time CABG (9·2% versus 2·4%).

Conclusion

Clinicians in primary care will encounter increasing numbers of patients having PTCA and CABG. The success of invasive coronary interventions depends on careful management of specific periprocedure problems in the short term and active control of risk factors for ischaemic heart disease in the long term in reducing restenosis and progression of native coronary artery disease.

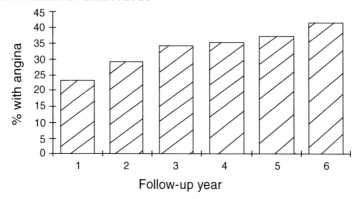

Fig 8.7   Prevalence of angina after coronary artery bypass surgery for the first six postoperative years (from *J Am Coll Cardiol* 1995; **26**: 896 with permission).

1 Society of Cardiothoracic Surgeons of Great Britain and Ireland:SCSGBI. London: *United Kingdom cardiac surgical register, 1992.*
2 British Cardiac Society. Council statement on the demand and need for cardiac services of the development of a waiting list strategy for cardiac disease. www http://bcs.rbh.nthames.nhs.uk.
3 Hubner PJB. Cardiac interventional procedures in the United Kingdom during 1990. *Br Heart J* 1992; **66**: 469–71.
4 Schomig A, Kastrati A, Mudra H *et al.* Four year experience with Palmaz-Schatz stenting in coronary angioplasty complicated by dissection with threatened or present vessel closure. *Circulation* 1994; **90**: 2716–24.
5 Serruys PW, de Jaegere P, Kiemeneij F *et al.* A comparison of balloon-expandable stent implantation with balloon angioplasty in treatment of coronary artery disease. *N Engl J Med* 1994; **331**: 489–95.
6 Currie P, Turnbull CM, Shaw TRD. Pseudoaneurysm of the femoral artery after cardiac catheterisation: diagnosis and treatment by manual compression guided by Doppler colour flow imaging. *Br Heart J* 1994; **72**: 80–4.
7 Medical Commission on Accident Prevention. *Medical aspects of fitness to drive.* London: HMSO, 1995.
8 Greunzig AR, King SB, Schlumpf M, Siegenthaler W. Long term follow up after percutaneous transluminal coronary angioplasty: the early Zurich experience. *N Engl J Med* 1987; **316**: 1127–32.
9 Fischman DL, Leon MB, Baim DS *et al.* A randomised comparison of coronary-stent placement and balloon angioplasty in the treatment of coronary artery disease. *N Engl J Med* 1994; **331**: 496–501.
10 Kimura T, Yokoi H, Nakagawa Y *et al.* Three years follow up after implantation of metallic coronary-artery stents. *N Engl J Med* 1996; **334**: 561–6.
11 Colombo A, Hall P, Nakamura S *et al.* Intracoronary stenting without anticoagulation accomplished with intravascular ultrasound guidance. *Circulation* 1995; **91**: 1676–88.
12 Schomig A, Neuman F-J, Kastrati A *et al.* A randomised comparison of antiplatelet and anticoagulant therapy after placement of coronary-artery stents. *N Engl J Med* 1996; **334**: 1084–9.
13 Serruys PW, Emanuelsson H, van der Giessen W *et al.* Heparin-coated, Palmaz-Schatz stents in human coronary arteries: early outcome of the Benestent II Pilot Study. *Circulation* 1996; **93**: 412–22.
14 Serruys PW, Herman J-P, Simon R *et al.* A comparison of hirudin with heparin in the prevention of restenosis after coronary angioplasty. *N Engl J Med* 1995; **333**: 757–63.
15 The EPIC Investigators. Use of a monoclonal antibody directed against the platelet glycoprotein IIb/IIIa receptor in high risk coronary angioplasty. *N Engl J Med* 1994; **330**:

456–61.

16 Schuster EH, Griffith LS, Buckley BH. Preponderance of acute proximal left anterior descending coronary artery lesions in fatal myocardial infarction: a clinical-pathological study. *Am J Cardiol* 1981; **49**: 1189–96.

17 Rahimtoola SH. Left main equivalence is still an unproven hypothesis but proximal left anterior descending coronary artery disease is a "high risk" lesion. *Am J Cardiol* 1984; **53**: 1719–21.

18 Goldman S, Copeland J, Moritz T. Improvement in early saphenous vein graft patency after coronary artery bypass surgery with antiplatelet therapy: results of a Veterans Administration cooperative study. *Circulation* 1988; **77**: 1324–32.

19 Varnouskas E, for the European Coronary Study Group. Twelve year follow-up of survival in the randomized European Coronary Surgery Group. *N Engl J Med* 1988; **319**: 332–7.

20 Yusuf S, Zucker D, Peduzzi P *et al.* Effect of coronary artery bypass graft surgery on survival: overview of 10 year results from randomised trials by the Coronary Artery Bypass Graft Surgery Trialists Collaboration. *Lancet* 1994; **344**: 563–70.

21 Loop FD, Lytle BW, Cosgrove DM *et al.* Influence of the internal mammary artery graft on 10 year survival and other cardiac events. *N Engl J Med* 1986; **314**: 1–6.

22 Cameron A, Davis KB, Green G, Schaff HV. Coronary artery bypass with internal-thoracic artery grafts – effect on survival over a 15 year period. *N Engl J Med* 1996; **334**: 216–19.

23 Cameron A, Davis K, Rogers W. Recurrence of angina after coronary artery bypass surgery: predictors and prognosis (CASS Registry). *J Am Coll Cardiol* 1995; **26**: 895–9.

24 Risum O, Abdelnoor M, Svennevig J *et al.* Risk factors of recurrent angina pectoris and of non-fatal myocardial infarction after coronary artery bypass surgery. *Eur J Cardiothorac Surg* 1996; **10**: 173–8.

25 Lorenz RL, Schacky CV, Weber M *et al.* Improved aortocoronary bypass patency by low-dose aspirin (100 mg). Effects on platelet aggregation and thromboxane formation. *Lancet* 1984; **i**: 1261–4.

26 Van der Meer J, Hillege HL, Kootstra GJ *et al.* Prevention of one-year vein-graft occlusion after aortocoronary-bypass surgery: a comparison of low-dose aspirin, low-dose aspirin plus dipyridamole, and oral anticoagulants. *Lancet* 1993; **342**: 257–64.

27 Garcia R, Jick H. Risk of upper gastrointestinal bleeding and perforation associated with individual non-steroidal anti-inflammatory drugs. *Lancet* 1994; **343**: 769–72.

28 Ehsanullah RS, Page MC, Wood JR. Prevention of gastroduodenal damage induced by non-steroidal anti-inflammatory drugs: controlled trial of ranitidine. *Br Med J* 1988; **297**: 1017–21.

29 Graham DY, White RH, Moreland LW *et al.* Duodenal and gastric ulcer prevention with misoprostol in arthritis patients taking NSAIDS. *Ann Intern Med* 1993; **119**: 257–62.

30a Roth S, Agrawal N, Mahowald M *et al.* Misoprostol heals gastroduodenal injury in patients with rheumatoid arthritis receiving aspirin. *Arch Intern Med* 1989; **149**: 775–9.

30b The Post Coronary Artery Bypass Graft Trial Investigators. The effect of aggressive lowering of low density lipoprotein cholesterol levels and low-dose anticoagulation on obstructive changes in saphenous vein coronary bypass grafts. *N Engl J Med* 1997; **336**: 153–62.

31 Blankenhorn DH, Nessim SA, Johnson RL *et al.* Beneficial effects of combined colestipol-niacin therapy on coronary atherosclerosis and coronary venous bypass grafts. *JAMA* 1987; **257**: 3233–40.

32 Sergeant P, Lesaffre E, Flameno W *et al.* The return of clinically evident ischaemia after coronary artery bypass. *Eur J Cardiothorac Surg* 1991; **5**(9): 447–57.

33 Kawasuji M, Sakakibara N, Hirofumi T *et al.* Coronary artery bypass grafting in familial hypercholesterolemia. *J Thorac Cardiovasc Surg* 1995; **109**: 364–9.

34 Betteridge DJ, Dodson PM, Durrington PN *et al.* Management of hyperlipidaemia: guidelines of the British Hyperlipidaemia Association. *Postgrad Med J* 1993; **69**: 359–69.

35 Peng MJ, Vargas FS, Cukier A *et al.* Post-operative pleural changes after coronary revascularization. *Chest* 1992; **101**: 327–30.

36 Kollef MC. Chronic pleural effusion following coronary artery revascularisation with the internal mammary artery. *Chest* 1990; **97**: 750–1.

37 Cochrane AD, Siddens M, Rosenfeldt R *et al.* A comparison of amiodarone and digoxin for

treatment of supraventricular arrhythmias after cardiac surgery. *Eur J Cardiothorac Surg* 1994; **8**: 194–8.

38 Thompson D, Bowman GS, Kitson AL *et al.* Cardiac rehabilitation in the United Kingdom: guidelines and audit standards. *Heart* 1996; **75**: 89–93.

39 O'Connor GT, Buring JE, Yusuf S *et al.* An overview of randomized trials of rehabilitation with exercise after myocardial infarction. *Circulation* 1989; **80**: 234–44.

40 Kirsh MV, Magee KR, Gago O *et al.* Brachial plexus injuries following median sternotomy. *Ann Thorac Surg* 1971; **11**: 315–19.

41 Fox K, Wray R. Are we using the right dose of ACE inhibitor? *Br J Clin Cardiol* 1995; **2**(10): 286–9.

42 Lakkis NM, Mahmarian JJ, Verani MS. Exercise thallium-201 single photon emission computed tomography for evaluation of coronary artery bypass graft patency. *Am J Cardiol* 1995; **76**: 107–11.

43 Bartel AG, Behar VS, Peter RH *et al.* Exercise stress testing in evaluation of aortocoronary bypass surgery. *Circulation* 1973; **48**: 141–8.

44 Mark DB, Shaw L, Harrell FE *et al.* Prognostic value of a treadmill exercise score in outpatients with suspected coronary disease. *N Engl J Med* 1991; **325**: 849–53.

184

9: Management strategies in atrial fibrillation

MM GALLAGHER, AG RAVI KISHORE AND
AJ CAMM

Atrial fibrillation is a common cardiac arrhythmia which occurs in 0·4% of the adult population and in as many as 2–4% of those 60 years or older.[1,2] In the Framingham Study, the overall incidence of atrial fibrillation was 2% and the incidence rose sharply with age.[3] Atrial fibrillation is a clinically important arrhythmia as it accounts for the largest number of days spent in the hospital, when the principal diagnosis is cardiac arrhythmia.[4] Yet until recently, atrial fibrillation has received much less attention than the other cardiac arrhythmias and its treatment remains difficult and poorly standardised. For the present day clinician, a bewildering array of pharmacological and non-pharmacological treatment options have become available. Optimum utilization of these modalities may help in developing better management strategies for patients with atrial fibrillation.

Introduction

In planning a treatment strategy for a patient with atrial fibrillation, it is important to consider the therapeutic endpoints. These will necessarily depend on the patient's symptomatology and the prognostic implications for the patient if the arrhythmia is allowed to persist or recur. The symptoms in a patient with atrial fibrillation can result from uncontrolled ventricular rate or from the loss of atrial contractile function. A fast and irregular ventricular rhythm results in the distressing symptom of palpitations. It also leads to increased myocardial oxygen demand and can precipitate a variety of ischaemic syndromes in predisposed individuals. Loss of atrial transport leads to a reduction in stroke volume by 20–40% and increase in left ventricular filling pressures.[5,6] These account for reduced work capacity, dyspnoea and can precipitate heart failure, especially in patients with diminished left ventricular function and other associated heart disease.

Atrial fibrillation has a significant impact on morbidity and mortality. In

185

the Framingham Study, atrial fibrillation was found to be associated with a doubled cardiovascular mortality and death due to all causes.[3] In the Manitoba Follow-Up Study (MFUS),[7] atrial fibrillation was associated with 1·7 times risk for total mortality and 2·4 times risk for cardiovascular death. Increased risk of thromboembolic events is probably the most important consequence of atrial fibrillation. Overall, after adjustment of age, gender and hypertension the risk of stroke is increased about fivefold by atrial fibrillation.[8] The risk of stroke in patients with lone atrial fibrillation is less clear, with a fourfold increase reported in Framingham Study[9] and no such association being reported by Kopecky *et al.*[10a] Even when the ventricular rate is well controlled, validated quality of life questionnaires reveal a significant impairment of quality of life associated with atrial fibrillation.[10b]

The prognostic importance of atrial fibrillation in the presence of congestive heart failure is variable (Figure 9.1). In patients with advanced heart failure, actuarial survival is significantly worse for patients with atrial fibrillation as compared to sinus rhythm patients (52% versus 71%).[11] The presence of atrial fibrillation, however, does not have any impact on the prognosis of patients with mild to moderate heart failure.[12] The impact of atrial fibrillation on the in-hospital and long term survival in patients after myocardial infarction is not clear, with conflicting observations being reported. The results of a large multicentre study suggest a lack of independent effect of atrial fibrillation on the in-hospital and long term survival after myocardial infarction.[13]

Finally it should be realised that, unlike ventricular tachycardia or

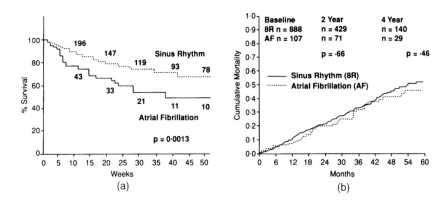

Fig 9.1 (a) Plots of actuarial one-year survival in patients with severe heart failure with sinus rhythm (n = 315, broken line) compared with those with atrial fibrillation (n = 75, solid line). (b) Cumulative mortality for atrial fibrillation versus sinus rhythm in patients with mild to moderate heart failure (the vasodilator heart failure trial II). p values are for two-year survival and overall mortality comparisons. Risk of mortality of patients with atrial fibrillation and mild to moderate heart failure.

fibrillation where a single recurrence might be fatal, this arrhythmia is basically benign. It is a nuisance arrhythmia, debilitating and incapacitating in some but not, except in rare circumstances, fatal. Thus it may not always be necessary to aim for total arrhythmia eradication and subject patients to potentially toxic antiarrhythmic therapy or expensive non-pharmacological interventions.

Considering these factors, the management decisions in atrial fibrillation must be individualised based on the clinical context. The broad treatment goals are restoration of sinus rhythm, maintenance of sinus rhythm and control of ventricular rate. Anticoagulant therapy, which forms an important treatment limb in atrial fibrillation, is discussed in Chapter 4.

Restoration and maintenance of sinus rhythm

Although sinus rhythm is preferable to atrial fibrillation, not all patients benefit from cardioversion. The need for sinus rhythm and the likelihood of immediate and long term success require individual consideration. Patients with recent onset atrial fibrillation should be considered for cardioversion, regardless of symptoms. For patients with sustained atrial fibrillation, however, the decision to cardiovert is generally based on the clinical setting (Table 9.1). It is important to consider not only the probability of successful cardioversion but also the likelihood of maintaining sinus rhythm thereafter. Up until now no clinically useful decision algorithms allowing for predictions concerning arrhythmia outcome have been established. Estimations of probability of conversion and postcardioversion success form an important guide in planning the management strategy in patients with atrial fibrillation.

Table 9.1   Indications and contraindications for cardioversion

---

Indications
Recent onset atrial fibrillation, even if asymptomatic
History of peripheral embolic episodes
Persistent AF, in spite of successful treatment of underlying disorder (e.g. thyrotoxicosis)
Rapid ventricular rate unresponsive to medical therapy
Persistent symptoms on medical therapy

Contraindications
Relative:
   Atrial fibrillation >2 years
   Left atrial dimension >50 mm
   NYHA class 3 or 4
   Left ventricular EF <25%
Absolute:
   Digitalis toxicity
   Patients with sinus node dysfunction and bradycardia-tachycardia syndrome, unless a
   pacemaker is implanted

Determinants of cardioversion and postcardioversion success

Duration of atrial fibrillation, type of underlying heart disease, patient's age, left ventricular function, and left atrial size are the factors studied by most workers. Duration of atrial fibrillation before attempted cardioversion appears to be an important prognostic indicator of both immediate and long term success. A duration of atrial fibrillation of more than one year resulted in a 48% recurrence rate at one month after successful cardioversion, compared to a 25% recurrence rate in those patients with atrial fibrillation of less than one year.[14] Underlying heart disease (especially rheumatic mitral valve disease),[15] associated pulmonary disease,[16] and patient age >50 years[17] have been associated with poor success rates. Conflicting reports are available with regard to the importance of left atrial size[16,18] and left ventricular dysfunction.[18,19] In a recent multivariant analysis, the only patient characteristics determining the chances of conversion were the arrhythmia duration and age of the patient.[20] The factors influencing maintenance of sinus rhythm were presence of mitral valve disease and a low precardioversion conversion functional class.[21a] Although most of the available data apply to external direct current cardioversion, the same factors may also influence results of other modes of cardioversion. Thus a careful analysis of the need for cardioversion and estimation of the probability of success may help to avoid unsuccessful cardioversions and improve the cost/benefit ratio.

Methods of cardioversion

Pharmacological cardioversion

Although electrical cardioversion is of proven efficacy and has stood the test of time, pharmacologial cardioversion can be attempted in stable patients with atrial fibrillation. It has the advantage of not requiring a general anaesthetic and high success rates have been reported with several drugs. The delay in the onset of action of drugs and risk of proarrhythmia, however, limits its utility to stable and low risk patients respectively. The drugs used for pharmacological cardioversion are shown in Table 9.2. There is some evidence that atrial contractile function recovers more quickly after pharmacological cardioversion than after DC shock.[10b,21b] This is balanced by a number of studies which suggest that the mechanical dysfunction is independent of the means of cardioversion.[21c,21d]

Digitalis Digoxin is still occasionally used for attempting to restore sinus rhythm. Weiner *et al.*, in an uncontrolled study, reported a high conversion rate with rapid intravenous digitalisation in 45 patients with recent onset atrial fibrillation.[21e] Reversion to sinus rhythm occurred in 40 of the 47 episodes within one to 96 hours after initiation of digitalis therapy. Falk *et al.*[22] in a randomised double blind trial involving 36 patients with recent

Table 9.2   Drugs used in atrial fibrillation

Drugs used primarily for controlling ventricular rate
Digitalis and other digitalis glycosides
β-blockers:
   Cardioselective – atenolol
   Partial agonists – pindolol, xamoterol
Calcium channel blockers:
   verapamil
   diltiazem

Drugs used in restoring sinus rhythm/maintenance of sinus rhythm
Increase atrial refractoriness and reduce conduction velocity:
   Quinidine
   Disopyramide
   Procainamide
   Morcsizine
Primarily reduce conduction velocity:
   Flecainide
   Encainide
   Propafenone
Primarily increase atrial refractoriness:
   Amiodarone
   Sotalol
   d-Sotalol
   Dofetelide
   Ibutelide
   E-4031

Anticoagulants and antiplatelet agents

---

onset atrial fibrillation, concluded that digitalisation was no more effective than placebo for reversion of atrial fibrillation to sinus rhythm. In conclusion, the data are limited, but suggest that digitalis is not effective in converting acute episodes of atrial fibrillation.

Quinidine   High oral loading doses (up to 1·5 g/day) are effective in restoring sinus rhythm in patients with atrial fibrillation. In a study comparing oral quinidine (up to 1·2 g) with intravenous flecainide (up to 2 mg/kg), Borgeat *et al.*[23] observed that both the drugs were equally effective in recent onset atrial fibrillation (80% versus 86% respectively) with quinidine being superior in patients with chronic atrial fibrillation (40% versus 22% respectively). Zehender *et al.*[24] compared the effects of intravenous amiodarone with quinidine and verapamil in patients with chronic atrial fibrillation. The combination of quinidine and verapamil restored sinus rhythm in 55% of patients as compared to 60% after amiodarone. Quinidine alone was, however, successful in only 25% of patients. A feature noted with the combination of quinidine and verapamil was a "rate smoothing" effect before conversion, which may confer a haemodynamic advantage in patients with atrial fibrillation. One of the major problems with quinidine is the incidence of both non-cardiac and cardiac side effects, particularly proarrhythmia. Provocation of torsade de

189

pointes and organisation of atrial fibrillation into atrial flutter have been reported.[25, 26] Its onset is unpredictable, unrelated to dosage and can occur within 48 hours of starting quinidine.

Procainamide Successful conversion of recent onset atrial fibrillation can be achieved with both oral loading (1·5 g) and intravenous infusion[27, 28] (15–20 mg/min up to a maximum of 1000 mg) of procainamide. With intravenous infusion, conversion is achieved in 40–60% of patients with no significant side effects.

Flecainide In spite of the general concerns regarding the use of flecainide after the publication of the CAST,[29] it is a useful atrial antiarrhythmic agent. Flecainide is effective in restoring sinus rhythm in patients with recent onset atrial fibrillation. Kingma *et al.*[30] reported an overall conversion rate of 86% with 2 mg/kg of IV flecainide, administered over 10 minutes (max. 150 mg). In patients with recent onset atrial fibrillation (<24 hours), the conversion rate was 96% and in those with long standing atrial fibrillation it was 67%. The success rate was clearly superior to intravenous propafenone and verapamil. Other workers have reported similar results.[31–34] Hohnloser *et al.* reviewed the literature and reported a 65% efficacy of flecainide for acute conversion in atrial fibrillation.[35] In another study Capucci *et al.*[36] reported restoration of sinus rhythm, within 24 hours, in 21 of 22 patients given 300 mg of flecainide as a single oral loading dose. No major adverse effects were reported. Crijns *et al.* reported that oral flecainide (up to 400 mg in three hours) was as effective as intravenous flecainide (up to 150 mg in 30 minutes).[34] It is, however, recommended that flecainide is best avoided in patients with severe left ventricular dysfunction and should always be administered with close electrocardiographic monitoring because transient adverse reactions on cardiac conduction system are common.[30]

Propafenone This is a class IC drug with mild β-blocking activity. Both intravenous (2 mg/kg over 10 minutes) and oral administration (600 mg as a single dose) have been shown to be effective for cardioversion.[30, 37, 38] Although less effective, propafenone has the advantage of having fewer adverse effects than intravenous flecainide.[30, 37] It has, however, been reported to cause a reversible low output state in patients already haemodynamically compromised and should probably be avoided in patients with severe cardiac failure.[37]

Amiodarone Amiodarone is also effective in reverting atrial fibrillation. There is, however, uncertainty regarding the appropriate dosing regimen. Success has been documented with both oral[39, 40] and intravenous routes.[24, 41–46] Intravenous administration is more effective. In a study comparing the efficacy of oral or intravenous amiodarone with DC

190

cardioversion for the restoration of sinus rhythm in atrial fibrillation, the success rates respectively were 29%, 64%, and 42%. When only first attempts at cardioversion were analysed, there was no difference between intravenous amiodarone and DC cardioversion.[46] Time to conversion has varied in different studies and ranges from 30 minutes to as long as four weeks, obviously depending on the route of administration, drug dosage, and patient characteristics.[24, 39–46] Successful conversion has been reported in recent onset[40–42, 45] as well as chronic atrial fibrillation.[24, 40, 44] Skoulargis et al.[39] reported a 77% conversion rate after four weeks of therapy with a high oral loading dose in patients with chronic atrial fibrillation. Bellandi et al.[45] reported an 81% efficacy in restoring sinus rhythm in 98 patients with recent onset stable atrial fibrillation after intravenous amiodarone. The mean conversion time was $11·2 \pm 4·3$ hours. Blevins et al.[47] reported the efficacy of amiodarone in patients with refractory atrial fibrillation (no response to two drug trials); eight of 40 patients reverted to sinus rhythm after intravenous amiodarone administered as an infusion. Brodsky et al.[48] reported successful cardioversion in 28 patients with chronic atrial fibrillation and a dilated left atrium (>45 mm). An uncommon but important side effect reported with intravenous amiodarone is severe bradycardia, mainly occurring during early infusion.This may require dose reduction or withdrawal of therapy.[44]

Sotalol   Uncontrolled studies have shown limited effectiveness of intravenous *d*-sotalol in terminating recent onset atrial fibrillation. In one study, intravenous sotalol (0·5 mg/kg in six minutes) caused arrhythmia in 4/11 patients with atrial flutter or fibrillation.[49a] Even at a dose of 1·5 mg/kg, conversion occurred in only two of 16 patients.[49b] Only in patients with atrial fibrillation of less than 24 hours duration does sotalol convert a significant proportion to sinus rhythm and even in this situation flecainide is far more effective.[49c]

Ibutilide   This newly developed class III drug is available only for parenteral use because of high first pass metabolism.[49d] It has a high efficacy in the acute conversion of atrial flutter, but converts only 31% of patients in atrial fibrillation.[49e] The lower efficacy in atrial fibrillation could not be attributed to the duration of the arrhythmia before attempted conversion. Administration of ibutilide was complicated by polymorphic ventricular tachycardia in 8·3% of cases.

Dofetilide   This is a new antiarrhythmic agent closely related to *d*-sotalol. It selectively prolongs refractoriness without any effects on conduction by blocking the delayed rectifier potassium channels.[50] Preliminary studies have confirmed a potent antiarrhythmic effect with minimum side effects.[51] In a recent open label dose ranging study,[52] dofetilide terminated atrial

191

fibrillation in 10/19 patients (53%). The mean time required for conversion was 40 ± 52 minutes and there were no significant side effects.

External direct current cardioversion

External cardioversion, introduced in 1962, is reported to restore sinus rhythm in approximately 90% of patients with chronic atrial fibrillation.[53] Little has changed in the technique since its introduction, although progress has been made in understanding the determinants of success.

There is some controversy regarding the optimal paddle position. Lown and colleagues[54] reported that the anteroposterior electrode position was more effective for cardioversion of atrial fibrillation than the anterior-anterior electrode position. In contrast, Kerber *et al.*[55] reported that electrode position made little difference to cardioversion success. For successful cardioversion, the current vector must transverse a critical mass of atrial muscle. The anteroposterior position fulfils this criterion best. Ewy[56] recommends the right anterior-left posterior position as the position of choice if the pathology involves both atria (i.e. atrial fibrillation due to atrial septal defect or diffuse cardiomyopathy) and the left anterior-posterior electrode position in patients with dominant left atrial pathology. This view has, however, not been tested in a controlled study. The anterior-anterior and apical-left posterior positions, are, however, not recommended as they probably do not provide optimal current vector and flow through the atria.

It is recommended that the shock be delivered in full expiratory phase of ventilation[57] with a firm electrode pressure.[58] Controversies exist regarding the optimum paddle area and the type of coupling agent used.[59] No clearcut recommendations can, however, be made. Chest size and the body weight of the patient[55] have been reported to influence the results of direct current cardioversion by their effects on transthoracic impedance. The negative effects of concomitant antiarrhythmic drug therapy are not clear; flecainide has been shown to increase the energy requirements for cardioversion.[60a] There is, however, no evidence to suggest whether this has any impact on the final result. Nevertheless, if cardioversion is unsuccessful in a patient receiving flecainide, it may be prudent to repeat the procedure after changing the drug. Amiodarone is reported to improve the probability of successful cardioversion,[60b] as is esmolol[60c] but not propafenone.[60d]

Constant current cardioversion

An important factor determining the success of electrical cardioversion is the amount of current reaching the heart muscle, which in turn is inversely related to the transthoracic impedance. Thus the traditionally used energy based cardioversion methods do not ensure the delivery of constant current. To obviate this disadvantage, a technique has been developed which allows selection of optimum energy levels in order to deliver a constant current. The energy requirements are decided depending on the transthoracic impedance which can be automatically measured. The development is still in the investigational phase and its superiority over traditional energy based cardioversion has to be confirmed in randomised trials.

High energy internal cardioversion

The technique, first described by Levy et al.[61] (Figure 9.2), involves delivering a 200–300 J shock between a free floating right atrial catheter (cathode) and an anodal back plate. Recently, results of a randomised comparison of external and internal cardioversion in 112 patients with sustained atrial fibrillation were reported.[62] The efficacy of internal cardioversion was significantly greater than that of external cardioversion (91% versus 67%) and it was equally safe. The recurrence rate of atrial fibrillation was, however, the same in both groups (63% at one year).

Several mechanisms have been postulated to explain the higher initial success with internal cardioversion.[63] As compared with external cardioversion, a greater proportion of the energy is delivered to the atria, the site of atrial fibrillation. Another explanation involves the barotrauma: the increased intracardiac pressures during endocavitary shocks are associated with stretch of cardiac structures and therefore modification of electrophysiological properties. High energy may be associated with alteration in transmembrane ion flux, leading to greater stability of myocardial cells and greater responsiveness to antiarrhythmic medication.

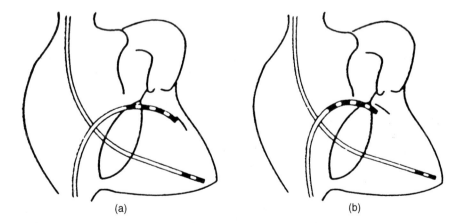

(a)   (b)

Fig 9.2 Schematic representation of the method used for high energy internal cardioversion. Defibrillation catheter electrodes are placed in at the apex of the right ventricle and the high right atrium.

Low energy internal cardioversion

In cases of persistent atrial fibrillation resistant to standard methods of cardioversion, administration of low energy biphasic shocks is emerging as a useful option. Electrodes are usually placed in the coronary sinus and right atrium (Figure 9.3). With this electrode configuration, defibrillation is usually achieved at energy levels of less than 4·5 J in recent onset atrial fibrillation.[64] In long standing cases, an energy of 7 J is sometimes required.[65a] Shocks delivered between the right atrium and pulmonary artery have also been used to cardiovert atrial fibrillation. This is associated with a higher defibrillation threshold,[65b] but the electrode position may be easier to obtain. Although the defibrillation threshold is far lower for internal than for transthoracic DC shocks, there is always some discomfort to the patient. In many cases sedation or analgesia is required[65c] but adjustment of the waveform of the defibrillating shock may overcome this.[65d]

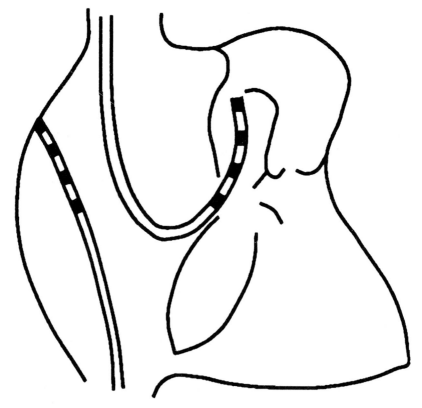

Fig 9.3 Schematic representation of the method used in low energy internal cardioversion. One defibrillation electrode is placed in the high right atrium and the other either in the coronary sinus or the pulmonary artery.

Oesothoracic cardioversion

The principal value of this technique is the close proximity between the oesophagus and the heart. There are scattered reports about trans-oesophageal cardioversion in atrial fibrillation. In a large series,[66] McKeown *et al.* reported a 79·5% initial success rate in patients with sustained atrial fibrillation. The majority responded to a shock of 100 J. A specially designed quadripolar electrode system was used to deliver the shocks.

Maintenance of sinus rhythm

This is the second major consideration in the management of atrial fibrillation. It may be required in patients with chronic atrial fibrillation following successful cardioversion or in those with paroxysmal atrial fibrillation to prevent recurrences. Several drugs have been tried for this purpose but the results are not very encouraging in the long term. In spite of high initial success rates only 20–60% of patients maintain sinus rhythm during the first year, irrespective of the institution of prophylactic antiarrhythmic drug treatment.

Quinidine Numerous studies are available documenting the efficacy of quinidine for maintaining sinus rhythm after cardioversion.[67-72] In controlled studies, quinidine prevented recurrences in 40–80% of patients during the first year. However, concerns regarding the safety of quinidine have been raised in a recent study by Coplen *et al.*,[73] in which a meta-analysis of previous randomised controlled trials of quinidine for prevention of atrial fibrillation was performed. Although quinidine treated patients had a two-fold chance of being in sinus rhythm at one year, as compared to controls, they demonstrated a nearly three-fold increase in mortality. These conclusions were, however, drawn from only 15 deaths from a total of 808 patients. The cause of death was known in only seven of the 12 quinidine treated patients and in only three was the death sudden. Another meta-analysis by the same group, this time also including the uncontrolled and non-randomised control trials, confirmed the previous observations: a crude mortality rate of 2·0% in the quinidine treated group as compared to 0·6% mortality in the controls. Sudden cardiac death was noted in 13/19 patients who died while on therapy.[74] Considering the usual problems of meta-analysis, these findings need to be verified in controlled prospective studies.

These safety concerns have been further extended with recent observations of an excess cardiac and arrhythmic mortality in patients with atrial fibrillation and congestive heart failure treated with antiarrhythmic drugs. Among patients with a history of congestive heart failure, those given antiarrhythmic medications had a relative risk of cardiac death of 4·7 compared with that of patients not so treated; the relative risk of arrhythmic

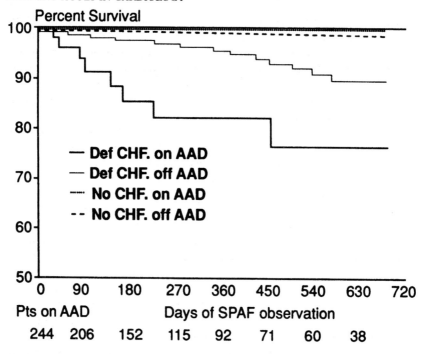

Fig 9.4 Survival to cardiac related death in patients with and without heart failure at entry. AAD = antiarrhythmic drug therapy; Def = definite history of; Pts = patients; SPAF = Stroke Prevention in Atrial Fibrillation.

death in the treated group was 3·7 (Figure 9.4). Quinidine was the commonest drug and class Ia the commonest group used in the study.[75]

Disopyramide Randomised trials have confirmed the efficacy of diso-pyramide, similar to quinidine, in maintaining sinus rhythm following successful cardioversion in patients with chronic atrial fibrillation.[76] The vagolytic action of disopyramide may confer a theoretical advantage in managing patients of paroxysmal atrial fibrillation (PAF), in whom the paroxysms are precipitated by vagotonia (pause dependent PAF).[77] Likewise, it may be disadvantageous in episodes triggered by sympathetic overactivity. Disopyramide has negative inotropic effects which limit its utility to patients with intact left ventricular function. Further, the general safety considerations involved in using class Ia drugs apply.[73–75]

Flecainide In addition to being an effective agent in terminating acute episodes of atrial fibrillation, flecainide is also effective in maintenance of sinus rhythm.[78–82] Most of the available studies involve patients with paroxysmal atrial fibrillation and structurally normal hearts. Anderson *et al.*[78] reported a multicentre double blind crossover study of flecainide and placebo in 64 patients with paroxysmal atrial fibrillation. The efficacy of the drug was judged by relief of symptoms as well as by intermittent transtelephonic monitoring. At the end of the study, 48 patients were found suitable for evaluation. These patients had undergone an average of 3·8 previous drug trials. The rate of symptoms and PAF attacks were significantly reduced by therapy. Flecainide also significantly prolonged the time to first attack and the interval between the episodes. In a recent review of literature, flecainide was found to be effective for long term therapy in 49% of the patients.[35] Leclercq et al.[79] reported a successful long term suppression of paroxysms in 38/53 (73%) with PAF. All these patients were previously resistant to quinidine. The success rate was slightly higher in patients with vagally induced PAF.

Safety issues of flecainide constitute the major concern, particularly after the CAST.[29] In the literature review reported by Hohnloser et al.[35] the risk of clinically significant adverse effects associated with the use of flecainide appeared to be small but not negligible. Clinically significant proarrhythmic events were reported in 3·5% of patients. Organisation of atrial fibrillation into flutter and life threatening ventricular arrhythmias related to vigorous exertion are some of the serious arrhythmias reported.[83-85] The overall incidence of the transformation of atrial fibrillation to flutter in patients receiving class Ic drugs is in the range of 3·5-5% and appears to be more common in patients with previous attacks of atrial flutter.[85, 86] The onset of atrial flutter is usually associated with 2:1 ventricular response (Figure 9.5) which is often aberrantly conducted with bizarre wide complexes. Rarely 1:1 AV nodal conduction can occur resulting in haemodynamic compromise. Concomitant use of digoxin, β-blockers or calcium blockers may be beneficial, especially in patients with previously documented atrial flutter, in order to control the ventricular rates if the complication does develop. All patients on flecainide should have exercise testing while on therapy to monitor for exertion related ventricular proarrhythmias. In another study, Pritchett et al.[87] compared the mortality of flecainide-encainide treated patients to that of a patient population seen at the research arrhythmia clinic. On Kaplan–Meier analysis, the estimated six-year survival function of these two patient populations did not differ significantly. The hazard ratio for the combined encainide-flecainide population relative to the control population was estimated to be 0·6. In conclusion, flecainide is an effective drug in the management of patients with PAF. However, it should be avoided in patients with ischaemic heart disease and heart failure and used with care in those with other structural heart disease.

Propafenone Few reports are available confirming the efficacy of propafenone in maintaining sinus rhythm in patients with PAF. Antmann et al.[88] studied the efficacy of long term oral propafenone for preventing PAF

197

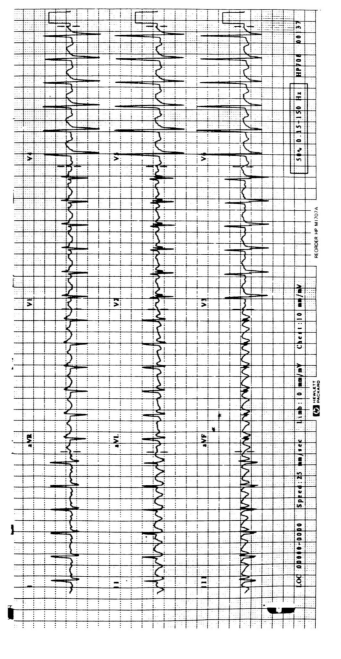

Fig 9.5 Atrial flutter with 2:1 conduction as a complication of flecainide therapy.

in 35 patients with drug refractory arrhythmia and for maintaining sinus rhythm in 21 patients with chronic atrial fibrillation following successful DC cardioversion; 40% of the patients were free from recurrences at six month follow-up. Similar results have been reported by other investigators.[89–90] Coumel and coworkers[90] reported on 17 patients with structurally normal hearts and neurally provoked atrial fibrillation or flutter (mean follow-up: 6·6 months). Propafenone was less effective in vagally dependent arrhythmias as compared to adrenergically mediated arrhythmias. Proarrhythmic complications similar to flecainide have been reported.[91]

Amiodarone   Several studies have confirmed the efficacy of amiodarone in maintenance of sinus rhythm following successful cardioversion in patients with chronic atrial fibrillation and in patients with PAF.[34, 35, 92–96] Reported success rates range from 53% to 97%. In the only comparative trial reported, Vitolo *et al.*[92] observed a higher success rate with amiodarone than with quinidine in maintaining sinus rhythm after electrical cardioversion (79% versus 46% respectively). It is especially useful in patients refractory to other drugs. In one of the largest experiences, Graboys *et al.*[93] have reported successful control of arrhythmia in patients resistant to an average of 3·2 previous drug trials. Complete suppression of arrhythmia was achieved in 74/95 patients (78%). In six patients the drug was partially effective (reduction in frequency of episodes). Brodsky *et al.*[48] have reported a moderate degree of success in 28 patients with dilated left atrium (>45 mm). In 25 patients earlier quinidine therapy had failed. After six months 21 patients were free of arrhythmia and after one year, complete suppression of arrhythmia was achieved in 10 patients. However, therapy failed in patients with LA dimension >60 mm. The non-cardiac side effect profile precluded the routine use of amiodarone. However, in a recent study involving 89 patients with chronic atrial fibrillation or flutter, Gosselink *et al.*[94a] used low dose amiodarone (mean dose 204±66 mg) for maintenance of sinus rhythm following successful cardioversion. Actuarially, 53% of patients were still in sinus rhythm after three years. Importantly, there was a low incidence of serious side effects and no proarrhythmia related mortality. The drug was even found to be useful in patients with left ventricular dysfunction. In conclusion, amiodarone is a useful drug for chronic suppression of atrial fibrillation. Incidence of serious adverse effects appears to be small when lower doses are employed and even at a dosage of 100 mg daily amiodarone has a higher efficacy than other agents.[94b]

Sotalol   Limited available data suggest that *d*-sotalol is an effective drug for maintenance of sinus rhythm postcardioversion. In a randomised trial comparing *d*-sotalol with quinidine for maintenance of sinus rhythm following successful cardioversion, both drugs showed similar effectiveness in maintaining sinus rhythm (52% versus 48% at six months). The incidence of proarrhythmic side effects was the same in both the groups. However, the sotalol group appeared to show better tolerance than the quinidine group, since the rates of adverse effects and withdrawal for drug intolerance were twice as low among the sotalol patients.[97] Efficacy has also been documented in preventing recurrences in patients with PAF.[98] A beneficial long term effect of d-sotalol has been demonstrated in a small group of patients,[99] but more trials are needed to confirm the safety and efficacy of sotalol in atrial fibrillation.

Digitalis Digoxin is still occasionally used in patients with PAF, for preventing recurrences or for control of the ventricular rate during the paroxysms. The available data, however, fail to confirm its efficacy. In a retrospective study of ambulatory ECG recordings from 72 patients with paroxysmal atrial fibrillation, Rawles et al.[100] observed that digoxin therapy did not significantly reduce the frequency of paroxysms, when compared to patients not receiving digitalis (60 versus 79 episodes respectively). More episodes lasting over 30 minutes occurred in patients taking digoxin compared to those not using this drug (13 versus four; $p > 0.01$). Analysis of Holter recordings from the recently conducted randomised, placebo controlled trial (CRAFT 1) showed that digoxin had no effect on the frequency or the mean heart rate in atrial fibrillation.[101] However, there was a trend towards a reduction in maximum heart rate during the episodes (on analysis of transtelephonically transmitted ECG) and a slight reduction in the number of symptomatic episodes in the treated individuals.[102] Retrospective data[67] on the role of digoxin therapy in preventing recurrence of atrial fibrillation after electrical cardioversion showed that digoxin when used alone, is ineffective. The data also suggest that digoxin may also reduce the antiarrhythmic effect of quinidine. Conflicting data are available regarding the efficacy of digoxin in preventing atrial fibrillation following cardiac surgery.[103, 104]

The lack of efficacy of digoxin in preventing atrial fibrillation could be explained by its effects on atrial myocardium. By shortening its refractory period and increasing the dispersion of refractoriness, digoxin increases the atrial irritability.[105] This could also explain the longer paroxysms of atrial fibrillation in patients receiving digitalis noted by Rawles et al.[100] and the reduced efficacy of quinidine when given along with digoxin.[67] Theoretically digoxin could also worsen vagally mediated atrial fibrillation.[77] In conclusion, the available data suggest that digitalis is not an effective drug for maintenance of sinus rhythm in patients with atrial fibrillation. However, it may indirectly contribute to restoration of sinus rhythm in patients with congestive heart failure by improving the haemodynamic variables, as a result of its positive inotropic effects.

β-blockers In general β-blockers are not effective therapy for reversion of atrial fibrillation or its prevention. It is likely that they may be beneficial in patients with exercise induced atrial fibrillation, since this may be induced by increase in sympathetic neural activity. Some studies have suggested that they may have a beneficial effect in patients after coronary artery bypass graft surgery,[106] another situation in which sympathetic activation may be important for occurrence of atrial fibrillation.

Although β-blockers have a limited role for reversion or prevention of atrial fibrillation when administered as a monotherapy, they may be important when used in combination with the conventional antiarrhythmic drugs. In one study, propranolol improved the efficacy of quinidine.[107] In selected patients, β-blockers have been shown to be effective in preventing the ventricular proarrhythmic effects of flecainide.[108] There are accumulating data that catecholamines and sympathetic stimulation may reverse the beneficial effects of antiarrhythmic drugs and β-blockers can prevent these catecholamine mediated changes.[109]

Proarrhythmic effects of atrial antiarrhythmic therapy

As in the case of patients with ventricular arrhythmias, pharmacologic treatment of atrial fibrillation may be associated with serious cardiac toxicity. The risk is probably less than with treatment of ventricular arrhythmias as the underlying heart disease is often less severe. Nevertheless, it is important to be aware of these potentially life threatening proarrhythmic responses. Table 9.3 shows the various forms of proarrhythmias that have been described with atrial antiarrhythmic therapy.

Control of ventricular rate in atrial fibrillation

Control of ventricular rate is the next important consideration in atrial fibrillation. Several factors determine the ventricular response in atrial fibrillation. These include refractory period of the AV node, the amount of concealed conduction within the node, the relative degree of vagal and sympathetic tone, and/or the level of endogenous catecholamines. The relative importance of AV nodal refractoriness and the amount of concealed conduction in determining the ventricular response is not clear, but it is likely that the former is the dominant factor.[110] The autonomic factors possibly play an important role in determining ventricular response during exercise, in acute situations, and at the onset of paroxysm in patients with PAF.

In addition to being responsible for the distressing symptom of palpitations and deleterious haemodynamic consequences, uncontrolled ventricular rate in atrial fibrillation has been reported to be responsible for left ventricular dysfunction. The most compelling evidence for this hypothesis comes from the data on catheter ablation of the AV junction, where four patients with atrial fibrillation and uncontrolled ventricular response had a rise in mean ejection fraction from 25% to 45% after a

Table 9.3 Proarrhythmias observed with atrial antiarrhythmic agents

Arrhythmia	Examples
Ventricular	
Toursade de pointes	Quinidine
	Sotalol
	Procainamide
	Amiodarone (rare)
Monomorphic VT	Flecainide
	Propafenone
Aberrant ventricular conduction	Flecainide
	Propafenone
Organisation into atrial flutter resulting in 2:1 conduction	Flecainide
	Propafenone
	Encainide
	Quinidine
Aggravation of atrial arrhythmia	Digitalis
Aggravation of sinus node disease	Digitalis
	β-blockers
	Calcium blockers
	Flecainide, amiodarone
AV block	Most drugs except class Ia

median follow-up of 28 months following ablation.[111a] Pharmacological methods form the mainstay of therapy for ventricular rate control. In resistant cases, AV junction ablation is an alternative option.

Drugs used in ventricular rate control

The choice of drugs generally revolves around three classes: digitalis, β-blockers and calcium channel blockers. Although all three classes have been in routine use for two decades, there is no consensus on the place of each in controlling the ventricular rate. Recent guidelines issued by the American Heart Association suggest that verapamil should be used in most cases.[111b] whereas the Canadian College of Cardiology recommend digoxin as the agent of first choice.[111c]

Digitalis The ventricular rate is decreased by digitalis through two synergistic pharmacologic actions: vagally mediated increase of the refractory period of the AV node, and more concealed AV nodal conduction due to higher frequency of atrial impulses.[105, 112] Since the predominant effect of digitalis is vagally mediated, it is hardly surprising that its action is blunted during exercise and in acute situations, when there is sympathetic hyperactivity. The use of digitalis for ventricular rate control can be considered in three clinical situations: for chronic rate control, rate control in acute situations and for rate control in PAF.

Digitalis is still the drug of first choice for rate control in patients with sustained atrial fibrillation. Although it significantly slows the resting heart rates in these patients, the effect is not maintained during exercise. In some patients during even mild effort (three minutes of exercise), digoxin doses of 0·5 mg day reduce the heart rate by a mean of only 8%.[113] Similar findings have been reported by other workers.[114] Therefore, if exertional symptoms persist after optimum therapy with digitalis, additional medications may have to be considered.

Delayed peak action, even on intravenous loading and antagonism by sympathetic overactivity, limits its use in acute situations.

The available data support the lack of efficacy of chronic digoxin therapy for preventing tachycardia during recurrences in patients with PAF. In their study of Holter ECG recordings, Rawles et al.[100] found no difference of ventricular rates at the onset of paroxysm in patients on digitalis as compared to untreated patients (140±25 versus 134±22). Similar observations have been made by other workers.[78, 97] Data from the CRAFT I, however, suggest a trend towards reduction in maximum heart rate during the episodes in patients receiving digitalis.

β-blockers Both intravenous and oral administration of β-blocking agents is effective for controlling a rapid ventricular response in atrial fibrillation. Intravenous infusion of esmolol, an ultra short acting β-blocker, has been successfully used for control of rapid ventricular rate. Although symptomatic hypotension was reported in 50% of patients by one group,[115] this complication was not observed in another study.[116] Generally, however, β-blocking agents are not used as first line therapy for acute rate control for fear of exacerbating unsuspected heart failure by their negative inotropic effects. An exception is atrial fibrillation associated with thyrotoxicosis, where β-blockade is the treatment of choice. In chronic atrial fibrillation, β-blockers significantly reduce the ventricular response to exercise. Several studies using a variety of β-blockers have demonstrated a heart rate reduction at all levels of exercise but have failed to show improvement in exercise tolerance. Some studies have shown a decreased exercise tolerance despite an adequate control of the excessive heart rate rise.[117, 118]

It is not clear from the available data whether β-blockers can control the ventricular rate at onset of paroxysm in patients with PAF. If the hypothesis[100] that sympathetic triggers predominate in PAF is accepted, then there is a theoretical basis for using β-blockers.

Xamoterol This is a unique agent with selective β1-adrenoreceptor partial agonist properties. It has been shown to be effective at controlling the ventricular rate in patients with atrial fibrillation. Xamoterol has positive inotropic effects and can be used in the treatment of mild heart failure.[119] In a placebo controlled study,[120] xamoterol was found to be more useful than digoxin in patients with atrial fibrillation with inappropriate bradycardia at rest, but with exertional tachycardia. Ventricular pauses and bradycardia were reduced by xamoterol as compared to digoxin and placebo. Similar beneficial effect when compared with verapamil was observed in another study.[121] However, the safety of this drug has been questioned after a large multicentre trial of xamoterol in heart failure reported an increased mortality[122] in the treatment group.

Pindolol This is a β-blocker with intrinsic sympathomimetic activity. It has been shown to markedly reduce the diurnal variation in heart rate in digitalised patients with atrial fibrillation, both ameliorating diurnal tachycardia and preventing nocturnal bradycardia and pauses.[123] In another study of elderly patients with atrial fibrillation, a combination of digoxin and pindolol reduced the maximum venricular rate without further depression of the minimum ventricular rate.[124] Pindolol also has the advantage of being less negatively inotropic when compared to other β-blockers.

Calcium channel blockers As with β-blockers, calcium channel blocking agents are effective in controlling the ventricular response in atrial fibrillation. Their lesser negative inotropism gives them a distinct advantage over β-blockers, especially when a rapid control of ventricular rate is required.

Intravenous verapamil is highly effective for slowing ventricular rate in atrial fibrillation. A maximal response is seen within 2–3 minutes and is independent of the level of sympathetic tone. Intravenous diltiazem is also effective, although its availability is restricted.[125]

In chronic atrial fibrillation, calcium channel blockers tend to reduce the resting heart rates slightly but significantly blunt the ventricular response to exercise. In contrast to β-blockers, many studies have reported a modest improvement in exercise tolerance[126, 127a] but several studies have shown that calcium channel blocking drugs, on their own or in combination with digoxin, provide no improvement in exercise capacity compared with digoxin alone.[127b, 127c, 127d, 128] One study failed to show improvement[128] but none has reported decreased tolerance, as is sometimes seen with β-blockers. Both verapamil and diltiazem seem to be equally effective for controlling ventricular response.[129] Diltiazem, however, has the advantage of not potentiating digoxin toxicity and having a lesser myocardial depressant activity. In a controlled trial, Roth *et al.*[127a] concluded that the combination of medium dose diltiazem (240 mg) and digoxin was as effective as a higher dose combination and more effective than any monotherapy.

Other drugs Although drugs such as *d*-sotalol, amiodarone, propafenone and flecainide have depressant effects on AV conduction and can effectively control ventricular rate, their long term use solely for the purpose of rate control is not justified.

Catheter ablation for control of ventricular rate

Transcatheter ablation of the AV node was first performed in 1982 using DC energy.[130] AV node ablation is now an established treatment for drug resistant atrial fibrillation (Figure 9.6). Radiofrequency energy has overtaken DC as the energy source of choice because of the lower incidence of side effects and the fact that it does not require the patient to be sedated.[131] Initial reports suggested that symptom control improves after AV node ablation[131] but there was an excess of sudden deaths in those in whom high energy DC ablation was used. Residual symptoms are reported, possibly due to ventricular ectopic activity.[132, 133a] Many patients show improved ventricular function after AV node ablation[133b] in keeping with the resolution of a ventricular myopathy induced by high ventricular response rate. Preliminary results of the 'Ablation and Pacing Trial' indicate that quality of life also improves.[133c]

Using radiofrequency energy it is possible to selectively ablate the atrial approaches to the AV node. Ablation in the anatomical area corresponding to the slow pathway produced a significant reduction in the ventricular response rate, at least in some cases.[133d, 133e]

Pacemaker therapy in patients with atrial fibrillation

The most common indication is drug induced symptomatic bradycardia. Other indications are sick sinus syndrome and the tachycardia-bradycardia syndrome. Antiarrhythmic therapy may fail to fully control the paroxysms and may aggravate posttachycardia pauses. Under these circumstances, permanent pacing facilitates treatment and abolishes pause related symptoms. Permanent pacing is also required following AV nodal ablation.

An evolving concept is whether atrial pacing can prevent episodes of paroxysmal atrial fibrillation. This has been reported to be possible in the subset of patients with vagally mediated atrial fibrillation where the paroxysms are triggered by relative bradycardia[134a] and in a small subset of patients in whom there is a long delay in inter- or intra-atrial, conduction in whom dual site atrial pacing may be indicated.[134b]

Choice of pacing mode

In patients with chronic atrial fibrillation and bradycardia, the choice is restricted to a ventricular demand pacemaker with either a fixed rate (VVI) or with rate modulating capabilities (VVIR), the latter being preferred. VVI pacemakers with hysteresis may still be satisfactory when reasonable rate response is preserved during exercise but pacing is needed because of long pauses or resting bradycardia. Older patients with chronic atrial fibrillation, with a low activity level, generally require only VVI pacing.

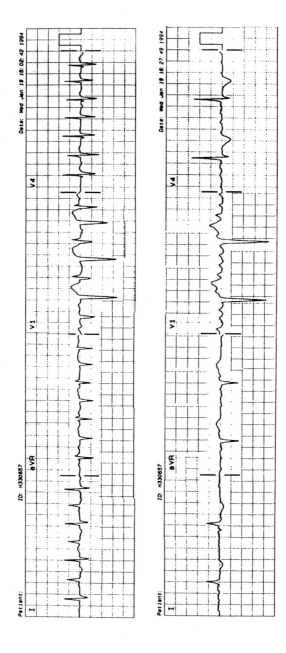

Fig 9.6   Recording of intracardiac electrogram, before and after radiofrequency catheter ablation of AV junction.

Paroxysmal atrial fibrillation was in the past considered a contra-indication for dual chamber pacing. It is, however, obvious from an enormous literature that progression to chronic atrial fibrillation is more common in patients with paroxysmal atrial fibrillation, who are paced with a ventricular system as compared to a dual chamber system.[135–138] The exact mechanisms associating the pacing mode and the prevention or development of chronic atrial fibrillation are not clear. In patients with ventricular pacing, progressive left atrial dilation due to loss of atrioventricular synchrony and modification of atrial refractoriness due to ventriculoatrial conduction have been incriminated. In patients with chronic atrial pacing, it has been hypothesised that elimination of sinus bradycardia allows homogenisation of atrial refractory periods and this prevents PAF from evolving into chronicity. However, Luck et al.[139] found that the abnormal refractoriness in patients with sick sinus syndrome did not improve after atrial pacing. Another theory is that the beneficial effect of atrial pacing lies in preventing reinitiation of arrhythmia by maintaining a high degree of exit block from all natural subsidiary atrial pacemakers.[140, 141]

One anticipated problem of DDD pacing in patients with paroxysmal atrial fibrillation is development of pacemaker mediated tachycardia or of tracking of fast atrial rhythms during attacks of tachycardia. Management requires antiarrhythmic therapy to control the atrial arrhythmias or programming of the pacemaker with a relatively long atrial refractory period (PVARP) and a low upper rate limit. Alternatively DDI mode may be selected in order to disable atrial triggering of ventricular stimulation.[142] Nevertheless, if reprogramming and pharmacologic measures still do not control this problem, the VVIR mode is the only choice. Recent developments in pacing technology have provided better alternatives.[143] One uses dual chamber systems with an automatic mode switch facility; during the episode of atrial fibrillation, the pacemaker automatically switches to DDI or VVI mode (Figure 9.7).

Implantable atrial defibrillator

Success in internal defibrillation in animal models of atrial fibrillation at low energy levels suggested that an implantable device might be used to terminate atrial fibrillation.[144–147] The technical problems with this approach include detection of AF, risk of proarrhythmia and patient discomfort due to shocks.[148a] The problems of sensing and proarrhythmia have been overcome and an implantable device is now available. Patient discomfort remains problematic but some patients find shocks only a mild nuisance.[148b]

Surgical approaches in atrial fibrillation

Despite its high prevalence atrial fibrillation has only recently been treated surgically. Standard map guided surgical techniques cannot be

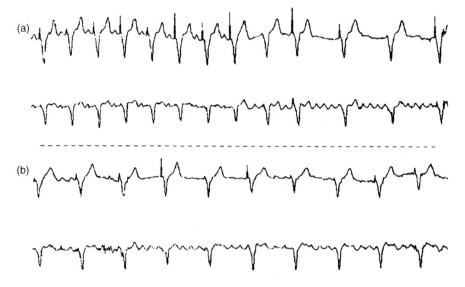

Fig 9.7   Illustration of mode switch function in dual chamber system. (a) Patient in sinus rhythm. (b) During an episode of atrial fibrillation, the pacemaker switches to VVI mode.

applied in atrial fibrillation because of the diffuse abnormalities in atrial electrophysiology. Despite this, surgical techniques have been developed and some results have been reported. The principle underpinning these techniques is the hypothesis that a critical mass of atrial tissue was required to sustain fibrillation.

The "Corridor" operation

The "corridor" operation is designed to maintain sinus rhythm by isolating the sinus node, a small corridor of connecting atrial tissue (the "corridor") and the AV node from the remaining atrial tissue (Figure 9.8). The hypothesis is that the corridor of atrial tissue would not be large enough to sustain atrial fibrillation, but would effectively conduct between the sinus node and the AV node. The operation maintains normal cardiac chronotropic function but not atrial mechanical function. The surgery has been successfully undertaken on patients with paroxysmal atrial fibrillation. A major complication is the development of postoperative sinus node dysfunction, requiring pacemaker implantation. This is probably related to pre-existent sinus node disease and might be avoided by proper case selection. The risk of systemic embolisation is not eliminated by this surgery. Results of the procedure in 20 patients with drug refractory paroxysmal atrial fibrillation were recently reported.[149] Of the 16 patients who had a successful procedure, there was no recurrence of PAF after a mean follow-up of 20 months. There was no operative mortality or any major morbidity. Postoperative sinus node dysfunction occurred in only two patients.

The "maze" operation

This operation[150] is more complicated than the "corridor" operation. In addition to maintaining sinus rhythm, it is designed to restore atrial mechanical function and obviate the need for anticoagulation. The surgery involves a series of carefully placed atrial incisions which create a "maze". Sinus node depolarisation then spreads through the atrium in a variety of directions following the maze. The maze pathways are sufficiently narrow that the depolarisation wave cannot turn back on itself and allow re-entry (Figure 9.9). Successful results have been reported in both chronic and paroxysmal atrial fibrillation. Perioperative death is uncommon, but temporary complications are frequent. Postoperative problems include sinus node dysfunction, requiring pacemaker implantation, and a tendency to fluid retention.

Cox *et al.* recently reported their five year experience with the maze procedure, involving 75 patients with paroxysmal or chronic atrial fibrillation and flutter.[151a] Postoperative atrial pacemakers were required in 30/75 patients. There was one procedure related mortality. Of the 65

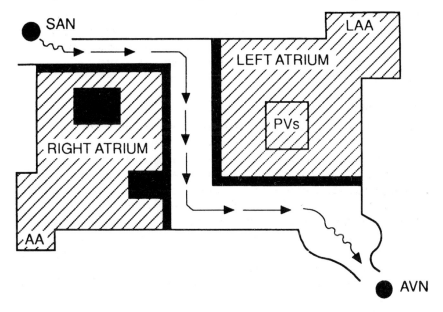

Fig 9.8 Schematic representation of the "corridor" operation. Most of the atrial myocardium is electrically isolated from the AV node by atrial incisions (heavy lines). The area which is isolated from the AV node includes both the right and left atrial appendages (RAA and LAA) and the pulmonary veins (PVs).

patients for whom the follow-up data were available at three months, 64 patients (98%) were in sinus rhythm and had preserved atrial transport function. The procedure was curative without the need for medications in 58/65 (89%) patients.

Catheter ablation of the atrial myocardium

The success of the surgical maze procedure has led clinical electrophysiologists to attempt to replicate this pattern of lines of conduction block in the atria using radiofrequency energy. There have been encouraging data from animal experiments[151b] and a small number of successful procedures in human subjects,[151c] but the procedure was too long to enter routine use as it now exists. In selected cases of atrial fibrillation, ablation of a focal source of excitation may prevent recurrence of paroxysmal atrial fibrillation.[151d]

Management strategies in atrial fibrillation

The management strategy in atrial fibrillation depends largely on the clinical presentation. The various methods of therapy which have already been discussed may be assembled to form overall strategies, for example a

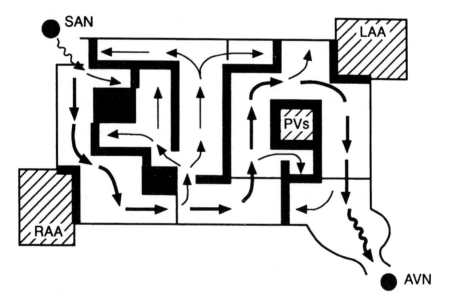

Fig 9.9 Schematic representation of the "maze" procedure. The right and left atrial appendages (RAA and LAA) are excised, and multiple incisions (heavy lines) are used to produce lines of conduction block. These isolate the pulmonary veins (PVs) from the remainder of the atrial myocardium and divide the remainder of the atrial myocardium into corridors too narrow to contain a re-entrant circuit.

strategy of striving to maintain sinus rhythm at any cost or a strategy of allowing atrial fibrillation to become permanent. No clinical trial has yet compared overall strategies of this type, but several such studies are under way. The American AFFIRM (Atrial Fibrillation Follow-up: Investigation of Rhythm Management) Trial, which will involve 5300 patients, and two smaller European trials, PIAF (Prognosis in Atrial Fibrillation) and RACE (Rate Control versus Electrical Cardioversion for Atrial Fibrillation), will compare the long term outcome with restoration and maintenance of sinus rhythm with control of ventricular rate. Until the results of these are available, management must be dictated by experience and common sense.

Recent onset atrial fibrillation

Most often the onset of atrial fibrillation is associated with symptoms that cause the patient to seek medical attention. The nature and severity of symptoms depend on several variables: ventricular rate, nature of precipitating illness, left ventricular function, etc.

The most important initial requirement is to control ventricular rate. Generally this is all that is necessary, as atrial fibrillation usually resolves with successful management of the precipitating illness. The drugs effective in controlling ventricular rates in atrial fibrillation are shown in Table 9.2. The agent selected and the mode of administration are dictated by the clinical presentation. For acute control, intravenous verapamil or β-blockers are effective. The latter should be avoided if heart failure is suspected. Digoxin, even with intravenous loading, takes several hours to reach its maximum effect and is therefore not a good drug in acute situations. However, if the patient is not acutely symptomatic, digoxin is the best initial drug, especially if there is concomitant heart failure. Addition of other drugs such as calcium channel blockers or β-blockers may be necessary depending on the clinical response.

Spontaneous conversion of atrial fibrillation occurs in 44–90% of the patients within 24 hours.[22, 152] In some cases this may be due to treatment of underlying cause and attempts to control the ventricular rate form the main aim of treatment. However, cardioversion should be considered if the ventricular rates are difficult to control medically, the patient is haemodynamically compromised and if the arrhythmia persists after treatment of precipitating factors. The success of cardioversion in recent onset arrhythmia is related to duration of the episode, with higher success rates in those with atrial fibrillation of onset <24 hours.[30] For patients in whom the duration of arrhythmia is more than 2–3 days or is unknown, the risk of embolisation from a left atrial thrombus is increased.[153, 154] The risk of embolic complication has to be weighed against the benefits of cardioversion. Embolic complication following cardioversion is especially likely in patients with mitral stenosis and severe heart failure. In such patients, it

211

would be prudent to continue drug treatment and plan an elective cardioversion, after adequate anticoagulation. Screening for left atrial clot, using transoesophageal echocardiography, lowers but does not eliminate the risk of postcardioversion embolic complications.[155]

Restoration and maintenance of sinus rhythm in sustained atrial fibrillation

Although all patients should ideally be in sinus rhythm, a balanced approach is required in this regard. As discussed in the previous section, the need for cardioversion and the probability of success (both immediate and long term) should be carefully assessed. It is generally considered safe to attempt cardioversion without anticoagulation if the duration of the arrhythmia is less than three days[153, 154] and there is no underlying mitral valve disease or history of previous thromboembolism. In all other cases, unless absolutely necessary, a minimum of four weeks of anticoagulation adequate to maintain an INR of 2·0–2·5 is required. Following successful cardioversion, it is imperative to continue anticoagulants for 4–12 weeks to allow for resumption of atrial mechanical activity. It is important to realise that pharmacological cardioversion does not eliminate the need for anticoagulation.

Pharmacological cardioversion obviates the need for general anaesthesia. Consistently high success rates have been reported with several antiarrhythmic agents. In recent onset atrial fibrillation, the best conversion rates are reported with intravenous flecainide, but its use should be restricted to patients without structural heart disease. Amiodarone and quinidine appear to be more useful than other drugs in converting chronic atrial fibrillation.[23, 24, 40, 44] Conventional antiarrhythmic drugs should be avoided in patients with severe left ventricular dysfunction and in ischaemic heart disease, particularly following acute myocardial infarction. External electrical cardioversion can be attempted primarily or if the drugs have failed. It has been reported that 90% of suitable patients with chronic atrial fibrillation[103, 104] are successfully converted to sinus rhythm with external cardioversion. Patients not reverting with external cardioversion can be considered for internal cardioversion as higher success rates have been reported with this modality.[73] Another strategy would be to repeat cardioversion on antiarrhythmic therapy.

Antiarrhythmic therapy before and after electrical cardioversion

Antiarrhythmic therapy following successful cardioversion improves the likelihood of maintaining sinus rhythm. This has been demonstrated in several trials with a variety of antiarrhythmic drugs. Following successful cardioversion, it may take at least three weeks until full atrial mechanical activity is restored.[156] It is therefore prudent to continue both the antiarrhythmic and the anticoagulant therapy at least until this period.

There is, however, no need for secondary long term prophylactic antiarrhythmic treatment after the initial cardioversion. Routine prophylaxis would lead to unnecessary exposure to potentially toxic drugs for many patients as 45% and 25% of patients remain in sinus rhythm three months and one year after cardioversion respectively, without prophylactic treatment.[73] Secondary prophylactic treatment is usually prescribed after repeat cardioversion. Long term antiarrhythmic therapy is also advised in patients with mitral valve disease, multiple previous episodes and in those with life threatening recurrences.[157] The other risk factors that have been reported to predict recurrent atrial fibrillation after successful cardioversion are history of coronary artery disease and female sex.[158]

It is, however, not clear whether prior administration of antiarrhythmic therapy improves the chance of successful cardioversion. Some recommend that the drugs be started after a successful procedure to avoid unpredictable proarrhythmic responses during cardioversion.[159] According to another view, prior administration of antiarrhythmic therapy helps in preventing very early recurrences following cardioversion. An added advantage quoted is that 10–20% of patients may revert with drug therapy alone.[157]

Control of ventricular rate in chronic atrial fibrillation

If sinus rhythm cannot be restored or sustained, the aim of therapy is to control the ventricular rates. There are no clearcut guidelines for defining the optimal rate control in patients with chronic atrial fibrillation. Using Doppler echocardiography, Rawles et al.[160] measured the relation between ventricular rate and cardiac output in 60 resting patients with atrial fibrillation. They concluded from this study that achieving a resting ventricular rate of 90 beats per minute in patients with atrial fibrillation would result in control with least compromise of cardiac output. A rate more than 140 beats per minute was always found to be excessive. The higher resting ventricular rate, compared to sinus rhythm, is required to compensate for the loss of effective atrial contraction.

Digoxin is often sufficient to achieve this goal. Whether one should aim for rigorous control of ventricular rates during exertion in all the patients is not clear. If the patient continues to be symptomatic, calcium channel blockers (verapamil or diltiazem) or β-blockers may be added. The therapy at this stage should be guided by ambulatory monitoring or exercise testing. Amiodarone is also a highly effective drug for this purpose but is generally restricted to resistant cases. In selected patients with inappropriate resting bradycardia and ventricular pauses but requiring rate control during exertion, xamoterol or pindolol may be an appropriate choice. Elderly patients may require permanent pacing to allow for optimal dosing of antiarrhythmic drugs. Patients not responding to drug therapy and having persistent symptoms should be considered for AV junction ablation.

213

Paroxysmal atrial fibrillation

This requires special consideration. The clinical characteristics are as yet not well defined. Some patients present with short lasting and fleeting paroxysms and others present with paroxysms lasting for hours to days (Figure 9.10). In minimally symptomatic patients reassurance is sufficient. In the other clinical groups, antiarrhythmic therapy is usually required and the goal of therapy is to reduce the frequency and/or severity (duration and ventricular rate) of the paroxysms. Patients with frequent long lasting paroxysms generally do not respond well to therapy and often require repeated cardioversions. Underlying thyrotoxicosis and other precipitating factors should be clearly identified.

Several drugs have been tried. Digoxin, although frequently given, does not appear to be very useful, although it has been reported to slightly reduce the number of symptomatic episodes.[102] The drugs which have been successfully used are quinidine, disopyramide, flecainide, propafenone, amiodarone, and sotalol. The proarrhythmic potential of flecainide,[35, 83-85] propafenone,[91] and sotalol[97] increased mortality shown with quinidine and related drugs[73-75] and the long term side effects of amiodarone require serious consideration before embarking on long term antiarrhythmic therapy. Flecainide and propafenone should be restricted to patients without structural heart disease. They should also probably be avoided in vigorously active individuals.[83] Low dose amiodarone is probably the best

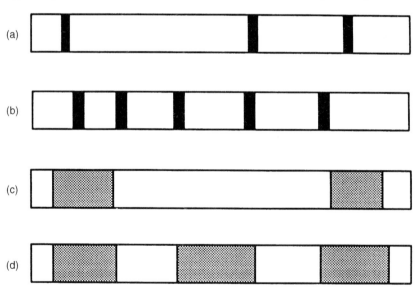

Fig 9.10   Clinical subsets of paroxysmal atrial fibrillation. (a) = brief paroxysms widely spaced; (b) = brief paroxysms occurring frequently; (c) = occasional but prolonged paroxysms; (d) = long periods of AF interspersed with sinus rhythm.

choice in the setting of structural heart disease. In patients with clearcut exercise related paroxysms, a trial of β-blockers would be indicated. In the so called "vagotonic" atrial fibrillation, amiodarone or flecainide (but probably not propafenone) may be particularly effective.[77, 90] Theoretically, drugs with vagolytic action (quinidine or disopyramide) could also be effective in these patients. It is possible that atrial pacing may benefit some of these patients with vagotonic atrial fibrillation.[134] For symptomatic arrhythmias unrelated to vagal triggers, the choice of sotalol, amiodarone, flecainide or propafenone may have advantage over quinidine as ventricular rate at time of recurrence is better controlled with these agents.[42, 107]

In the subset of patients with recurrent episodes of sustained atrial fibrillation requiring cardioversion, it is important to consider the feasibility of attempting pharmacological cardioversion on an outpatient basis. Such an option would be welcome from both the patient and health resources viewpoint. The risk of thromboembolism would not be a consideration if the time of onset of paroxysm has been clearly noted. Successful cardioversion can be achieved with oral flecainide, propafenone, quinidine, and procainamide. Quinidine, because of its dose related proarrhythmic effects, definitely requires supervised administration. Until larger trials have confirmed the safety of other orally administered drugs, their administration cannot be recommended without supervision. In patients having recurrences while on antiarrhythmic therapy, addition of β-blockers at the onset of paroxysm may aid in control of symptoms and also improve the efficacy of the antiarrhythmic agent.[107, 109]

Refractory atrial fibrillation

In patients refractory to conventional antiarrhythmic therapy, the options are limited. One strategy recommended is a "tiered" therapy – sequential use of different antiarrhythmic drugs; the rationale for this strategy is that the arrhythmogenic mechanism may vary between patients, leading to varied responses to different drugs. For example, therapy can be initiated with a membrane stabilising drug and if there is no response, it can be replaced with drugs which would slow the conduction velocity and later with drugs which increase the refractoriness. A similar strategy has been successfully used in patients with refractory atrial fibrillation.[161, 162] Another option is to try drug combinations; a combination of flecainide with amiodarone was reported to be particularly effective.[79] A pharmacologic interaction between the two drugs requires a reduction in dosage of flecainide by 25–33%.[163, 164] This combination can, however, cause severe sinus bradycardia requiring pacemaker implantation. Propranolol has been reported to improve the efficacy of quinidine in maintaining sinus rhythm.[107] Verapamil has also been reported to improve the efficacy of quinidine.[24] AV junction ablation may have to be used in several of these patients. Improvement in surgical results and development of an implantable atrial defibrillator may improve the therapeutic options in severely symptomatic patients.[148]

Aggressive treatment strategies for maintaining sinus rhythm are probably not justified in most patients, in view of the risks of proarrhythmia and the lack of evidence of benefit of this strategy when compared with simple control of ventricular rate. Anticoagulation to reduce the thromboembolic risk and attempts at rate control may probably be sufficient in most of the patients with refractory atrial fibrillation.

Conclusions

Atrial fibrillation is a common arrhythmia which, although generally considered benign, is associated with an increased morbidity and mortality. Although the most prevalent arrhythmia, its therapy has been neglected. The role of digoxin and the importance of anticoagulation in atrial fibrillation have become clear only recently. Acute onset of atrial fibrillation is easily converted to sinus rhythm in most cases. Although many chronic cases of atrial fibrillation may be converted, safe and effective agents for long term maintenance of sinus rhythm are not yet available. Unfortunately, the patients who are most likely to benefit from antiarrhythmic therapy are also the most susceptible to the risks of treatment. It is also not clear whether aggressive treatment to maintain sinus rhythm is superior to simple control of ventricular rates. Paroxysmal atrial fibrillation can cause significant symptoms and cannot be easily treated. None of the available antiarrhythmic agents have a proven long term efficacy and safety record. At least in some of these patients, non-pharmacological therapeutic approaches may have a significant application in future.

1 Ostrander LD Jr, Brandt RL, Kjelsberg MO, Epstein FH. Electrocardiographic findings among the adult population of a total natural community. Tecumseh, Michigan. *Circulation* 1965; **31**: 888–98.

2 Peterson P, Godtfredsen J. Atrial fibrillation – a review of course and prognosis. *Acta Med Scand* 1984; **216**: 5–9.

3 Kannel WB, Abbott RD, Savage DD, McNamara PM. Epidemiologic features of atrial fibrillation: the Framingham study. *N Engl J Med* 1982; **306**: 1018–22.

4 Bialy D, Lehmann MH, Schumacher DN, Steinman RT, Meissner MD. Hospitalisation for arrhythmias in the United States: importance of atrial fibrillation (abstract). *J Am Coll Cardiol* 1992; **19**: 41A.

5 Orlands JR, Von Herick R, Aronow WS *et al.* Hemodynamics and echocardiograms before and after conversion of atrial fibrillation to normal sinus rhythm. *Chest* 1979; **76**: 521–5.

6 Lau C, Leung WH, Wong CK *et al.* Hemodynamics of individual atrial fibrillation: a comparative assessment of sinus rhythm, atrial and ventricular pacing. *Eur Heart J* 1990; **11**: 209–14.

7 Krahn DA, Manfreda J, Tate BR, Mathewson FAL, Cuddy TE. Prognosis of atrial fibrillation in men. Manitoba Follow-up Study (MUFS) (abstract). *J Am Coll Cardiol* 1993; **21**: 478A.

8 Wolf PA, Abbot R, Kannel W. Atrial fibrillation as an independent risk factor for stroke: the Framingham study. *Stroke* 1991; **22**: 983–8.

9 Brand FM, Abbot RD, Kannel WB, Wolf PA. Characteristics and prognosis of lone atrial

fibrillation: 30 year follow-up in the Framingham study. *JAMA* 1985; **254**: 3449–53.

10a Kropecky SL, Gersh BJ, McGoon MD *et al*. The natural history of lone atrial fibrillation: a population based study over three decades. *N Engl J Med* 1987; **317**: 669–74.

10b Jenkins LS, Ellenbogen K, Kay N *et al*. Quality of life in patients with symptomatic atrial fibrillation. *Circulation* 1995; **92**(8): I–490.

11 Middlekauff HR, Stevenson WG, Stevenson LW. Prognostic significance of atrial fibrillation in advanced heart failure. A study of 390 patients. *Circulation* 1991; **84**: 40–8.

12 Carson PE, Johnson GR, Dunkman WB, Fletcher RD, Farrel L, Cohn JN. The influence of atrial fibrillation on prognosis in mild to moderate heart failure. The V-HeFT studies. The V-HeFT VA cooperative studies group. *Circulation* 1993; **87** (Suppl): VI102–10.

13 Goldberg RJ, Seely D, Becker RC *et al*. Impact of atrial fibrillation on the in-hospital and long term survival of patients with acute myocardial infarction: a community wide perspective. *Am Heart J* 1990; **119**: 996–1001.

14 Szekely P, Sideris D, Batson G. Maintenance of sinus rhythm after atrial fibrillation. *Br Heart J* 1970; **32**: 741–6.

15 Brodsky MA, Allen BJ, Capparelli EV, Luckett CR, Morton R, Henry WL. Factors determining maintenance of sinus rhythm after cardioversion in chronic atrial fibrillation with left atrial dilatation. *Am J Cardiol* 1989; **63**: 1065–8.

16 Dittrich CH, Erickson JS, Schneiderman T, Blacky R, Savides T, Nicod PH. Echocardiographic and clinical predictors for outcome of elective cardioversion of atrial fibrillation. *Am J Cardiol* 1989; **63**: 193–7.

17 Waris E, Kreus KE, Salokannel J. Factors influencing persistence of sinus rhythm after DC shock treatment of atrial fibrillation. *Acta Med Scand* 1971; **189**: 161–6.

18 Ewy G, Ulfers L, Hager W *et al*. Response of atrial fibrillation to therapy: role of aetiology and left atrial diameter. *J Electrocardiol* 1980; **13**: 119–24.

19 Flugelman MY, Hasin Y, Katznelson N, Krivsky M, Shefer A, Gotsman MS. Restoration and maintenance of sinus rhythm after mitral valve surgery for mitral stenosis. *Am J Cardiol* 1984; **54**: 617–19.

20 Hall JI, Wood DR. Factors affecting cardioversion of atrial arrhythmias with special reference to quinidine. *Br Heart J* 1968; **30**: 84–90.

21a Van Gelder IC, Crijns HJ, Van Gilst WH, Verwer R, Lie KI. Prediction of uneventful cardioversion and maintenance of sinus rhythm from direct current electrical cardioversion of chronic atrial fibrillation or flutter. *Am J Cardiol* 1991; **68**: 41–6.

21b Manning WJ, Silverman DI, Katz SE *et al*. Temporal dependence of the return of atrial mechanical function on the mode of cardioversion of atrial fibrillation to sinus rhythm. *Am J Cardiol* 1995; **75**: 624–7.

21c Mobarek S, Harjai K, Cheirif J, Murgo J, Revall S, Abi-Samra F. Electrical cardioversion is associated with greater atrial mechanical dysfunction than chemical cardioversion for atrial fibrillation (abstract). *PACE* 1996; **19**: 642.

21d Falcone RA, Morady F, Armstrong WF. Transoesophageal echographic evaluation of left atrial appendage function and spontaneous contrast formation after chemical or electrical cardioversion of atrial fibrillation. *Am J Cardiol* 1996; **78**: 435–9.

21e Weiner P, Bassan MM, Jarchovsky J, Lusim S, Plavnick L. Clinical course of acute atrial fibrillation treated with rapid digitalization. *Am Heart J* 1983; **103**: 223–7.

22 Falk RH, Knowlton AA, Bernard SA, Gotlieb NE, Battinelli NJ. Digoxin for converting recent onset atrial fibrillation to sinus rhythm. A randomized double blinded trial. *Ann Intern Med* 1987; **106**: 503–6.

23 Borgeat A, Goy JJ, Maendly R, Kaufman V, Grbic M, Sigwart W. Flecainide versus quinidine for conversion of atrial fibrillation to sinus rhythm. *Am J Cardiol* 1986; **58**: 496–8.

24 Zehender M, Hohnloser S, Muller B, Meinertz T, Just H. Effects of amiodarone versus quinidine and verapamil in patients with chronic atrial fibrillation: results of a comparative study and a 2 year follow-up. *J Am Coll Cardiol* 1992; **19**: 1054–9.

25 Roden DM, Woosley RL, Primm RK. Incidence and clinical features of quinidine associated long QT syndrome: implications for patient care. *Am Heart J* 1986; **111**: 1088–93.

26 Cheng TO. Atrial flutter during quinidine therapy of atrial fibrillation. *Am Heart J* 1956;

217

52: 273–89.

27 Halpern SW, Elrodt G, Singh BN, Mandel WJ. Efficacy of intravenous procainamide infusion in converting atrial fibrillation to sinus rhythm: relation to left atrial size. *Br Heart J* 1980; **44**: 589–94.

28 Fenster KE, Comess KA, Marsh R, Katzenberg C, Hager WD. Conversion of atrial fibrillation to sinus rhythm by acute intravenous procainamide infusion. *Am Heart J* 1983; **106**: 501–4.

29 Cardiac Arrhythmia Suppression Trial (CAST) Investigators. Randomized trial of arrhythmia suppression after myocardial infarction. *N Engl J Med* 1989; **321**: 406–12.

30 Kingma JH, Suttorp MJ. Acute pharmacologic conversion of atrial fibrillation and flutter: the role of flecainide, propafenone and verapamil. *Am J Cardiol* 1992; **70**: 56A–61A.

31 Nathan AW, Camm AJ, Bexton RS, Hellestrand KJ. Intravenous flecainide acetate for the clinical management of paroxysmal tachycardia. *Clin Cardiol* 1987; **10**: 317–22.

32 Goy JJ, Grbic M, Hurnie M *et al.* Conversion of supraventricular arrhythmias to sinus rhythm using flecainide. *Eur Heart J* 1985; **6**: 518–24.

33 Crijns HJ, Van Wijk LM, Van Gilst WH, Kingma JH, Van Gelder IC, Lie KI. Acute conversion of atrial fibrillation to sinus rhythm: clinical efficacy of flecainide acetate. Comparison of two regimes. *Eur Heart J* 1988; **9**: 634–8.

34 Donovan DK, Dobb JG, Coombs JL *et al.* Efficacy of flecainide for the reversion of acute onset atrial fibrillation. *Am J Cardiol* 1992; **70**: 50A–55A.

35 Hohnloser SH, Zabel M. Short and long term efficacy and safety of flecainide acetate for supraventricular arrhythmias. *Am J Cardiol* 1992; **70**: 3A–10A.

36 Capucci A, Lenzi T, Boriani G *et al.* Effectiveness of loading oral flecainide for converting recent onset atrial fibrillation to sinus rhythm in patients without organic heart disease or with only systemic hypertension. *Am J Cardiol* 1992; **70**: 73–7.

37 Bianconi L, Boccadamo R, Papalardo A, Gentili C, Pistolezi M. Effectiveness of intravenous propafenone for conversion of atrial fibrillation and flutter of recent onset. *Am J Cardiol* 1989; **64**: 335–8.

38 Cappuci A, Lenzi T, Boriani G *et al.* Efficacy of propafenone to convert atrial fibrillation to sinus rhythm: a controlled study comparing acute intravenous infusion versus oral loading (abstract). *Circulation* 1993; **88**: I–445.

39 Skoularigis J, Rothlisberger C, Studicky D, Essop MR, Weisenbaugh T, Sareli P. Effectiveness of amiodarone and electrical cardioversion for chronic rheumatic atrial fibrillation after mitral valve surgery. *Am J Cardiol* 1993; **72**(5): 423–7.

40 Kopelman HA, Horowitz LN. Efficacy and toxicity of amiodarone for the treatment of supraventricular arrhythmias. *Prog Cardiovasc Dis* 1989; **5**: 355–66.

41 Stasberg B, Arditti A, Scarovsky S, Lewin RF, Buimovici B, Agmon J. Efficacy of intravenous amiodarone in the management of paroxysmal or new atrial fibrillation with fast ventricular response. *Int J Cardiol* 1985; **7**: 47–55.

42 Cowan JC, Gardiner P, Reid DS. A comparison of amiodarone and digoxin in the treatment of atrial fibrillation complicating suspected acute myocardial infarction. *J Cardiovasc Pharm* 1986; **8**: 252–6.

43 Kadish A, Morady F. The use of intravenous amiodarone in the acute therapy of life threatening arrhythmias. *Prog Cardiovasc Dis* 1989; **4**: 281–94.

44 Sannia L, Frau G, Dore L. Pharmacologic conversion with intravenous amiodarone. *Boll Soc Ital Cardiol* 1980; **26**: 553–8.

45 Bellandi F, Cantini F, Pedone T, Dabizzi RP, Palchetti R. Efficacy of intravenous propafenone and amiodarone in conversion of recent onset atrial fibrillation, and efficacy of oral therapy at one year follow-up. *G Ital Cardiol* 1993; **23**(3): 261–71.

46 Horner SM. A comparison of cardioversion of atrial fibrillation using oral amiodarone, intravenous amiodarone and DC cardioversion. *Acta Cardiol* 1992; **47**: 473–80.

47 Blevins RD, Kerin NZ, Benaderet D *et al.* Amiodarone in the management of refractory atrial fibrillation. *Arch Intern Med* 1987; **147**: 1401–4.

48 Brodsky MA, Allen BJ, Walker CJ III, Casey TP, Luckett CR, Henry WL. Amiodarone for maintenance of sinus rhythm after conversion of atrial fibrillation in the setting of a dilated left atrium. *Am J Cardiol* 1987; **60**: 572–5.

49a Levy S, Rovini JC, Metge M *et al.* Intravenous sotalol in the acute treatment of supraventricular tachycardia. *Arch Mal Coeur* 1986; **79**: 1781–5.

49b Sung RJ, Tan HL, Karagounas L *et al.* Intravenous sotalol for the termination of supraventricular tachycardia and atrial fibrillation and flutter: a multicenter, randomised, double-blind, placebo-controlled study. *Am Heart J* 1995; **129**: 739–48.

49c Reisinger J, Gatterer E, Kuehn P, Slaney J. Flecainide versus sotalol for immediate conversion of atrial fibrillation (abstract). *J Am Coll Cardiol* 1997; **29**: 471A.

49d Buchanan LV, Thompson DD, Hsu CL, Walters RR, Gibson JK. Antiarrhythmic and electrophysiological effects of sublingual ibutilide fumarate. *Drug Dev Res* 1995; **34**: 322–8.

49e Stambler BS, Wood MA, Ellenbogen KA *et al.* and the Ibutilide Repeat Dose Study Investigators. Efficacy and safety of repeated intravenous doses of ibutilide for rapid conversion of atrial fibrillation and flutter. *Circulation* 1996; **94**: 1613–21.

50 Sedgewick M, Rasmussen HS, Walker DK, Cobbe SM. Pharmacokinetic and pharmacodynamic effects of UK-68-798, a new class 3 antiarrhythmic drug. *Br J Clin Pharmacol* 1991; **32**: 429–32.

51 Rasmussen HS, Allen MJ, Blackburn KJ, Butrous GS, Dalrymple HW. Dofetilide, a novel class III antiarrhythmic agent. *J Cardiovasc Pharmacol* 1992; **20**: S96–105.

52 Suttorp MJ, Polak PE, Van't Hof A, Rasmussen HS, Dunselman PH, Kingma JH. Efficacy and safety of a new class III antiarrhythmic agent Dofetilide in paroxysmal atrial fibrillation or flutter. *Am J Cardiol* 1992; **69**: 417–19.

53 Lown B, Amarasingham R, Neuman J. New method for terminating cardiac arrhythmias. *JAMA* 1962; **182**: 548–55.

54 Lown B, Kleiger R, Wolf G. The technique of cardioversion. *Am Heart J* 1964; **67**: 282–4.

55 Kerber RE, Jensen SR, Grayzel J, Kennedy J, Hoyt R. Elective cardioversion: influence of paddle electrode location and size on success rates and energy requirements. *N Engl J Med* 1981; **305**: 658–62.

56 Ewy GA. Optimum technique for electrical cardioversion of atrial fibrillation. *Circulation* 1992; **86**: 1645–7.

57 Ewy GA, Hellman DA, McClung S, Tare D. Influence of ventilation phase on transthoracic impedance and defibrillation effectiveness. *Crit Care Med* 1980; **8**: 164–6.

58 Kerber RE, Grayzel J, Hoyt R, Marcus M, Kennedy J. Transthoracic resistance in human defibrillation: influence of body weight, chest size, serial shocks, paddle size and paddle contact pressure. *Circulation* 1981; **63**: 676–82.

59 Aylward PE, Kieso R, Hite P, Charbonnier F, Kerber RE. Defibrillator electrode-chest wall coupling agents: influence on transthoracic impedance and shock success. *J Am Coll Cardiol* 1985; **6**: 682–6.

60a Van Gelder IC, Crijns HJGM, Van Gilst WH, DeLangen CDJ, Van Wijk LM, Lie KI. Effects of flecainide on atrial defibrillation threshold. *Am J Cardiol* 1989; **63**: 112–14.

60b Newby KH, Waugh R, Hardee M, Henderson PH, Mertz J, Natale A. Amiodarone decreases defibrillation threshold in patients undergoing elective cardioversion for atrial fibrillation (abstract). *Circulation* 1996; **94**: I-667.

60c Niebauer M, Chung MK, Holmes D, Van Wagoner DR, Tchou P. Esmolol reduces atrial defibrillation thresholds: a randomised, placebo-controlled study (abstract). *J Am Coll Cardiol* 1997; **29**: 292A.

60d Bianconi L, Mennuni M, Lukic V, Castro A, Chieffi M, Santini M. Effects of oral propafenone administration before electrical cardioversion of atrial fibrillation: a placebo controlled study. *J Am Coll Cardiol* 1996; **28**: 700–6.

61 Levy S, Lacombe P, Cointe R, Bru P. High energy trans-catheter cardioversion of chronic atrial fibrillation. *J Am Coll Cardiol* 1988; **12**: 514–18.

62 Levy S, Lauribe P, Dolla E *et al.* A randomized comparison of external and internal cardioversion of chronic atrial fibrillation. *Circulation* 1992; **86**: 1415–20.

63 Levy S. Direct current cardioversion of established atrial fibrillation. *Clin Cardiol* 1992; **15**: 445–9.

64 Murgatroyd F, Slade AK, O'Farrell DM *et al.* Low-energy internal cardioversion. *J Am Coll Cardiol* 1994; **23**: 126A.

65a Keane D, Sulke N, Cooke R, Jackson G, Sowten E. Endocardial cardioversion of atrial flutter and fibrillation (abstract). *Pace* 1993; **16**: 928.

65b Alt EU, Ammer RM, Putter KE, Schmitt CM. Internal cardioversion of atrial fibrillation with a new, single lead, balloon-guided catheter system (abstract). *Circulation* 1996; **94**: I–71.

65c Murgatroyd FD, Slade AK, Sopher SM, Rowland E, Ward DE, Camm AJ. Efficacy and tolerability of transvenous low energy cardioversion of paroxysmal atrial fibrillation in humans. *J Am Coll Cardiol* 1995; **25**(6): 1347–53.

65d Ammer R, Alt G, Lehmann G *et al*. Pain threshold for internal cardioversion with low or no sedation (abstract). *J Am Coll Cardiol* 1997; **29**: 113A.

66 McKeown PP, Croal S, Allen DJ, Anderson J, Adgy JAA. Transoesophageal cardioversion. *Am Heart J* 1993; **125**: 396–404.

67 Grande P, Sonne B, Pederson A. A controlled study of digoxin and quinidine in patients DC converted reverted from atrial fibrillation to sinus rhythm (abstract). *Circulation* 1986; **74**: II–101.

68 Hall JI, Wood DR. Factors affecting cardioversion of atrial arrhythmias with special reference to quinidine. *Br Heart J* 1968; **30**: 84–90.

69 Radford MD, Evans DW. Long term results of DC reversion of atrial fibrillation. *Br Heart J* 1968; **30**: 81–3.

70 Sodermark T, Jonsson B, Olsson A *et al*. Effect of quinidine in maintaining sinus rhythm after conversion of atrial fibrillation or flutter. A multicenter study from Stockholm. *Br Heart J* 1975; **37**: 486–92.

71 Boissel JP, Wolf E, Gillet J *et al*. Controlled trial of a long acting quinidine for maintenance of sinus rhythm after electroversion of chronic atrial fibrillation. *Eur Heart J* 1981; **2**: 49–55.

72 Hartel G, Louhija A, Kontinen A, Halone PI. Value of quinidine in maintenance of sinus rhythm after electric cardioversion of atrial fibrillation. *Br Heart J* 1970; **32**: 57–60.

73 Coplen SE, Antman EM, Berlin JA, Hewit P, Chalmers TC. Efficacy and safety of quinidine therapy for maintenance of sinus rhythm after cardioversion. A meta-analysis of randomized controlled trials. *Circulation* 1990; **82**: 1106–16.

74 Reimold SC, Chalmers TC, Berlin JA, Antman EM. Assessment of safety and efficacy of antiarrhythmic therapy of chronic atrial fibrillation; observations on the role of trial design and implications of drug related mortality. *Am Heart J* 1992; **124**: 924–31.

75 Flaker GC, Blackshear JL, McBride R, Kronmal RA, Halperin JL, Hart RG. Antiarrhythmic drug therapy and cardiac mortality in atrial fibrillation. The stroke prevention in atrial fibrillation investigators. *J Am Coll Cardiol* 1992; **20**: 527–32.

76 Karlson BW, Torstensson I, Abjorn C, Yansson GO, Peterson LE. Disopyramide in maintenance of sinus rhythm after electroversion of atrial fibrillation – a placebo controlled one year follow up study. *Eur Heart J* 1988; **9**: 284–90.

77 Coumel P. Neural aspects of paroxysmal atrial fibrillation. In: Falk RH, Podrid PJ. eds. *Atrial fibrillation. Mechanisms and management.* New York: Raven Press, 1992.

78 Anderson JL, Gilbert EM, Alpert BL *et al*. and the Flecainide Supraventricular Study Group. Prevention of symptomatic recurrences of paroxysmal atrial fibrillation in patients initially tolerating antiarrhythmic therapy. A multicenter, double blind, crossover study of flecainide and placebo with transtelephonic monitoring. *Circulation* 1989; **80**: 1557–70.

79 Leclercq JF, Chouty F, Denjoy I, Coumel P, Slama R. Flecainide in quinidine resistant atrial fibrillation. *Am J Cardiol* 1992; **70**: 62A–65A.

80 Anderson JL, Jolivette DM, Fredell PA. Summary of efficacy and safety of flecainide for supraventricular arrhythmias. *Am J Cardiol* 1988; **62**: 62D–66D.

81 Pritchett ELC, DaTorre SD, Platt ML, McCarville SE, Hougham AJ, for the Flecainide Supraventricular Study Group. Flecainide acetate treatment of supraventricular tachycardia and paroxysmal atrial fibrillation: dose–response study. *J Am Coll Cardiol* 1991; **17**: 297–303.

82 Pietersen AH, Helleman H. Usefulness of flecainide for prevention of paroxysmal atrial fibrillation and flutter. Danish-Norwegian Flecainide Multicenter Study Group. *Am J Cardiol* 1991; **67**: 713–17.

83 Falk RH. Flecainide induced ventricular tachycardia and fibrillation in patients treated for atrial fibrillation. *Ann Intern Med* 1989; **111**: 107–11.

84 Sihm I, Hansen FA, Rasmussen J *et al*. Flecainide acetate in atrial flutter and fibrillation. The arrhythmogenic effects. *Eur Heart J* 1990; **11**: 145–8.

85 Feld GK, Chen PS, Nicod P *et al*. Possible proarrhythmic effects of class IC

antiarrhythmic drugs. *Am J Cardiol* 1990; **66**: 378–83.

86 Falk RH. Proarrhythmic responses to atrial antiarrhythmic therapy. In: Falk RH, Podrid PJ. eds. *Atrial fibrillation. Mechanisms and management*. New York: Raven Press, 1992.

87 Pritchett EL, Wilkinson WE. Mortality in patients treated with flecainide and encainide for supraventricular arrhythmias. *Am J Cardiol* 1991; **67**: 967–80.

88 Antman EM, Beamer AD, Cautillon C, McGowan N, Goldman L, Friedman PL. Long term oral propafenone therapy for suppression of refractory symptomatic atrial fibrillation and atrial flutter. *J Am Coll Cardiol* 1988; **12**: 1005–11.

89 Pritchett EL, McCarthy EA, Wilkinson WE. Propafenone treatment of symptomatic paroxysmal supraventricular arrhythmias. A randomized placebo controlled cross over trial in patients tolerating oral therapy. *Ann Intern Med* 1991; **114**: 539–44.

90 Coumel L, Leclerq JF, Assayag P. European experience with antiarrhythmic efficacy of propafenone for supraventricular and ventricular arrhythmias. *Am J Cardiol* 1984; **54**: 60D–64D.

91 Murdock CJ, Kyles AE, Yeun-Lai-Wah JA, Qi A, Vorderbrugge S, Kerr CR. Atrial flutter in patients treated with atrial fibrillation with propafenone. *Am J Cardiol* 1990; **66**: 755–7.

92 Vitolo E, Tronci M, Larovere MT, Rumolo R, Morabito A. Amiodarone versus quinidine in the prophylaxis of atrial fibrillation. *Acta Cardiol* 1981; **36**: 431–44.

93 Graboys TB, Podrid PJ, Lown B. Efficacy of amiodarone for refractory supraventricular tachyarrhythmias. *Am Heart J* 1983; **106**: 870–6.

94a Gosselink AM, Crijns HJ, Isabelle CVG, Hillige H, Wiesfeld ACP, Lie KI. Low dose amiodarone for maintenance of sinus rhythm after cardioversion of atrial fibrillation or flutter. *JAMA* 1992; **267**: 3289–93.

94b Acquati F, Forgione F, Caico S *et al*. Prophylaxis of atrial fibrillation following electrical cardioversion. A prospective randomised study comparing low-dose and very low-dose amiodarone to propafenone: preliminary results (abstract). *J Am Coll Cardiol* 1997; **29**: 112A.

95 Gold RL, Haffajee CL, Charos G, Solan K, Baker S, Alpert JS. Amiodarone for refractory atrial fibrillation. *Am J Cardiol* 1986; **57**: 124–7.

96 Horowitz LN, Spielman SR, Greenspan AM *et al*. Use of amiodarone in persistent and paroxysmal atrial fibrillation resistant to quinidine therapy. *J Am Coll Cardiol* 1985; **6**: 1402–7.

97 Jull-Moller S, Edvardsson M, Rehnqvist AN. Sotalol versus quinidine in the maintenance of sinus rhythm after direct current conversion of atrial fibrillation. *Circulation* 1990; **82**: 1932–9.

98 Reimold SC, Cantillon CO, Freidman PL, Antman EM. Propafenone versus sotalol for suppression of recurrent symptomatic atrial fibrillation. *Am J Cardiol* 1993; **71**: 558–63.

99 Sahar DI, Raffel JA, Bigger JT Jr, Squarito A, Kidwell GA. Safety and tolerance of *d*-sotalol in patients with refractory supraventricular tachyarrhythmias. *Am Heart J* 1989; **117**: 562–8.

100 Rawles JM, Metcalfe MJ, Jennings K. Time of occurrence, duration and ventricular rate of paroxysmal atrial fibrillation: the effect of digoxin. *Br Heart J* 1990; **63**: 225–7.

101 Murgatroyd FD, Xie B, Gibson SM, Ward DE, Malik M, Camm AJ. The effects of digoxin in patients with paroxysmal atrial fibrillation: analysis of Holter data from the CRAFT-I trial (abstract). *J Am Coll Cardiol* 1993; **21**: 203a.

102 Murgatroyd FD, O'Nunain S, Gibson SM, Poloneicki JD, Ward DE, Camm AJ. The results of the CRAFT-I: a multi-center, double blind, placebo-controlled crossover study of digoxin in symptomatic paroxysmal atrial fibrillation (abstract). *J Am Coll Cardiol* 1993; **21**: 478.

103 Johnson LW, Dickstein RA, Freuhan CT. Prophylactic digitalization for coronary artery bypass surgery. *Circulation* 1976; **53**: 819–22.

104 Tyras DH, Stothert JC, Kaiser GC. Supraventricular tachyarrhythmias after myocardial revascularization: a randomized trial of prophylactic digitalization. *J Thorac Cardiovasc Surg* 1979; **77**: 310–14.

105 Engel TR, Gonzalez AD. Effects of digitalis on atrial vulnerability. *Am J Cardiol* 1978; **42**: 570–6.

106 Stephenson LW, MacVaugh H, Tomasello DN, Josephson ME. Propranolol for

221

prevention of post-operative cardiac arrhythmias: a randomized study. *Ann Thorac Surg* 1980; **29**: 113–16.

107 Fors WJ, Vanderark CR, Reynolds LW. Evaluation of propranolol and quinidine in the treatment of quinidine resistant arrhythmias. *Am J Cardiol* 1971; **27**: 190–4.

108 Myerburg RJ, Kessler KM, Box MM *et al*. Reversal of proarrhythmic effects of flecainide acetate and encainide hydrochloride by propranolol. *Circulation* 1989; **80**: 1571–9.

109 Niazii I, Naccarelli G, Dougherty A, Rinkenberger R, Tchou P, Akhtar M. Treatment of atrioventricular nodal reentrant tachycardia with encainide: reversal of drug effect with isoproteranol. *J Am Coll Cardiol* 1989; **13**: 904–10.

110 Toivonen L, Kadish A, Kou W, Morady F. Determinants of the ventricular rate during atrial fibrillation. *J Am Coll Cardiol* 1990; **16**: 1194–200.

111a Abbot JA, Schiller NB, Ivento JB *et al*. Catheter ablation of atrioventricular conduction may improve left ventricular function and cause minimal aortic valve damage. *Pace* 1987; **10**: 411.

111b Prystowsky EN, Benson DW, Fuster V *et al*. Management of patients with atrial fibrillation. A statement for healthcare professionals from the committee on electrocardiography and electrophysiology, American Heart Association. *Circulation* 1996; **93**: 1262–77.

111c Gardner MJ, Gilbert M. Heart rate control in patients with atrial fibrillation. *Can J Cardiol* 1996; **12**: 21A–23A.

112 Meijler FL. An "account" of digitalis and atrial fibrillation. *J Am Coll Cardiol* 1985; **5** (Suppl A): 60A–68A.

113 Lang R, Klein HO, Weiss E *et al*. Superiority of oral verapamil therapy to digoxin in treatment of chronic atrial fibrillation. *Chest* 1983; **83**: 491–9.

114 Beasley R, Smith DA, McHaffie DJ. Exercise heart rates at different serum digoxin concentration in patients with atrial fibrillation. *Br Med J (Clin Res)* 1985; **290**: 9–11.

115 Anderson S, Blansky L, Byrd R *et al*. Comparison of the efficacy and safety of esmolol, a short acting beta-blocker, with placebo in the treatment of supraventricular arrhythmias. The esmolol vs placebo multicenter study group. *Am Heart J;* 1986; **111**: 42–8.

116 Shettigar UR, Toole JG, Appun DO. Combined use of esmolol and digoxin in the acute treatment of atrial fibrillation and flutter. *Am Heart J* 1993; **126**: 368–74.

117 Atwood JE, Sullivan M, Forbes S *et al*. Effects of beta adrenergic blockade on exercise performance in patients with chronic atrial fibrillation. *J Am Coll Cardiol* 1987; **10**: 314–20.

118 Di Bianco R, Marganroth J, Freitag RJ *et al*. Effects of nadolol on the spontaneous and exercise provoked heart rate in patients with chronic atrial fibrillation receiving stable doses of digoxin. *Am Heart J* 1984; **108**: 1121–7.

119 Molajo AO, Coupe MO, Bennet DH. Effect of Corwin (ICI 118,587) on resting and exercise heart rate and exercise tolerance in digitalized patients with chronic atrial fibrillation. *Br Heart J* 1984; **52**: 392–5.

120 Ang E, Chang WL, Cleland JGF *et al*. Placebo controlled trial of Xamoterol versus digoxin in chronic atrial fibrillation. *Br Heart J* 1990; **64**: 256–60.

121 Lundstrom T, Moore E, Ryden L. Differential effects of xamoterol and verapamil on ventricular rate regulation in patients with chronic atrial fibrillation. *Am Heart J* 1992; **124**: 917–23.

122 The Xamoterol in Severe Heart Failure Study Group. Xamoterol in severe heart failure. *Lancet* 1990; **336**: 1–6.

123 James MA, Channer KS, Papouchado M, Rees JR. Improved control of atrial fibrillation with combined pindolol and digoxin therapy. *Eur Heart J* 1989; **10**: 83–90.

124 Wang R, Camm AJ, Waed D, Washington H, Martin A. Treatment of chronic atrial fibrillation in the elderly, assessed by ambulatory electrocardiographic monitoring. *J Am Geriatr Soc* 1980; **28**: 529–34.

125 Salerno DM, Dias VC, Kleiger RE *et al*. Efficacy and safety of intravenous diltiazem for treatment of atrial fibrillation and flutter. The diltiazem atrial fibrillation/flutter study group. *Am J Cardiol* 1989; **63**: 1046–51.

126 Lang R, Klein H, Segni E *et al*. Verapamil improves exercise capacity in chronic atrial fibrillation: double-blind cross-over study. *Am Heart J* 1983; **105**: 820–5.

127a Roth A, Harrison E, Mitani G, Cohen J, Rahimtoola SH, Elkayem U. Efficacy and safety of medium and high dose diltiazem alone and in combination with digoxin for control of heart rate at rest and during exercise in patients with chronic atrial fibrillation. *Circulation* 1986; **73**: 316–24.

127b Lewis RV, Lakhani M, Moreland TA, McDevitt DG. A comparison of verapamil and digoxin in the treatment of atrial fibrillation. *Eur Heart J* 1987; **8**: 148–53.

127c Lewis RV, Laing E, Moreland TA, Service E, McDevitt DG. A comparison of digoxin, diltiazem and their combination in the treatment of atrial fibrillation. *Eur Heart J* 1988; **9**: 279–83.

127d Lewis RV, Irvine N, McDevitt DG. Relationships between heart rate, exercise tolerance and cardiac output in atrial fibrillation: the effects of treatment with digoxin, verapamil and diltiazem. *Eur Heart J* 1988; **9**: 777–81.

128 Atwood JE, Myers JN, Sullivan MJ, Forbes SM, Pewes WF, Froelicher VF. Diltiazem and exercise performance in patients with chronic atrial fibrillation. *Chest* 1988; **93**: 20–5.

129 Lundstrom T, Ryden L. Ventricular rate control and exercise performance in chronic atrial fibrillation: effects of diltiazem and verapamil. *J Am Coll Cardiol* 1990; **16**: 86–90.

130 Scheinmann MM, Morady F, Hess DS, Gonzalez R. Catheter induced ablation of atrioventricular junction to control refractory supraventricular arrhythmias. *JAMA* 1982; **248**: 851–5.

131 Olgin JE, Scheinmann MM. Comparison of high energy direct current and radio-frequency catheter ablation of the atrioventricular junction. *J Am Coll Cardiol* 1993; **21**: 557–64.

132 Evans GT, Scheinmann MM, Zipes DP. The Percutaneous Cardiac Mapping and Ablation Registry: final summary of results. *Pace* 1986; **9**: 923–6.

133a Rosenqvist M, Lee MA, Moulinier L *et al.* Long term follow up of patients after transcatheter direct current ablation of the atrioventricular junction. *J Am Coll Cardiol* 1990; **16**: 1467–74.

133b Edner M, Caidahl K, Bergfeldt L, Darpo B, Edvardsson N, Rosenqvist M. Prospective study of left ventricular function after radiofrequency ablation of atrioventricular junction in patients with atrial fibrillation. *Br Heart J* 1995; **74**: 261–7.

133c Ellenbogen KA, Kay GN, Guidici M *et al.* and the ATP Trial Investigators. Radiofrequency ablation of the AV junction improves functional status in patients with congestive heart failure: results from the APT trial (abstract). *Circulation* 1996; **94**: I–682.

133d Feld GK, Fleck RP, Fujimura O, Prothro DL, Bahnson TD, Ibarra M. Control of rapid ventricular response by radiofrequency catheter modification of the atrioventricular node in patients with medically refractory atrial fibrillation. *Circulation* 1994; **90**: 2299–307.

133e Williamson BD, Ching-Man K, Daoud E, Niebauer M, Strickberger A, Morady F. Radiofrequency catheter modification of atrioventricular conduction to control the ventricular rate during atrial fibrillation. *N Engl J Med* 1994; **331**: 910–17.

134a Coumel P, Fricourt P, Mugica J, Attuel P, Leclercq JF. Long term prevention of vagal arrhythmias by atrial pacing at 90/min. Experience with 6 cases. *Pace* 1983; **6**: 552–60.

134b Saksena S, Prakash A, Hill M *et al.* Prevention of recurrent atrial fibrillation with chronic dual-site right atrial pacing. *J Am Coll Cardiol* 1996; **28**: 687–94.

135. Feur JM, Shandling AH, Messenger JC. Influence of cardiac pacing mode on long term development of atrial fibrillation. *Am J Cardiol* 1989; **64**: 1376–9.

136 Zanini R, Facchinetti AI, Gallo G, Cazamalli L, Bonadi L, Dei-Cas L. Morbidity and mortality of patients with sinus node disease: comparative effects of atrial and ventricular pacing. *Pace* 1990; **13**: 2076–9.

137 Sgarbossa EB, Pinski SL, Maloney JD *et al.* Chronic atrial fibrillation and stroke in paced patients with sick sinus syndrome. Relevance of clinical characteristics and pacing modalities. *Circulation* 1993; **88**: 1045–53.

138 Camm AJ, Katritsis D. Ventricular pacing for sick sinus syndrome – a risky business? (editorial) *Pace* 1990; **13**: 695–9.

139 Luck JC, Engel TR. Dispersion of atrial responsiveness in patients with sinus node dysfunction. *Circulation* 1979; **60**: 404–12.

140 Page P. Sinus node during atrial fibrillation: to beat or not to beat? *Circulation* 1992; **86**: 334–6.

141 Kirchoff CJHJ, Allessie MA. Sinus node automaticity during atrial fibrillation in isolated rabbit hearts. *Circulation* 1992; **86**: 263–71.

142 Sutton R. Pacing in atrial arrhythmias. *Pace* 1990; **13**: 1823–6.

143 Van Wyhe G, Sra G, Rovang K *et al.* Maintenance of atrioventricular sequence after His bundle ablation for paroxysmal supraventricular rhythm disorders: a unique use of the fall back mode in dual chamber pacemakers. *Pace* 1991; **14**: 410–14.

144 Mower MM, Mirowski M, Denniston RH. Assessment of various models of acetylcholine induced atrial fibrillation for study of internal arterial cardioversion (abstract). *Clin Res* 1972; **20**: 388.

145 Dunbar DN, Tobler HG, Fetter J, Gornick CC, Benson DWJ, Benditt DG. Intracavitary electrode catheter cardioversion of atrial tachyarrhythmias in the dog. *J Am Coll Cardiol* 1986; **7**: 1015–27.

146 Cooper RAS, Alferness CA, Smith WM, Ideker RE. Internal cardioversion of atrial fibrillation in sheep. *Circulation* 1993; **87**: 1673–86.

147 Kumagai K, Yamanouchi Y, Tashiro N, Hiroki T, Arakawa K. Low energy synchronous transcatheter cardioversion of atrial flutter/fibrillation in the dog. *J Am Coll Cardiol* 1990; **16**: 497–501.

148a Levy S, Camm AJ. An implantable atrial defibrillator. An impossible dream? *Circulation* 1993; **87**: 1769–71.

148b Lau CP, Tse HF, Lee K *et al.* Initial clinical experience of a human implantable atrial defibrillator (abstract). *Pace* 1995; **19**: 625.

149 DeFauw JJ, Guiraudon GM, Van Hemel NM, Vermeulen FE, Kingma JH, de Bakker JM. Surgical therapy of paroxysmal atrial fibrillation with the "corridor" operation. *Ann Thorac Surg* 1992; **53**: 564–70.

150 Cox JL, Schuessler RB, D'Agostino HJ *et al.* The surgical treatment of atrial fibrillation. III. Development of a definitive surgical procedure. *J Thorac Cardiovasc Surg* 1991; **101**: 569–83.

151a Cox JL, Boineau JP, Schuessler RB, Kater KM, Lappas DG. Five year experience with the maze procedure for atrial fibrillation. *Ann Thorac Surg* 1993; **56**: 814–24.

151b Elvan A, Pride H, Eble JN, Zipes DP. Radiofrequency catheter ablation of the atria reduces inducibility of atrial fibrillation in dogs. *Circulation* 1995; **91**: 2235–44.

151c Swartz JF, Pellersels G, Silvers J, Patten L, Cervantez D. A catheter based curative approach to atrial fibrillation in humans (abstract). *Circulation* 1994; **90**: I-335.

151d Jais P, Haissaguerre M, Shah DC *et al.* A focal source of atrial fibrillation treated by discrete radiofrequency ablation. *Circulation* 1997; **95**: 572–6.

152 Buscarini L, Imberti D. Increased incidence of spontaneous conversion to sinus rhythm in patients with paroxysmal atrial fibrillation. *G Ital Cradiol* 1991; **22**: 949–52.

153 De Silva RA, Graboys TB, Podrid PJ, Lown B. Cardioversion and defibrillation. *Am Heart J* 1980; **100**: 881–95.

154 Laupacis A, Albers G, Dunn M, Feinberg W. Antithrombotic therapy in atrial fibrillation. *Chest* 1992; **102** (Suppl 4): 426S–33S.

155 Black IW, Hopkins AP, Lee LCL, Walsh WF. Evaluation of trans-oesophageal echocardiography before cardioversion of atrial fibrillation and flutter in non-anti-coagulated patients. *Am Heart J* 1993; **126**: 375–81.

156 Manning WJ, Leeman DE, Gotch PJ, Come PC. Pulsed Doppler evaluation of atrial mechanical function after electrical cardioversion of atrial fibrillation. *J Am Coll Cardiol* 1989; **13**: 617–23.

157 Falk RH, Podrid PJ. Electrical cardioversion of atrial fibrillation. In: Falk RH, Podrid PJ. eds. *Atrial fibrillation. Mechanisms and management.* New York: Raven Press, 1992.

158 Suttorp MJ, Kingma JH, Koomen EM, Van't Hof A, Tijssen JG, Lie KI. Recurrence of paroxysmal atrial fibrillation or flutter after successful cardioversion in patients with normal left ventricular function. *Am J Cardiol* 1993; **71**: 710–13.

159 Lundstrom T, Ryden L. Chronic atrial fibrillation. Long term results of direct cardioversion. *Acta Med Scand* 1988; **223**: 53–9.

160 Rawles JM. What is meant by a "controlled" ventricular rate in atrial fibrillation? *Br Heart J* 1990; **63**: 157–61.

161 Crijns HJ, Van Gelder IC, Van Gilst WH, Hillege H, Gosselink AM, Lie KI. Serial antiarrhythmic drug treatment to maintain sinus rhythm after electrical cardioversion for

chronic atrial fibrillation or flutter. *Am J Cardiol* 1991; **68**: 335–41.

162 Antman EM, Beamer AD, Cantillon C, McGowan M, Freidman PL. Therapy of refractory symptomatic atrial fibrillation and flutter: a staged care approach with new antiarrhythmic drugs. *J Am Coll Cardiol* 1990; **15**: 698–707.

163 Shia P, Lal R, Kim SS, Schechtman K, Ruffy R. Flecainide and amiodarone interaction. *J Am Coll Cardiol* 1986; **7**: 1127–30.

164 Leclercq JF, Denjoy I, Menter F, Coumel P. Flecainide acetate dose concentration relationship in cardiac arrhythmias: influence of heart failure and amiodarone. *Cardiovasc Drug Ther* 1990; **4**: 1161–6.

10: Implementing cardiovascular management strategies in hospital practice

JR McEWAN

Cardiovascular disease accounts for more than 50% of all occupied bed days in hospital.[1] Only a minority of these patients will be under the care of or even reviewed at any time by a consultant with a particular interest in cardiovascular disease. The 1992 survey by the British Cardiac Society[2] revealed that there were still 44 districts in the UK without a physician with an interest in cardiology and 34 large districts (greater than 250,000 population) which had only one rather than the two recommended by the fourth report of the Joint Committee of the Royal Colleges.[3] The 1994 survey showed that there had been an increase of 6·3% in whole time equivalent (WTE) cardiologists since 1993 but at a total of 417·5 WTE cardiologists, this is still below the one cardiologist per 100,000 population which is recommended.[4]

The scarcity of this resource means that many cardiologists deal with less common areas of their specialty and common problems, some of which have been discussed in the foregoing chapters, fall within the remit of general physicians involved in the care of acute emergency admission. Debate about the contribution of a cardiologist to the emergency management of acute myocardial infarction[5] is academic when almost all patients who suffer a myocardial infarction never see a cardiologist. A survey of generalists, family practitioners and cardiologists in the USA confirmed that cardiologists there are more informed about key advances in the treatment of myocardial infarction than are their generalist colleagues.[6] In the USA a study of 8241 elderly patients with an acute myocardial infarction demonstrated a 12% reduction in mortality when they were under the care of a specialist cardiologist rather than a primary care physician (a general physician or family practitioner).[7]

The results of the recent clinical trials should be having a major impact on current clinical practice and this becomes particularly relevant with the emerging pressures for auditing treatment and outcomes.[8] Some of the reviews of management guidelines have been published in specialist journals[9] so a major role for the cardiologists in the UK at the present time is to work with their generalist colleagues in interpretation and implementation of effective management policy.

A useful tool for guiding such policy is a local acute cardiology handbook. An example of one such document is given in the Appendix on page 228. The booklet illustrated is produced in a "Filofax" size, so as to fit into such pocket books, and is generated and stored on a computer to allow updates at six monthly intervals. Brief didactic instructions are supplemented by algorithms on cardiac arrest and arrhythmias published by the European Resuscitation Council. A major advantage of such a locally produced document is the incorporation of local drug policy. Most hospitals now have hospital formularies and local therapeutic policy groups. This serves to rationalise the number of medicines stocked in the pharmacy, examines carefully the evidence of any new therapy and has the advantage of economic control. For this reason the drugs indicated in the Appendix are recommended as those on the formulary of the institution where I hold my appointment. Class specific events are assumed in such areas as β-blocker and ACE inhibitor therapy, so locally approved drugs could be substituted.

Not only acute management guidelines but also checklists for secondary preventive measures can be incorporated. The ASPIRE Study has highlighted the variation in how individual patients may be treated or advised, notably on lipid lowering, use of β-blockers and aspirin.[10]

Such a handbook allows the widespread dissemination of the often sparse input of cardiologists to acute medicine. Specialist knowledge and generalist experience need to be combined to produce guidelines which can be followed with ease. Instructing the junior staff in interpretation and adjudication where decisions are clearly difficult are roles for both cardiologist and generalist. An essential aspect of the consultant role is the teaching of the junior doctor on how to assess the patient with cardiovascular disease and other medical problems, rather than a "trial subject". Where possible the guidelines should be supplemented by a joint ward round of a representative of the cardiology service of specialist grade with the admitting team to rapidly assess all new cardiovascular admissions. The guidelines can be reinforced and new junior staff rapidly initiated into the approved system. Patients felt to be at high risk can be identified and transferred for specialist investigations.

Not all areas of medicine (even cardiological) have been examined in clinical trials so in some areas treatment is not yet evidence based. What follows is a personal interpretation which is revised and updated according to new evidence and perceived wisdom every six months. It is written from

227

the standpoint of a cardiologist in a tertiary centre with immediate access to all interventional facilities, but also with a service commitment to acute coronary admissions such as are seen in any district general hospital. The pace of progress is such that it is likely to be out of date by the time of publication. However, it provides a starting point for others to design their own handbook of protocols, in keeping with local policy and drug use.

1 Data on file. National Casemix Office, Winchester.
2 Chamberlain D, Parker J, Balcon R *et al.* Eighth survey of staffing and cardiology in the United Kingdom 1992. *Br Heart J* 1994; 71: 492–500.
3 Fourth Report of a Joint Cardiology Committee of the Royal College of Physicians of London and the Royal College of Surgeons of England. Provision of services for the diagnosis and treatment of heart disease. *Br Heart J* 1992; 67: 106–16.
4 Data on file. British Cardiac Society, London.
5 Gwiltt DJ. Cardiologists in casualty (commentary). *Lancet* 1995; 346: 1571–2.
6 Ayarian JZ, Hauptman PJ, Guadagnoli E *et al.* Knowledge and practices of generalist and specialist physicians regarding drug therapy for acute myocardial infarction. *N Engl J Med* 1994; 331: 1136–42.
7 Jollis JG, Delong ER, Peterson ED *et al.* Outcome of acute myocardial infarction according to the specialty of the admitting physician. *N Engl J Med* 1996; 335: 1880–7.
8 Report of a Workshop of the Joint Audit Committee of the British Cardiac Society and the Royal College of Physicians. The management of acute myocardial infarction: guidelines and audit standards. *J Roy Coll Physicians London* 1994; 28: 312–17.
9 The Task Force on the Management of Acute Myocardial Infarction of the European Society of Cardiology. Acute myocardial infarction: prehospital and in hospital management. *Eur Heart J* 1996; 17: 43–63.
10 ASPIRE Steering Group. A British Cardiac Society survey of the potential for the secondary prevention of coronary disease: ASPIRE (Action of Secondary Prevention through Intervention to Reduce Events). *Heart* 1996; 75: 334–42.

Appendix

Admissions to CCU

1. Patients with ECG signs of acute infarction. Event presumed to have occurred in the previous 24 h.
2. Rhythm and conduction disorders requiring therapeutic intervention or monitoring.
3. Unstable angina (chest pain *and* ECG changes, e.g. T wave changes, intermittently at rest).
4. Other cardiovascular emergencies (dissecting aneurysm, malignant hypertension, pulmonary oedema, pulmonary embolism, cardiogenic shock, **but consider ITU**).
5. **Chest pain of uncertain aetiology** if two main symptoms or signs plus one other main or subsidiary sign from those in the following list.

Main

(a) Pain located at least in part in the retrosternal area.
(b) Chest oppression ("squeezing", "weight on chest", "constriction").
(c) Pain severe enough to require opiate analgesia.

Subsidiary

(d) Nausea or vomiting (prior to opiates).

(e) Perspiration (cold and clammy skin).

(g) Tachycardia or bradycardia (<50; >120).

(h) Hypotension SBP, <100 mmHg.

The chest pain triage nurse may admit patients directly to the CCU on her own judgement. The administration of thrombolytics requires prescription by a doctor.

One of our aims is an admission, assessment and administration of thrombolytics time of less than 30 minutes for acute infarction.

Discharges

1. **Uncomplicated infarction**: transfer to general ward if pain free 24–48 h after onset of symptoms. All patients with acute infarcts should have a submaximal predischarge exercise test prior to discharge usually 5–7 days postinfarction. Those with angina and/or ischaemia on exercise will go on to coronary arteriography. Those without pain or ischaemia predischarge should be booked for review and a maximal exercise test at six weeks postinfarction.

2. Patients with **complicated infarcts** will be retained in the CCU until the complication (arrhythmia, heart failure, etc.) has resolved and the patient has been stable for 24 h.

3. **Unstable angina**: patients with documented intermittent ischaemic changes on ECG will be transferred for further investigations at the earliest opportunity.

4. Patients in whom the diagnosis is unclear will have a maximal or submaximal exercise test within 24 h of admission.

5. Where a "non-cardiac" diagnosis is made the patient will be discharged home, with appropriate referral or follow-up, or maintained in the care of the "take" team.

6. Other cardiovascular emergencies will be stabilised and referred on as appropriate.

There is a *daily* round of all acute coronary admissions, with cardiology service input at 8 am. The RMO and HP have responsibility for the care and treatment of *all* CCU patients and the duty registrar or consultant cardiologist is happy to advise. Teams with patients on CCU and those commencing emergency take *must* attend the round which should last *no more* than 30 minutes.

Management of acute myocardial infarction

Thrombolytic agents should be administered to patients with an *unequivocal* acute MI who have no specific contraindications to their use *without delay*. ECG changes are ST elevation or LBBB when history good.

229

Routine investigations

On admission: 12 lead ECG (+RV4 when indicated), portable chest X-ray (on CCU), FBC, U&E, glucose (urgent), dipstick urinalysis.

Cardiac enzymes: if doubt or need to assess size of inarct, CK on admission *and* next and following day with CK isoenzymes if IM injection given.

Cholesterol: with admission bloods.

Daily: U & E (creatinine first routine), ECG.

Management

Thrombolysis (see below) *and:*
1. *IV line* (twice daily saline flush while in CCU).
2. *Analgesia:* diamorphine 2·5–5 mg IV and repeat as required with metoclopramide 10 mg initially.
3. *Oxygen* by face mask if patient tolerates it and no history of COAD.
4. 150 mg soluble *aspirin* immediately and daily thereafter.
5. *β*-blocker: atenolol 5 mg IV and then 50 mg daily, *except:*
(a) bradycardia (rate <50 bpm)
(b) hypotension (systolic BP <90 mmHg)
(c) heart block (1st, 2nd or 3rd degree)
(d) asthma/COAD
(e) symptomatic heart failure.
6. *Thrombolysis:* Streptokinase unless specifically contraindicated. Discuss rTPA admin with cardiology registrar on call. We recommend recombinant tissue plasminogen activator (rPTA) only for anterior MI presenting within 6h or
(a) streptokinase 5 days to 54 months previously
(b) systolic BP <100 mmHg
(c) cardiogenic shock
(d) recent (1 month) streptococcal infection.

rTPA contraindicated:
(a) >6h after first symptom
(b) age >75y (use streptokinase)
(c) absence of diagnostic ECG changes.

Thrombolytic protocol
Indications: diagnosis of MI beginning in the past 12 h.
Contraindications: (discuss with cardiac reg, ?PTCA):
(a) trauma, major surgery or CVA in recent weeks
(b) proven GI bleed in recent months
(c) systolic BP >200 mmHg
(d) actively proliferative diabetic retinopathy (relative CI to be balanced

against infarct size and site)

(e) recent (hours) central venous or arterial line

(f) prolonged external cardiac massage.

Doses:

(a) streptokinase 1·5 M units in 100 ml 5% dextrose over 60 min (note: no heparin)

or

(b) rTPA 15 mg over 1–2 min, then 0·75 mg/kg over 30 min (max. 50 mg), then 0·5 mg/kg over 1h (max. 35 mg), then, 4h after start of thrombolysis, heparin 5000 U IV then at rate to keep KCCT at 1·5–2×control (about 12,000 U 12 hly) for 24 h.

7. *Heparin*: IV if large infarcts, heart failure, etc. KCCT 1·5–2×control (about 12,000 U 12 hly)

8. *Magnesium sulphate*: we feel this is no longer merited.

9. *Nitrates*: for heart failure or recurrent ischaemia glyceryl trinitrate IV. Take 50 mg in 10 ml and dilute to 50 ml in N saline then administer at 1–10 ml/h to relief of symptoms or fall in SBP to 100 mmHg.

10. *Angiotensin converting enzyme inhibitors*: Begun the day after admission in all MI patients other than limited small inferior MI. Particularly with signs or symptoms of failure. Start with ramipril 2·5 mg then increase as tolerated. If on loop diuretics beware of hypotension (treat with colloids). Review requirement at six week follow-up (2Decho useful).

11. *Angiography and angioplasty*: it is **imperative** that the cardiology registrar is told immediately a patient in shock or with a large anterior MI is admitted (?PTCA or other invasive support). Discuss patient with the cardiology registrar on call before instigating thrombolysis in the following situations (bloods before transfer: FBC, U&E, Gp and save, coag screen, HepBV):

(a) large anterior infarcts

(b) patients with cardiogenic shock

(c) unstable angina (see below)

(d) recurrent ischaemia (new pain/ECG changes)

(e) failure of reperfusion

(f) patients in whom thrombolysis is contraindicated.

12 *Associated conditions*:

(a) diabetes mellitus: IV insulin for blood glucose 4–10 mmol/L **(stop oral hypoglycaemics)**

(b) hypertension: relieve pain and anxiety and treat with β-blockers, IV nitrates, calcium channel blockers as appropriate.

Complications of MI

1. Pulmonary oedema: treat with nitrates (as above) and frusemide 40 mg IV. **Alert ITU staff and cardiology reg on call.**

2. Cardiogenic shock (?RV infarct, signs of mitral regurgitation, VSD):
(a) use rTPA as thrombolytic
(b) give oxygen
(c) **Alert ITU staff and discuss with cardiology registrar** re urgent 2Decho, Swann-Ganz catheter, urgent angiocardiography, PTCA, emergency CABG, intra-aortic balloon counter pulsation
(d) dobutamine 2–20 μg/kg/min IV (preferably through central line)
(e) dopamine 2–5 μg/kg/min IV
(f) frusemide 40 mg IV.
3. Non-recanalisation despite thrombolysis or reocclusion. No resolution of ECG signs and patient symptoms within 90 min of thrombolysis or recurrence of ECG signs or symptoms after initial improvement. **Alert ITU staff and discuss with cardiology registrar.**
4. Arrhythmias (see below).

Other CCU admissions

Unstable angina: angina at rest (usually called crescendo angina if rapidly decreasing exercise tolerance) but episodic. Get an ECG during pain and check cardiac enzymes. Refer to cardiologists as soon as possible for early investigation/catheterisation.

Treatment: bed rest and observe. If diagnosis likely (i.e. ECG changes transiently), aspirin, heparin IV (full anticoagulation), IV GTN 1–10 mg/h, β-blockade if not previously given, calcium ch blocker (e.g. diltiazem 60 mg tds).

Unless known coronary disease, if no ECG changes and pain gone do not give IV drugs, just aspirin and oral nitrates and oral antianginal meds but observe.

Aortic dissection: chest/back pain in absence of ECG changes of infarction though MI may occur because of coronary dissection. If suspected organise spiral CT and refer to cardiologists as soon as possible. Transoesophageal echo may be indicated. Keep SBP < 110 mmHg with IV nitroprusside 0·5–8 μg/kg/min *and* labetolol 1 mg/min.

Malignant hypertension: severe hypertension (DBP > 120 mmHg in adults) *and* haemorrhages and exudates bilaterally on fundoscopy. Admit CCU or ITU. Intra-arterial BP monitoring. Oral atenolol (or IV nitroprusside if encephalopathic). Aim for *slow* fall in BP to diastolic of 100–110 mmHg in 24 h.

Rehabilitation from MI/cardiac surgery

We have a rehab course for patients postinfarct and after cardiac surgery.

IMPORTANT

Some consultants do not have junior staff on the site so the patient must remain under the care of the admitting team while on the site, even if transfer for urgent investigation under the cardiologists is planned. We are very happy to confer regularly about any sick patient and will endeavour to send someone to CCU to help with a specific procedure or to review a problem.

Management of arrhythmias

Remember you are treating the patient, not the ECG.

Bradycardias: not uncommon after inferior MI but a sign of poor prognosis after acute anterior MI.

Sinus bradycardia

Treatment: none unless hypotension, then atropine 600 μg IV (repeat up to total of 2·4 mg, then pace).

Sinoatrial arrest/sinoatrial block (pause >2 sec)

Treatment: atropine or transvenous pacing if prolonged or symptomatic.

First degree AV block (PR interval >0·20 sec)

Treatment: none; observe, check drug treatment for β-blockers, Ca channel blockers, etc.

Second degree heart block

(a) Mobitz type I (Wenckebach) AV block
(PR increasing then dropped beat).
Treatment: if symptoms, then atropine but if after anterior MI then temporary transvenous pacemaker.
(b) Mobitz type II (2:1, 3:1, etc.)
Treatment: temp transvenous pacemaker but atropine and isoprenaline infusion (2 mg in 500 ml dextrose, give 1 μg/min) in interim if symptomatic.

New bifascicular block RBBB + L axis deviation, LBBB + R axis deviation

or *trifascicular block*, bifascicular block and long PR
Treatment: prophylactic temp pacemaker

Complete heart block (3rd degree AV block)

Dissociated atrial and ventricular activity. Treatment: atropine and isoprenaline temporarily or external pacemaker if severely bradycardic, hypotensive and reduced consciousness then transvenous temp pacemaker (almost always required if CHB after anterior MI).

Pacemaker: if PM is anticipated (rhythm disturbance on presentation)

233

someone with wide experience of central lines should gain central venous access via external jugular (ask ITU team) before thrombolysis. The alternative is access through a femoral or antecubital vein.

Temp pacing in acute MI

Rate/conduction disturbance	Indication
Sinus brady, without hypotension	
ventric ectopics, angina, LVF, syncope	–
Sinus brady with any of the above	+
despite atropine	
Accelerated idioventricular rhythm	–
Idioventricular rhythm with rate <45	+
and/or hypotension	
Recurrent sinus pause >2 sec	+
Toursade de pointes	+
First degree AV block	–
Second degree AV block	
Wenckebach (unless hypotension)	–
Wenckebach with hypotension/bradycardia	+
Mobitz II (dropped beats)	+
Complete heart block	+
Isolated left anterior hemiblock, left posterior	
hemiblock or RBBB	–
New LBBB	+
New bifascicular block (alternating RBBB	
and LBBB, RBBB with LAD, RBBB with RAD)	+
Trifascicular block (BBB with PR prolonged)	+
Asystole	+

Junctional rhythms: narrow or wide complex regular rhythm with PR interval short (retrograde conduction) or lost in the QRS complex. After infarct is usually slow and is associated with high vagal tone. If fast (>150/min) is another form of SVT.
Treatment: often none; if hypotensive, try atropine.

Atrial flutter: "saw-tooth" baseline rate about 300/min. Variable degree of block. If ventricular response is fast, carotid massage or IV adenosine (see below) may increase block and unmask the flutter waves.
Treatment: if hypotensive and unwell, then urgent DC cardioversion.
If ventricular rate fast (>100/min) consider amiodarone ± elective cardioversion in all patients after starting IV heparin.

234

Atrial fibrillation: if haemodynamically compromised and of recent onset then consider DC cardioversion (heparinise). If well tolerated then heparinise, arrange 2Decho and plan elective cardioversion (DC or pharmacological flecainide (if ventricular function good) or amiodarone (if not)). If chronic and well tolerated then control ventricular response with digoxin ± verapamil or a β-blocker. Anticoagulate for all but emergency cardioversion. Avoid digoxin in Wolff Parkinson White syndrome (suspect if ventricular response > 200/min and aberrant conduction).

Digitalisation: for long standing AF. If haemodynamically unstable then IV verapamil or β-blocker. Digoxin loading with 0·5 mg orally, then 0·25 mg after 4h, then 0·25 mg after further 4h. Maintenance is 0·25 mg/day or 0·125 mg/day in elderly. The maintenance dose will have to be reduced in those with renal failure.

Supraventricular tachycardia: regular, narrow complex tachycardia, rate about 150/min.
Includes:
sinus tachycardia
paroxysmal atrial tachycardia (PAT)
atrial flutter (2:1 block)
atrial fibrillation (almost regular response)
parox. AV nodal tachycardia (AVNRT)
AV re-entrant tachycardia (AVRT) through accessory pathway.
Diagnose by ECG ± carotid sinus massage, Valsalva or IV adenosine.
Treatment as appropriate for diagnosis (AF, etc.) or by interrupting re-entrant circuit. If patient shocked or haemodynamically compromised then DC cardioversion, 50, 200, 300 J, less if patient digoxin toxic.

IV adenosine: monitor ECG and give fast boluses of incremental doses, e.g. 1, 3, 6, 12 mg.

IV verapamil: boluses of 5 mg at 15 min intervals to max of 20 mg. May aggravate hypotension. Avoid in patients already on a β-blocker. If adenosine and verapamil are ineffective then reconsider the diagnosis; is patient septic or haemorrhaging?
Other drugs: esmolol, 40 mg IV.

Discuss other intervention/drugs with cardiology team, e.g. flecainide 2 mg/kg over 30 min to max of 150 mg then 1·5 mg/kg/h for 1 h, then 0·1–0·25 mg/kg/h for next 24 h if good LV.

Ventricular arrhythmias

Isolated VEs (ectopics) are broad QRS complexes, not preceded by p waves. No treatment unless immediately postinfarction and R on T. Check serum K^+. Treat with IV lignocaine 50–100 mg bolus then 2 mg/kg/min.

Treat ischaemia.

Monomorphic VT: more than five consecutive broad QRS complexes, regular rate (>100/min, if 60–100/min=accelerated idioventricular rhythm). Treatment: if shocked/hypotensive then DC cardioversion. Correct electrolyte abnormalities, e.g. potassium and magnesium (8 mmol over 20 min).

Drugs: *lignocaine* IV bolus 75–100 mg over 2 min, then 1–4 mg/min. If ineffective then IV *amiodarone* **by central line** (phlebitis) 300 mg over 60 min (BP may fall), then 1200 mg/24 h.

If resistant to both drugs and recurring after DC cardioversion then consult cardiologist. Other drugs to consider include the following but may get into problems with proarrhythmic polypharmacy:

Flecainide 2 mg/kg over 30 min then 1·5 mg/kg/h for one hour then 100–250µg/kg/h, max 600 mg in 24 h.

Mexilitine: 100–250 mg at 25 mg/min followed by infusion of 250 mg (0·1% sol) over 1 h, 125 mg/h for 2 h then 500µg/min.

Sotalol: 20–60 mg bolus over 2–3 min.

Bretylium: 5–10 mg/kg over 8–10 min to 30 mg/kg (dilute to 10 mg/ml in 5% dextrose), then 1–2 mg/min.

Procainamide: 100 mg IV over 5 min up to max. of 5 times then 40 µg/kg/ min.

Polymorphic VT/torsade de pointes: frequently patient has an underlying bradycardia. It is often initiated by "late" VE. Often self terminating but recurrent. QT prolongation may predispose. Treat hypokalaemia, and give magnesium, pace bradycardic patients and stop drugs which may predispose by prolonging QT, e.g. sotalol and interactions of antihistamines, etc. Isoprenaline or adrenaline IV may be useful initially.

Differential diagnosis of broad complex tachycardias

If there is a history of ischaemic heart disease then >95% of broad complex tachycardias are VT. **If in doubt treat as VT.** Do not try verapamil.

If an SVT with aberrant conduction (usually RBBB and <160 msec duration) is strongly suspected then IV adenosine should be tried.

Index